THE REDIRECTION OF PSYCHOLOGY
Essays in Honor of Amedeo P. Giorgi

Une édition du
(An Edition of the)

Cercle interdisciplinaire de recherches phénoménologiques (Cirp)
(Interdisciplinary Circle of Phenomenological Research)

Université du Québec à Montréal
(University of Quebec in Montreal)

Thomas F. Cloonan & Christian Thiboutot,
responsables de l'édition
(Editors)

THE REDIRECTION OF PSYCHOLOGY
Essays in Honor of Amedeo P. Giorgi

Contributors

Christopher M. Aanstoos, Ph.D.	University of West Georgia (United States)
Marc Applebaum, Ph.D.	Saybrook University (United States)
Thomas F. Cloonan, Ph.D.	Marymount College of Fordham University (Emeritus) (United States)
Larry Davidson, Ph.D.	Yale University (United States)
Magnus Englander, Ph.D.	Malmö University (Sweden)
Barbro M. Giorgi, Ph.D.	Saybrook University (United States)
Steen Halling, Ph.D.	Seattle University (United States)
Mufid James Hannush, Ph.D.	Rosemont College (United States)
Bernd Jager, Ph.D.	University of Quebec in Montreal (Canada)
George Kunz, Ph.D.	Seattle University (United States)
Bertha Mook, Ph.D.	University of Ottawa (Canada)
James Morley, Ph.D.	Ramapo College (United States)
Richard Rojcewicz, Ph.D.	Point Park University (United States)
David L. Smith, C.S.Sp., Ph.D.	Duquesne University (United States)
Les Todres, Ph.D.	Bournemouth University (United Kingdom)
Frederick Wertz, Ph.D.	Fordham University (United States)
Akihiro Yoshida, Ph.D.	Shukutoku University & Tokyo University (Emeritus) (Japan)

Thomas F. Cloonan & Christian Thiboutot, Editors

Cirp – Cercle interdisciplinaire de recherches phénoménologiques
(Interdisciplinary Circle of Phenomenological Research)
Département de psychologie
Université du Québec à Montréal
C.P. 8888, Succursale Centre-Ville
Montréal, Québec
H3C 3P8

Les Collectifs du Cirp
(The Collective Works of the Cirp)

ISBN 978-0-9866654-1-7
(Online version: www.cirp.uqam.ca)

10 9 8 7 6 5 4 3 2 1

Dedication

While these essays were written to honor Amedeo Giorgi, the book itself is dedicated to the memory of his beloved wife, Barbro Giorgi (1957-2007), who was his most significant inspiration and critic and whose untimely death has left all of us and the phenomenological world that much poorer.

While this book went to press we received the sad news of the death of Tom Cloonan, the first editor and tireless promoter of this volume. Without his initiative and constant support this publication would not have seen the light of day. That he may rest in peace.

Christian Thiboutot, Co-Editor

Note From the Publisher's Editor

The publication of *The Redirection of Psychology: essays in honor of Amedeo P. Giorgi* marks an important turning point in the history of the Cirp (le "Cercle interdisciplinaire de recherches phénoménologiques") and the Department of Psychology at the University of Quebec at Montreal (UQAM). With this first English title in the scientific repertoire of the *CIRP*, phenomenological psychology at UQAM takes an important step on the international scene.

This original publication wants to honor Professor Amedeo Giorgi, both as a world-renowned and innovative psychologist and as an eminent former colleague, who, more than a decade ago, reinforced and expanded phenomenological psychology in UQAM. In the ensuing years the university has attracted a growing number of gifted teachers and students whose interests coalesced around the idea of a *human* science of psychology that would no longer model itself exclusively on the natural sciences but that would draw its main inspiration from the experience of concrete living. Today these psychologists form a unique and fertile group of professors and students within the university's psychology department.

The contributors to this bundle of essays live and work in all corners of the world, from England, Canada and the United States to Sweden, South Africa and Japan. What the authors have in common is that they all are former students and colleagues of Professor Amedeo Giorgi. The essays collected in this volume are meant to express their appreciation and gratitude for Amedeo Giorgi's tireless teaching, for his great scholarship and erudition and, last but not least, for his unfailing collegiality and loyal friendship.

Finally, I want to thank my colleague Professor Tom Cloonan, who not only conceived the idea of this book, but also solicited and collected the manuscripts and did the substantial editing of them, and then entrusted their publication to the CIRP that did the further required publisher's editing of the material. I also thank my colleague Professor Bernd Jager for his steady encouragement and his editorial advice.

Christian Thiboutot, Ph.D.
Codirector of the Cirp

Preface

Our book, *The Redirection of Psychology*, is a Festschrift. Literally, that German word means "a writing in celebration". For us, it is a celebratory piece of writing in honor of Amedeo P. Giorgi for his accomplishments of scholarly writing and of research and direction of others' research as well as for his conceptualization of the Simon Silverman Phenomenology Center that was established at Duquesne University in 1980. In addition, we honor Amedeo's instrumentality in the foundation of the International Human Science Research Conferences (IHSRCs) through the hosting of its first meeting at Duquesne University in 1983.

Another accomplishment of Amedeo's lifework also deserving of our honoring of him through this Festschrift is the *Journal of Phenomenological Psychology*, published by Brill. It is the flagship journal of phenomenological psychology and it is on its way to its half-century anniversary, 2020, since Amedeo's founding of it in 1970.

There are 17 of us who have written essays that constitute this book celebrating Amedeo. The topics and styles of the essays are as individualistic as their authors. The common denominator is the human science focus. We hope through our essays to educate and to advocate the importance and urgency of psychology as human science. There can be no better celebration of Amedeo than this.

Finally, a term in academia that has sometimes been used in lieu of Festschrift is Liber Amicorum, a Book of Friends. This Latin term is as appropriate as Festschrift is for the book, a book that has been written by colleagues and former students, all of whom are his friends. In our circle of friends most certainly are Professor Christian Thiboutot and his colleagues of CIRP and the Department of Psychology at the University of Quebec at Montreal. Without their friendship and cooperation, this book's conception with its 17 essays would still be waiting for its birth.

Thomas F. Cloonan, Ph.D., Editor of the Essays

Table of Contents

INTRODUCTION

Thomas F. Cloonan, Ph.D.

Marymount College of Fordham University (Emeritus)
United States

The focus that envelops the essays within this book is the redirection of psychology to a human science psychology. The occasion for declaration of this focus is the celebration of the contributions of Amedeo P. Giorgi to the discipline of psychology. These contributions have been at the forefront of psychology's human science redirection.

The "spirit" of human science redirection unifies the diversity of the essays. Within the diversity, there are natural clusterings that give structure to the book. These clusters constitute Parts of the book, which are four in number. They are: Part I, history of human science and biography of Amedeo Giorgi; Part II, psychotherapy; Part III, themes; and Part IV, philosophical connections.

Part I

In this Part, the opening essay by Christopher M. Aanstoos presents to the reader the progressive emergence of the historical and holistic antecedents of human science psychology. Aanstoos' essay describes three waves of the human science sensibility; (1) the classical period of Greek thought within which intimations of human science first become expressed, (2) the Renaissance whose retrievals of original texts of the classical period in effect facilitated a new era of philosophical thought in which the individual moves front-center for attention; and (3) the contemporary situation that has had its definition with the human science psychology and its holistic program for psychology promoted by Ludwig Binswanger, Medard Boss, J. H. van den Berg and R. D. Laing in Europe, and by Carl Rogers, Abraham Maslow, Rollo May, and Amedeo Giorgi in the Western hemisphere.

The second essay of Part I picks up on Giorgi's name from this history. David L. Smith, C.S.Sp., outlines the earlier and formative years of Amedeo Giorgi's biography and his first major academic commitments that were at Duquesne University. Smith's documentation is thorough. One can appreciate how these twenty-four years of Giorgi's life naturally segue into the additional, significant years of his academic profession and research at *l'Université du Québec à Montréal* and at Saybrook University.

Part II

Part II highlights human science contributions to psychotherapy. In her essay on the application of the descriptive phenomenological research method to the field of clinical research, Barbro M. Giorgi, the late and lamented wife of Amedeo, points to the disparity between the empirical research on psychotherapy and the experiences of psychotherapists. She suggests that the chasm of this disparity, "can be bridged by phenomenological research strategies that are experientially congruent and based upon the discovery of lived meanings derived from the concrete descriptions of the participants, whether therapists or clients". Barbro M. Giorgi's arguments, backed by her investigation's findings, are apposite to the controversy issuing from evidence-based research and its ascendancy in clinical research.

The second essay in this psychotherapy Part of the book is by Mufid James Hannush. In his essay, Hannush presents his application of "an existential-dialectical-phenomenological (EDP) method toward understanding two so-called case histories, which in reality are self-analyses, in the works of Rollo May". Hannush's essay, a report of self-analysis done by a master human science psychotherapist, is interesting to study. Hannush, furthermore, underlines how May's descriptions of "a pivotal passage" is anticipatory of his later contributions to existential-humanistic psychology.

Bertha Mook in her essay offers a "hermeneutic phenomenological foundation for psychotherapy as a human science". Mook's contribution is a response to the current situation in which psychotherapy either is founded on the natural science paradigm or follows social constructionism. Mook critiques this situation and she addresses the relationship between hermeneutic phenomenology and psychotherapy in general. In connection with the Continental Philosophy tradition, she makes specific references to Hans-Georg Gadamer's concepts of play and to Paul Ricoeur's theory of narrative structure as they relate to correlative parts of psychotherapy.

Les Todres' essay explores, "how caring practices in applied disciplines such as psychotherapy or nursing benefit from a research approach that "goes back to the things themselves". It [particularly emphasizes] the importance of embodied knowing in both research and practice". Embodiment, embodied subjectivity, is a priority theme of phenomenological and existential psychotherapy and research. Todres argues well that, "phenomenologically-derived qualitative research findings can facilitate "embodied relational understanding" and judgment-based care by focusing more attention on the ways in which we express and disseminate our findings, and also by focusing more attention on the potential educative role that such findings may play in supporting the holistic development of the person of the practitioner engaged in caring practices".

The fifth essay of this psychotherapy Part of the book is by Larry Davidson. In his essay, Davidson reviews and critiques the position that psychology assumes "the existence of the natural world" and that it should "remain in this way transcendentally naïve". Davidson argues that "for psychology to be grounded in phenomenology it must constitute a *return* to naïve positivity from the transcendental rather than stop short of taking the transcendental turn". In his spotlighting of Edmund Husserl's presentation of the "transcendental reduction", Davidson affirms a depth dimension to Husserl's transcendental phenomenology that has been obscured by the larger profile of Martin Heidegger's existential phenomenology in the human science world. Davidson underlines the efficacy of Husserl's transcendental turn in the treatment of psychosis. Davidson's essay straddles the world of psychotherapy and the world of transcendental phenomenology with naturalness and with achievement.

Part III

In this part of the book, the essayists address issues, topics, or perspectives of mainstream and human science psychology. They are all together called "themes". There are five essays here.

Marc Applebaum is the first contributor presented here. His themes are "scientism" and "relativism" and the relationship of Giorgi's work to them. Applebaum lays out the map of the phenomenological tradition broadly as twofoldly characterizable; that of "descriptive or Husserlian perspectives" and that of "the interpretive (hermeneutic) perspectives articulated by Heidegger, Gadamer, and Ricoeur". He alludes to the significance of the tension between these two perspectives that constitute the phenomenological tradition. Against the background of this tradition and its tension, Applebaum in his essay seeks, "to situate Giorgi's body of work *vis-à-vis* hermeneutic approaches in order to highlight the uniqueness of his contribution to the field". Giorgi's work, Applebaum says, is the alternative to the scientism of psychology conceived as positive science and to the relativism implicit in many of the research approaches based upon hermeneutic or postmodernist philosophy.

Magnus Englander's themes in his essay are subjectivity and memory and their optimal accessibility through Giorgi's qualitative method. Englander points out the continuing failure of natural scientific psychology to address the issue of subjectivity in a meaningful way. Referring to the phenomenon of memory, Englander highlights "the notion of subjectivity in Giorgi's method as it applies to human science". His concern is with, "the overall phenomenological dialogue on the intricate relationship between the phenomena of the body, memory, and self". The connections are well-made.

Truth is the theme of Steen Halling's essay, the third one. Halling declares that, "the truths that researchers search for are elusive and can be spoken of in a multitude of ways. Truths in human life are elusive not because they are abstract or unreal but because they transcend us even as they touch us deeply". Embodied truths with reference to instances of qualitative research along with everyday life examples are at the core of Halling's quite worthwhile essay.

In his essay, Bernd Jager redirects the attention of psychology to the being of *homo habitans* that inheres in and is fulfilled in a human and divine cosmos, away from the human being as merely *homo sapiens*, who inhabits only a natural and material universe. This is his theme. Jager says, "a psychology that draws its inspiration from festive encounters and that allies itself with the arts and the humanities will be able to fully explore a human and divine cosmos and thereby evoke the festive appearance of *homo habitans*". The *sui generis* style of Jager's essay is itself expressive of the relatedness and cogency of the arts and humanities to human science psychology.

In the fifth essay of this Part of the book, Akihiro Yoshida presents for the reader's consideration a specific situation in the human science of education. He "explicates the implicit meanings of a Japanese master teacher's practices of teaching literary works of art". Specifically, Yoshida draws out the prominence of what he terms as the "Why-question" and the "What-question" that are addressed to students for the behaviors and experiences of characters in novels. Yoshida, in addition, advances the parallel of the two types of questions to the Explanation and Understanding dimensions of knowledge that are so often discussed by human science psychologists and philosophers. The theme of Yoshida's essay, therefore, is the reciprocal relevance of human science perspective and of the teaching of literary works of art to each other. The essay is one of sensitivity and subtlety.

Part IV

The five essays of the fourth Part of the book directly engage philosophers of the Continental tradition. (In previous Parts, of course, essayists have made reference to these philosophers.) George Kunz' "philosopher of choice" from this tradition is Emmanuel Levinas, who was a student of Edmund Husserl. In Kunz' essay, "it is proposed that Levinas' major distinctions between, for example, *totality* and *infinity*, *need* and *desire*, *self-initiated/self-directed* and *invested freedom*, and between the *there is* and *the face*, have significant and ethical relevance to mainstream psychology." Kunz makes reference to a communication from Giorgi to him that Levinas was a "philosopher of action" and not a challenge to Husserl, the "philosopher of experience"." Kunz presents us an essay with the important perspectives of Levinas.

Richard Rojcewicz, a philosopher, in his essay takes on Jacques Derrida's criticism of the phenomenological theory of signs. He presents a refutation of the critique. However, success of the refutation, Rojcewicz points out, does not connote for phenomenology a return to ascendency in the realm of philosophy. Rojcewicz interestingly considers the connection of this scene in philosophy to developments in the world of art. Just as the school of Impressionist art, according to Rojcewicz, is one of the portents of phenomenology, so also is Pop Art a portent of deconstruction, the movement in philosophy for which Derrida was articulator. Whether eliciting agreement from the reader or not, Rojcewicz' thoughts provoke serious consideration on relevancies to human science psychology.

James Morley's essay speaks to the procedure of Husserl's epoché whose characterization in phenomenological philosophy and psychology has been as "rigorous and disciplined." Morley refers to, "current scholarship that restores Husserl's understanding of transcendental subjectivity as always an embodied subjectivity adhered to the lifeworld – not at all a transcendentalism. Furthermore the essay comments on how mundane versions of the epoché permeate everyday life and how the methodological epoché shares elements in common with contemplative meditation traditions across cultures."

Frederick J. Wertz' essay is, "a review of Husserl's ideas about free imaginative variation and the intuition of essences as they developed throughout his career… Examination is made of how Husserl used his method to determine the essences of 'psychological phenomena,' and of the demands his insights into the essence of the subject matter of psychology make on the discipline. There is attention to Husserl's directives for the sciences, especially psychology, about their use of the phenomenological method." Wertz considers the nature and use of eidetic intuition in the, "light of post-modern critiques of essentialism and of skepticism concerning 'essences.' Finally, the implications of these clarifications of the method of eidetic intuition for our understanding of phenomenological psychological research are spelled out." Wertz' essay on these central themes of Husserl's philosophy is scholarly and important. It is, in effect, a resource article for phenomenological psychologist researchers.

In his essay, Thomas F. Cloonan contends that, "artistic experiences and aesthetic experiences may instigate changes in the psychological character of existence by way of ontological re-structurings of the person." Cloonan's conclusion comes from the study of Maurice Merleau-Ponty's writings on art and his last work posthumously published, *The Visible and the invisible*

(1964/1968). He makes references to Giorgi's research on the psychology of imagination. Mainstream psychology of art conceptualizations and vocabulary are inadequate to the appreciation of the fundamental contributions of Merleau-Ponty to a psychology of art that expresses itself in terms of flesh and the visible and invisible. Cloonan's essay is an attempt to bridge the gap – however quixotic that task may seem to be.

The unity of the essays with their distribution into the four Parts above lays in their redirection of psychology to psychology as a human science. It is fitting that the concern for honoring the contributions of Amedeo P. Giorgi occasions the essays' publication. Giorgi is expounder *par excellence* of the phenomenological psychology portion of the human science of psychology. All the contributors are academic and practitioner advocates of human science. The influence of Amedeo Giorgi is present at least implicitly, when not explicitly, in their work.

HOLISTIC FOUNDATIONS OF PSYCHOLOGY IN HISTORICAL PERSPECTIVE

Christopher M. Aanstoos, Ph.D.

University of West Georgia
United States

Abstract

In ancient Greece we encounter the first sense of how humanistic thought was founded on a holistic view, such that the profound Greek grasp of the meaning, fate and destiny of being human was grounded within an even more encompassing context of the non-dual presencing of Being. Second, during the Renaissance, scholars emphasized the irreducibility of the human experience. Finally, as part of a larger shift in the Zeitgeist, *a reform movement emerged within European and American psychology in the 1960s. Inspired by previous developments in existential-phenomenological philosophy, psychologists on both sides of the Atlantic began to revision the basic presuppositions of elementism and mechanism, and a new wave of humanistic thought emerged. Key figures included Binswanger, Boss, van den Berg and Laing, from Europe, and May, Rogers, Maslow, and Giorgi in the United States. In the examination of these three "waves", this chapter presents the thesis that holism is no merely current fad. It is the deepest taproot of our civilization and the gift of 2500 years of humanism. As the philosophical heirs to this legacy, the contemporary human sciences have the opportunity, and responsibility of bringing this vision of wholeness to fulfillment – precisely when it is most needed.*

The Inspiration of Amedeo Giorgi : A Personal Prologue

Amedeo Giorgi was my dissertation advisor and my mentor, shepherding my still raw novice thinking about psychology into a capacity for deeper reflection on its possibilities. But more than that, for a generation Giorgi has been an inspiration for an entire wing of psychology, through his penetratingly sustained analysis of the limitations of psychology's traditional foundations, and the prospects of an alternative human science approach (Aanstoos, 1996; Wertz & Aanstoos, 1999). He has heroically led this reform movement for almost half a century, yet has done so with profound humility and respect. Repeatedly, he has humbly reminded us that the work is "only one percent done, ninety-nine percent to be worked out". And he has always respected the individualized pathways taken by his colleagues on the journey. As a result of the multifarious creativities of his cohorts, the movement has been both less and more than he imagined.

As the various chapters of this book amply demonstrate, Giorgi's leadership has been inspirational, not doctrinaire. But if there is one unifying theme that he has indelibly contributed to this movement, it has been to appreciate the real, phenomenological fullness – "the full range" (Giorgi, 1970, p. XII) – of human psychological life, and the correlative need for a psychology that can be "comprehensive" of that scope (Giorgi, 1984a, p. 27). Giorgi (1984a, pp. 22-25) sees psychological reality as being both "paraphysical" and "paralogical" – that is, as being a reality in between the purely physical and the logical, reducible to neither. In the face of a small-minded psychology that reduces the human to one or the other and so fails to capture this full scope, Giorgi's retort has always been to remind us that "we are more than that". Yes, we are. And so, my contribution to this collective honoring of Amedeo Giorgi is an exploration of just how big we really are.

The Holistic Vision : A Thematic Prologue

Giorgi's critique (e.g., 1970, 1976, 1981, 1984b, 1985, 1994, 2006, 2007, 2008, 2009) is contemporaneous with a larger a dissident movement that arose within western psychology in the latter third of the twentieth century, in order to emphasize the neglected significance of specifically human being. Lacking a single vision, a variety of movements – such as humanistic, transpersonal, existential, phenomenological – developed and remained largely marginalized vis-à-vis the mainstream. I can see that these variegating branches do share an implicit core vision, whose articulation is vitally important for our times; and that Giorgi's work contributes powerfully to that prospective unity. This core vision is that of holism, understood especially in contrast to the dominant vision of dualism.

The term "holism" has become much more common in the past decade in popular culture, largely on account of its increasing usage to indicate innovative approaches to healing (as "holistic medicine"). It remains uncommon in psychology, however, despite its having been introduced to the field even before its current usage in medicine. For example, in 1939 Kurt Goldstein's book *The Organism: A Holistic Approach to Biology Derived from Pathological Data in Man*, appeared, with its mission of understanding biological data holistically, that is, in terms of their psychological context. In 1965 a posthumous collection of the papers of Andras Angyal was published as *Neurosis and Treatment: A Holistic*

Theory. The title reflected Angyal's approach to the person as a holistic system. In his own early major work, *Psychology as a Human Science*, Giorgi (1970) presciently employed the term "holistic" in both his critique of what traditional approaches in psychology lacked, and in his call for what was urgently needed: "psychology must take the problem of "holistic phenomena" seriously" (1970, p. 84).

With Giorgi, I am convinced that the essential core a psychology adequate to its phenomena is holism: an approach to the person as a whole, non-reducible and contextually situated within a larger, interdependent whole. Indeed, I am convinced that holism is the timely defining idea for the future, not merely of psychology, but for all the human sciences, and really for the future of humanity, faced with the now acute dilemmas that are our heritage of centuries of reductionistic, elementistic and dualistic thinking.

This vision is not only contemporary, but also timeless. Holism has infused and guided humanistic thought throughout history. Giorgi (1992, p. 424) once noted that a reason humanistic psychology did not become more influential was its failure to "link their concept of "human" to the strong humanistic traditions of antiquity or of the Renaissance". I think that's a very astute observation, so to recover a holistic vision, I looked to these previous eras, during which the use of a holistic vision reached a critical mass that, for a while, became a leading paradigm and so was able to proverbially "move the culture".

By means of that historical analysis of holism (Aanstoos, 2007, 2009a, 2009b, 2009c), I found this holistic vision is built upon a long tradition in western intellectual history[1]. For the most part, it has been the "counter-tradition" to other, more mainstream viewpoints. Whether these mainstreams originated in religion or natural science, they have been elementistic rather than holistic, indeed usually the crude elementism of an empiricism that presupposes reductionistic, dualistic, and mechanistic relations among the elements. But there have been "peak periods" in which the "wave" of holistic thought crests and becomes manifest as a "critical mass" able, for a time, to advance a decisively transformational vision. There have been three such periods: the first occurred around 600-300 B.C.E. in ancient Greece, the second during 1300-1600 in the European Renaissance, and the third in the late 20th century in the United States. In ancient Greece we encounter the first sense of how humanistic thought was founded on a holistic view, such that the profound Greek grasp of the meaning, fate and destiny of being human was grounded within an even more encompassing context of the nondual presencing of Being. Second, during the Renaissance, scholars emphasized the irreducibility of the human experience. Finally, the 20th century rise of the human sciences was carried forth on such a wave. As part of a larger shift in the *Zeitgeist*, a reform movement emerged within European and American psychology, and coalesced in the 1960s. Inspired by previous developments in existential-phenomenological philosophy, psychologists on both sides of the Atlantic began to revision the basic presuppositions of elementism and mechanism, and a new wave of humanistic thought emerged. A careful examination of each of these waves will reveal key insights of foundational value to the development of a truly holistic psychology.

The First Wave. Being and Logos *: The Greek Roots of Humanism*

Let us first consider the wave of humanism from ancient Greece. Here we encounter the first sense of how reflecting on the being of human being was founded on a holistic view. The Greeks profoundly grasped that the meaning, fate and destiny of being human was grounded within an even more encompassing context. So let's reflect on the origins of that vision in the realm of Greek antiquity. Ancient Greek thought flowered in that millennium between the 7th century BCE through the 3rd century CE. During that time it shifted through three phases: the pre-Socratic, the classical, and the neo-Platonic. It is the first phase, the pre-Socratic period of the 7th through 4th centuries BCE, I want to examine here, as having provided the original and earliest roots of holistic thought. A more usual standard for scholars is to focus instead on the "classical" period, the "golden age" of Athens – roughly 500-300 B.C.E., especially on the major philosophers: Socrates, Plato, Aristotle; supplemented by the major dramatists: Sophocles, Euripides, Aeschylus. And this approach does offer the human sciences a rich yield at the hands of skilled classicists (such as Hamilton, 1930; or Dillon, 2008). But I think that Heidegger's (1975; Seidel, 1964) insight about the significance of earlier Greek thinking is even more crucial for our inquiry into the holistic roots of the human sciences. Heidegger found these earlier Greek philosophers had understood the human in relation to a very deep grasp of wholeness at a profound, ontological level (Heidegger, 1992; Heidegger & Fink, 1979). So let us follow him there, to articulate this holistic vision by searching into these ancient Greek roots of western humanism.

But it is not easy to think with these ancients – to leap across millennia and all the subsequent conceptual encrustations. And, of course, any effort to slice into the past and locate a "beginning" is a pretense, and an always futile gesture, since any historical age necessarily owes the roots of its own understanding to an even earlier period. And certainly this is true of the pre-Socratic thought of ancient Greece. So, allow first a very brief excurses into its antecedent roots in the archaic age that preceded this period.

The earliest Greeks – the Hellenes – migrated between 2000-1000 BCE into an area already settled by an even older culture, the Mycenaean, then already is disrepair, which itself was the outgrowth of the earlier Minoan civilization, centered on Crete, but extending through the Aegean islands and coastline. This preceding Minoan culture was itself the blend of the Levantine (likely Phoenician) and Egyptian – racially similar to the Phoenician and artistically resembling Egyptian. The now excavated ruins of elaborate palaces and cities indicate a previous high level of development for the Minoans, which was likely ultimately brought down by a series of devastating earthquakes and volcanic eruptions in the 12th century BCE, leaving them vulnerable to conquest, and subsequent absorption by the migrating Hellenes (Durant, 1939; Fox, 2006).

This prehistory of Greek society is important because of what the Minoans contributed to the Greek mind, for the Minoans were the last surviving matriarchal culture in the west. In Minoan culture, the status and possibilities of women were relatively more equal to that of men in both public and private life – a characteristic shared by the other two waves of holistic thought as well (in the Renaissance and in the 20th century). And so, as in earlier matriarchal cultures, the divine power – the power to create new life – was imaged as feminine. As the Hellenes conquered the Minoans, the Minoans' feminine deities of the earth – Mother Nature – married the male sky-gods of the Greeks. A marriage that richly contributed to the emerging Greek vision of holism. For the early Greeks, the divine was not some entity residing in some remote redoubt off behind the clouds. Oh no – the gods dwelt amidst the people, right here on earth. And the voices of the gods and goddesses were heard everywhere, in the babbling of the brook, in the sound of the wind, in the swaying of the tree (von Hildebrand, 1966). The Naiads, fresh water nymphs, could be heard amidst the churning waves, just as the river gods could be heard in the rushing waters, cascading over the rocks. The Dryads, or tree goddesses, were heard whenever the wind rustled the branches. The earth itself was lushly full of divinity, just as Persephone returned to her mother from the underworld each Spring with the new blossoms. Indeed, so co-extensive was the world of mortals and the world of the divine, that the land itself was sensed as having eyes, living eyes, in flowers, trees, water. "So crowded full is the air with them", wrote one poet of the time, "that there is no room to put in the spike of an ear of corn without touching one" (MacGregor, 1959, p. 1).

The gods "were not simply up in heaven… gloating over human suffering. Greek life was lived with a sense of their potential presence, in the clamour of storms or the stresses of sickness, in the dust-clouds of battle or on distant hillsides […] Greeks saw around them […] gods crowding their public spaces […] they seemed to stand beside' them as "manifest helpers" […] gods and goddesses […] made love […] to […] mortals" (Fox, 2006, pp 49-50). Gods and goddesses lived nearby, had human forms, and consorted with human friends and rivals. To the Greeks of this archaic age, the experience of wholeness was very palpable. Heaven and earth were not yet bifurcated. As the poet Hesiod wrote in the 8th century BCE in his *Theogony*, earth and sky were originally one, and were never fully separated. Rather, the subsequent oppositions are understood as polarities, kin, familial relationships (Robinson, 1968, pp. 3-12).

This core mythical-religious vision continued to exert its influence on the stirrings of pre-Socratic philosophy in the subsequent three centuries. Its guiding insight was that not only were human and divine one whole fabric, but – even more generally – each and every thing was seen in relation to the whole. As Anaxagoras in the 5th century BCE said, "the beings we perceive as separate and distinct from one another are simply different kinds of seeds [...] Everything has a share in everything" (in Cahill, 2003, p. 148). The temple, for example, was not perceived as an independent entity, but sited in relation to the land, the hill, the sky and the sea (Hamilton, 1930, pp. 221-248; also cf. Heidegger, 1960/1971; Steiner, 1979, pp. 134-135; Scully, 1979). Individual actions are seen nested within their larger, fateful historical context. Even the transient and the eternal wrapped round one another like a Mobius loop. Mind and spirit, the manifest and the hidden, the finite and the infinite, the human and the divine, go together. Or, as Heraclitus wrote in his *Fragments*: "That which differs with itself is in agreement: harmony consists of opposing tension, like that of the bow and the lyre". We can distinguish, but not separate, for we deal with polarities, not opposites.

To the great pre-Socratic philosophers, this vision of a unified whole guided their questioning about the nature of reality, about the nature of Being itself. They knew this interrogation was no merely analytical exercise, in which the whole is to be taken apart, an then re-assembled so as to discover what it is made of. No! They knew to approach the whole in terms that would be appropriate. Their approach was wonder and play. Their aim was to know. Their methods were oracular, visionary, lyrical, mythical, epic, dramatic.

From the start, pre-Socratic philosophy understood that Being presenced as a whole. For Thales, the first philosopher (7th century BC), there was no fundamental distinction between the immanent and the transcendent, between mortality and immortality – all things are alive, and all are full of gods, and the gods are blended with all things. For his follower, Anaximander (6th century BC), this immanent/transcendent unity was infinite and boundless. He called it the "*apeiron*". But it was for the next two generations, those of Heraclitus and Parmenides, that this wholeness of reality would be articulated. For them, it was clear that reality, as *Physis*, or Being, presences. Yes! For the Greeks, *Being itself presences*! And *we* are capable of knowing Being, of knowing what it means to be, of being the sheltering place for the unconcealment of Being. That is our human potential. And our human responsibility. Our destiny – and the destiny of Being itself. For with this presencing of Being, says Heraclitus, "the fateful occurs: One unifying All" (Heidegger, 1975, p. 75). The *presencing* of Being. The *worlding* of the world.

This obviously is holism in the very big sense of that word – human/ Being as an ontological whole. But it is also quite a riddle to our contemporary ears. And it was not easy for the ancient Greeks either! For, ultimately, as Heidegger points out, their effort to articulate this presencing of Being, this very coming-forth-into-appearance of Being, this worlding of the world, lent itself to a basic misunderstanding, one which, over time, gradually rent that unified whole. Over the three centuries from Thales to Aristotle, the effort to articulate this presencing came more and more to take the form of a two-fold: "the presencing" itself and "that-which-presences" through such presencing. Over time, "that-which-presences" came more and more to resemble "beings" – that is, objects, entities, separate things. And the "presencing" itself a more and more abstract notion. Plato was the last to try to hold together the creative tension of this two-fold, but his already dualistic sense of it led directly to his student Aristotle's simple reversal of his teacher's idealistic view of it into an empirical one. And with it, to a fateful fissuring of Being – a legacy that, in the hands of the subsequent Roman synthesis of the Hebraic and the Hellenic, became the seedling of the dualistic western tradition. As Heidegger wrote, "the lightning abruptly vanished. No one held onto its streak of light and the nearness of what it illuminated" (Heidegger, 1975, p. 78).

To summarize so far, pre-Socratic Greek philosophy was premised upon an insight about an intrinsic unity, an intrinsic unity between the timely and the timeless, between the immediate perceptual world and a world of eternal or infinite meaning, between the individual and the whole, between the timely and the timeless, the immanent and the transcendent, the human and divine, the historical and the mythological. Heidegger hoped that, by retrieving the insight underlying that worldview, we could overcome the nihilistic metaphysics of duality that bedeviled western thought ever since. So he wanted to recover those origins in order to rebuild anew the holistic understanding that he saw there.

How did that forgetting of that truth of Being take place? As he points out, the seeds for that forgetting must have already been there for that to happen. Certainly if we compare the span from Anaximander to Aristotle, we can see how during those three centuries there was a shift, so by the time we get to Aristotle we're not talking about Being anymore; we're talking about beings. *Physis* has come to be understood as nature, taken as the sum total of all beings. But once you slide one into the other, what gets forgotten is the ontological difference between Being and beings. The difference between Being and thing. For the pre-Socratics – Parmenides, Heraclitus and Anaximander – as contrasting as their ideas are about Being, they all understood that Being is not a thing, but the very presencing itself – a process, a verb, not a noun, not an entity.

Now we do have to ask: what is the relationship between Being and beings? Being is presencing. But notice how easy it is to slide into a certain metaphysic such that when you start looking for Being, what you are looking for in this presencing are the things that are present. And, we get already a weird kind of premonition of the splitting in the way that we speak about this eventing of Being as a presencing and as that-which-presences. To say, for example, "there is a chair that presences" easily leads us to implicate what Heidegger calls a "two-fold". And this sense of "two-fold" is the beginning of a later splitting apart. Because once you have a presencing and that-which-presences, you can start looking at that-which-presences and identify the types of things that they are. And, as we focus on identifying what kinds of things are present, the presencing itself becomes an additional sort of quasi-thing. Being – some mysterious ultra – or abstract thing behind or at the back of these actual things. ("It's God" the theists say, unawarefully compounding its characterization as an entity.) Or, it just becomes too abstract and unreal to talk about it anymore. It's the sort of embarrassment that gives philosophy a bad reputation in our thing-centered culture. And something the human sciences ought not get too close to, for fear of contamination.

But instead of slinking away, let's go back and recoup what Heidegger got from the Greeks on this point as a way to recover from such destructive entity-metaphysics. Recall that for the Greeks Being is originally called presencing. And presencing, as far back as Anaximander, is an enduring *here* in unconcealment *now*, and *for a while*. In other words, a bringing forth of unconcealment in and as the present moment. But when depicting the presencing by the word Being, we are already beginning to slide into trickier and nebulous terminology. The verb "to be" is a later and more abstract way of thinking. What does it mean "to be"? What do we mean when you say that that table *is*? That they <u>are</u> having an affair? What does this verb "to be" really mean here? Heidegger says that to name this upsurging presencing "Being" is both an effort to articulate the eventing and at the same time laying the seeds for that later metaphysical dualism, as "Being" becomes defined by "beings" and that which is present becomes focused upon rather than the presencing itself.

How did the original pre-Socratic understand this relation of this two-fold, of the worlding of the world, of the presencing and that which is presenced?

What is the relation? *Logos*. Heraclitus says "listen not to me, but to the *logos*. It is wise to say, that according to the *logos*, all is one". Listen to the *logos* of Being. And what do you hear? The *logos* of Being unconceals or manifests that all is one. In other words, that-which-presences is not just scattered random stuff. *Logos* – the term for that non-randomness – Heidegger (1975, p. 59) sometimes translates as "meaning", "meaningfulness", or in the original Greek sense: "gathering". The *logos* is a gathering, a bringing meaningfully together, of that-which-presences. As such, it is a work of recollection (Levin, 1985) – an understanding that this isn't merely stuff; it is no-thing-ness; this is the manifestation of Being. Heidegger, in his remarkable 1966 seminar with Eugen Fink on Heraclitus (Heidegger & Fink, 1970/1979, esp. pp. 84-86) devotes considerable attention to this "coming-forth-into-appearance" using Husserl's notion of "constitution" as a clue, trying as always, to cut between the dualistic and reductionistic notions that meaning is either to be "found out there" as an objectivity, or "created in here" as a subjectivity. Rather, this old Greek sense of *logos* cuts between and beneath these antimonies of realism and idealism, opening exactly the space for phenomenology and the human sciences.

Now of course the word *logos* has been trampled by so many different traditions that modern thought no longer understands what Heraclitus meant. For modern thought *logos* just means the power to put something into words. But what the Greeks meant by *logos* was much more powerful than merely "word". It only came to mean word by the much later Aristotelian metaphysics of Being. Remember Aristotle's famous definition of the human is "*zoon logon echon*": Man is the rational animal. By Aristotle's time, the power to logos becomes the power of rationality. The power to identify, and classify and name the things – that's what he saw *logos* as.

But for Heidegger "*zoon logon echon*" means something very different than just rationally classifying the categories of things. With Heidegger, we could re-translate Aristotle's phrase as: Man is the being that has the power to *logos* (Murray, 1975). *Logos*, Heidegger (1975, p. 76) tells us is our capacity to "breathe things into existence" – "the laying that gathers [...] that which gathers all present beings into presencing and lets them lie before us". To let Being be. Heidegger develops this translation of *logos* from the double sense of the Greek verb form *legein* which means both "to speak" and "to lay" – "in the sense of bringing things to lie together, collecting them, gathering them together" (Sallis, 1975, p. 7). It is both a "planting" (as a donating) and a harvesting (as an accepting). Thus, when you let Being be, it is a way of "being with" not a "challenging forth". *Physis* as *Poesis* – which I think is not a bad mantra for the human sciences.

What these Greeks understood is that human being is the place of the unconcealment of Being. As Heidegger was fond of putting it, we are the *anwesen* – the lighted clearing – of Being. In that way of unconcealing, we are gathering the eventing of Being itself. And, human being then is that which gathers all present beings into presencing and lets them lie before us [...] in *the presencing*. This is the human responsibility as human being.

A very shorthand answer to the question "what are we here for?": to let Being be. If you're looking at this answer from a dualistic metaphysics, you'd naturally react: "what hubris to think, you let Being be! How full of pride the human is". But that's only if you hypostatize Being as if it were some quasi-thing – over there, like a trained monkey, and you're in charge of it. But that leaves you with a mere pile of entities. You can't find Being in that. When entities are taken to be the hallmark and basis of reality, then meaning is squeezed out. Not an object, it becomes a mere epiphenomenal, something added "merely subjectively" on top of the "objective" reality of things. But therein lies the rub – for once meaning is stripped away, it cannot then be subsequently added back since, as Merleau-Ponty (1945/1962) long ago showed, you cannot derive intrinsic meaning from the extrinsic meaninglessness.

But that's not what the Greeks sought. That kind of degeneration, when the metaphysics of things has come to see beings as entities, is not at all the relation of *logos* to *physis* that the Greeks understood. How do we let Being be? How does human being manifest the truth, the unconcealment, of Being? If our destiny, if our responsibility is to let Being be, how do we fulfill this charge? How are we to be the place of the presencing of Being? How do we *let Being be*? Such a task refers to a deeper, holistic relationship, an anterior or preconceptual or non-mediated relationship to Being, that lets Being be, and that's what Heidegger means by truth as *aletheia* –truth as the unconcealment of Being. Truth in this sense does not equal a correspondence between proposition A and object B, whereby A is true if it corresponds to thing B. On the contrary, to be the place of the unconcealment of Being – to let Being be – isn't to make statements about the objectivity of things. How then do we *let Being be*?

The Greek sense is that human existence is open to Being-as-a-whole. The here and now of my life – of living in *this* place at *this* time – is interpenetrated by the whole of Being. Oedipus was not just a story of some guy that lived 2,400 years ago. It's *both* mythological *and* psychological. It's both personal *and* general. The plays of Euripides and Sophocles, the poetry of Aeschylus and the fables of Aesop, the love poems of Sappho, these were not just about historical characters, they were about your life. In other words, the timeless and the timely, the infinite and the finite, together form a synthesis, an intrinsic unity. The immediately given perceptual and the timeless meanings are manifesting in *our* everyday lives *here* and *now* – *here* and *now*. Being presences whenever we bring awareness. *Right here. Right now.* The present moment is saturated with Being. The everyday is fraught with meaning.

This very deep point can be well illustrated with a story about Heraclitus that Heidegger (1947/1977) is fond of repeating. When Heraclitus was old, and renowned throughout Greece as a celebrated thinker, a group of foreigners came to see him. Having arrived at his house, they found him stooped over his stove, warming himself. At this disappointing spectacle of a shivering old man, the visitors lost their interest in coming any closer and indeed are on the verge of leaving, when Heraclitus encouraged them to enter by saying "here too the gods are present".

Or, to use another idiom, as Jesus replied to his apostles' question of where to find the kingdom of heaven, "split the wood, and I am there. Lift the rock, and I am there". But, as he added, it is "only when you make the two as one, the above as the below, that you enter the kingdom" (cf., Pagels, 1979; Pagels & King, 2007). Or, as the Tibetan Buddhists are long fond of noting, the jewel of enlightenment, *nirvana*, is right here, at our feet, in these very weeds.

That's the holistic vision I've sought to recover from the Greeks. And that's why, as Tarnas (1991, p. 72) wrote, "for the Greeks it's as if heaven and earth have not yet been fully rent asunder". Rather, in the wholeness of the un-bifurcated ever-present moment, there is a freshness "as of the world lit by a kind of six o'clock in the morning light and the due imperishably on the grass" (Tarnas, 1991, p. 72). It is this sense of unvarnished wonder and awe in the face of the actually lived world that Husserl summoned in his followers with his injunction to "return to the things themselves".

The Second Wave. Renaissance Humanitas : The Irreducibility of Human Experience

But as the classical worldview was swept away, replaced eventually by a medieval worldview, this heritage was lost, though not forever. Rather, it lay dormant beneath a medieval cosmology that very sharply divided earth from heaven, this life and the next, the temporal from the eternal, the true faith from the damned. Wholeness waited for a re-awakening, a renaissance. This occurred in Italy in the late 14th century, and spread through Europe, deeply infusing the western tradition, for a while, with a re-invigorated sense of humanism. And, once again, this sense of humanism had a taproot in a profoundly holistic vision.

Many different influences sparked this renaissance, from the Bubonic Plague to the new mobility of money derived from commerce rather than land. But most of all it was the impact of ancient Greek texts that inspired a new generation of thinkers and artists. The artifacts and ruins of Greco-

Roman antiquity had lain buried for a millennium in virtually every farmer's field in Italy, but with the discovery and faithful translation of original texts by a small band of humanist thinkers, a renewal in our conception of ourselves was launched: an enlarged conception that re-integrated the "voiceless zone" (Hale, 1991) of that previous medieval era. These new voices included: women (who could now be scholars, orators, poets, politicians); "the heart" (in contrast to the abstract Scholastic tradition whose mental gymnastics had nothing to contribute to real life); and "the pagan" (those *pre-* and *non-*Christian scholars whose texts now came into prominence once more.

A new vision was emerging: the world itself came to be seen, not as the Devil's playground of temptation and sin, but as enchanted. Likewise, the human was understood not as a hopelessly befouled creature, but a worthy emanation of the divine. Human and world, possessing a divine spark (Tarnas, 1991). Perhaps the clearest example of Renaissance humanism was Pico della Mirandola's *Oration on the Dignity of Man*. He argued that the greatness of human being is our freedom to choose our own way, and that can we attain this ambition responsibly through knowledge and love. He then grounded this claim in scriptural sources from the New Testament, then from the Old, and then from pre-Christian sources, Greek and Asian. His *tour de force*, synthesizing the worlds of Christianity and antiquity set a clear tone for the holistic aims of the Renaissance.

This mending of the rupture between the Christian worldview of medieval Europe with the "pagan" world of antiquity brought with it an enlarged vision of the organic, indeed seamless, intertwining of the previous dualism of human/divine. The work of Marsilio Ficino may stand as a particularly shining example. His Theologia Platonica de immortalitate animorum (1469-1474/2006), a multi-volume study of Plato and the key neo-Platonists, especially Plotinus, was an effort to show that in fact that Platonism was the intellectual root of Christianity, but of a particularly non-dual vision of spirituality (c.f., Kristeller, 1964; Mahoney, 2006). This holistic vision was rooted in the concrete, natural order of actual life. The interrelatedness of human/divine Ficino expressed most poignantly in his understanding of the human soul:

> This is the greatest of all miracles in nature. All other things beneath god are always one single being, but the Soul is all things together. It possesses the images of the divine things on which it depends itself and the concepts and originals of the lower things [...] since it is the center of all things, it has the forces of all. Hence it passes into all things. And since it is the true connection of all things, it goes to the one without leaving the others. It goes into an individual thing and

> always deals withal. Therefore it may be rightly called the center of nature, the middle term of all things, the series of the world, the face of all, the bond and the juncture of the universe. (as translated in Kristeller, 1964, p. 120)

What medieval theology had rent asunder, Renaissance scholars, guided by a spirit of "determined decompartmentalization" (Tarnas, 1991, p. 230), were now putting back together: the contrapuntal, the paradoxical harmonized within an enlarged whole. Painting lends us many fine examples. Early on, Botticelli's two most famous paintings: The *Birth of Venus* and *Primavera* brought together the Christian and pagan. But perhaps Raphael's *School of Athens* will best exemplify this point. Commissioned by the Pope, and painted as a fresco on the wall of the *Stanza della Signatora*, the room in the Vatican where the pope signed key documents, it faced on the opposite wall his fresco *Disputa del Sacramento* – a vision of the glories of the Christian church through an assemblage of dozens of its historical and Biblical figures. To face this august religious assembly, Raphael now chose to paint "the glorification of philosophy":

> [...] half a hundred figures summing up rich centuries of Greek thought, and all gathered in an immortal moment under the coffered arch of a massive pagan portico... Plato... Aristotle... Socrates... Pythagoras... Heraclitus... Diogenes... Archimedes... Ptolemy... Zoroaster... all in all, such a parliament of wisdom had never been painted, perhaps never been conceived before. And not a word about heresy, no philosophers burned at the stake here; here, under the protection of a Pope too great to fuss about the difference between one error and another, the young Christian has suddenly brought all these pagans together, painted them in their own character and with remarkable understanding and sympathy, and placed them where the theologians could see them and exchange fallibilities, and where the Pope, between one document and another, might contemplate the co-operative process and creation of human thought. This painting and the *Disputa* are the ideal of the Renaissance – pagan antiquity and Christian faith living together in one room and in harmony. (Durant, 1953, p. 459-460)

But, in contrast to the theological, the humanistic viewpoint does not have a similarly univocal legitimating authority; surely not only a weakness but also its source of innovativeness and range of topics (Bullock, 1985) – namely the whole human experience. As the great French Renaissance scholar, Montaigne, pointed out, everything we know comes through our experience and so the key is to be fully human, to cultivate our actual experience. Modernism and postmodernism have both incorrectly identified the Renaissance with the maxim that "man is the measure of all tings" (e.g., by Barnes, 1937). But that maxim (actually derived from Protagoras) is a decisive mis-characterization of the true Renaissance project: that the proper study of mankind is man (from a poem by Alexander Pope in 1870 and linked to the Renaissance by many, e.g., Durant, 1953).

Emphasizing this primacy of experience, the humanists of the Renaissance redirected the focus from the abstract metaphysical questions of medieval scholasticism to the practical concerns of actual life: "the art of living". As Petrarch, an early Renaissance humanist, argued, people have a right to concern themselves with their actual human life, to enjoy an open delight in the here and now, and to augment its beauties, and to seek fulfillment in it (Barzun, 2000; Durant, 1953). Renaissance writers provided books of advice on good living, such as Marsilio Ficino, who's contribution, *Three Books on Life* (1489), recommended sleeping well, not repressing sexual desire, and laughing and being merry as often as one can. Other notable treatises on how to live well included Francesco Barbaro's *Concerning Marriage* (1414), Leon Battista Alberti's *On the Family* (1433), Matteo Palmieri's *On Civil Life* (1435-1438), and especially Lorenzo Valla's (1433) *On Pleasure*. (c.f., Nauert, 1995). Even minor Renaissance scholars, such as Bartolommeo della Fonte, whose orations in the 1480s vigorously sought to defend the value of humanism in all its branches, from rhetoric to philosophy, did so in terms of its contributions to the concord of the individual and civic life of the community – to the arts of civilization (c.f., Trinkaus, 1960). Summing up this impact, Stinger (1988, pp. 176-177) demonstrated that humanism "contributed answers to moral issues Florentines confronted in the conduct of their daily lives, and it inspired the exercise of creative intelligence in the pursuit of human virtue and fulfillment". Renaissance humanists were "urbane and lusty spirits [...] who feed and live on this legacy of mental freedom, esthetic sensitivity, embracing its joys of sense, mind, and soul; and hearing ever in their hearts, amid hymns of hate and above the cannon's roar" (Durant, 1952, p. 728). An all-embracing ode to Joy.

They brought philosophy back down to earth by re-introducing the old Greek question of how to live a good life. But what, exactly, does it mean to „live a good life"? For the humanists of the Renaissance, this question involved much more than merely frivolity or good-natured conduct. They understood that people are actively embedded within a world, understood as inclusive of a social world, civil world and a natural world. Their answer to this question was that one lives a good life by an active involvement in the world and that men and women, through education (as *paidagogia* – the old Greek sense of education), could sharpen and use their curiosity, their imagination, their will, their creative and free power to transform themselves and to affect their fate and aspire to the highest excellence.

The key to the good life was to develop one's capacity for awareness. But awareness of what? Ultimately, of one's self and of one's situation, one's context, one's relation to the world. To wake up, to become aware, for them, meant understanding these world-relations. Regarding one's self, the depth of one's own engaged, worlded consciousness became a key discovery.

In the literary arts, many key examples abound. From Boccaccio's *Decameron* to Machiavelli's *Mandragola*, to More's *Utopia*, Renaissance fiction displayed the rough and tumble of lives lived within the contexts of their worlds, with the all-too-human dilemmas of relationships of love and loss, played out within the even wider contexts of plague and political intrigue. Nonfiction literature likewise took very seriously the importance of contextual analysis. For example, Colet's 1496 lectures at Oxford on St. Paul's *Epistles*, took them in their original Greek, and located Paul clearly in his own time and place, and so "enabled Paul to speak almost as directly to the students at Oxford as he had spoken to the Corinthians" (Hale, 1994, p. 196). Likewise, Erasmus's analysis of St. Jerome's letters portrayed Jerome as a human being, alive in his own place and time, stripped of all the confabulating conventions that had stripped Jerome of his historical credibility (Rice, 1988, pp. 19-20). Rabil (1988b, p. 170) notes that the Renaissance civic humanists "introduced a historical consciousness that has ever since characterized western thinking". They replaced notions of "immobility, monarchy, authority, eternity, hierarchy" that had dominated political writing with ideas of "progress, patriotism, equality, liberty, and utopia". Furthermore, they understood that the role of fate in human destiny can be mitigated by one's own wise and skillful action.

The visual arts likewise offer many excellent examples. A telling implication of this insight came through the development of the new use of perspective in Renaissance art. Alberti systematized the theory of perspective which Brunelleschi had begun. Perhaps the best illustration of the use of perspective can be seen in the bronze cast panels on the doors on the Baptistery of San Giovanni in Florence, sculpted by Lorenzo Ghiberti. These magnificent panels offered a revolutionary new vision, in two respects. First, through the use of innovative techniques in gradation of relief, a sense of perspective is achieved, so that the standpoint of the beholder is implicated, thus achieving in bronze casting the effect newly developed by Renaissance painters. Furthermore, what the viewer is invited to stand in relation to is also unprecedented. In contrast to previous pictorial relief work, in which solitary figures were immersed in a hazy and vague atmosphere, an undefined and indefinable space, these panels portrayed not merely isolated figures, but astonishingly complete situations, including their background. The narrative complexity of each panel was far more comprehensive and coherent than anything previously envisaged. In these ways, Renaissance art disclosed the humanistic conception of people existing within the world of their involvements, rather than as detached figures lacking any intrinsic relatedness.

This same grasp of our human situatedness was also being utilized in architecture. Palladio's buildings are still masterpieces for their excellence in this regard, such as his La Rotonda and the Villa Poiana near Vincenza, and the Basilica in Venice. By placing the person in the world, humans acquire an awareness not only of the world, but of themselves as participants in this world. This holistic grasp of self, this conscious self-awareness is the basis for the Renaissance call to fulfill the potential of human being. Hickey calls Palladio's house "a house undivided" and credits Palladio with "the science of happiness". He adds:

> An aura of sweet self-consciousness [...] less critical or ironic than joyfully self-aware [...] rescues his buildings from the vice of pretension by the simple stratagem of not pretending [...] Palladio is never impersonating classical architecture, he is performing it [...] the real benison of Palladio's performances is the good-natured permission they grant us to take the stage he has provided and perform with commensurate self-conscious elegance. (Hickey, 2003, p. 69)

So, human experience is accorded its full due as awakened consciousness being-in-the-world, and is accorded its due as the proper study mankind, a study that synthesizes its philosophical interest in the profound meaning of being human with the practical affairs of everyday life. This Renaissance impetus may be best exemplified by Leonardo da Vinci's masterpiece: the Mona Lisa. Here is Durant's (1953, p. 212) description of da Vinci's "engaging merger of painting and philosophy":

> This, then, is the face that launched a thousand reams upon a sea of ink. Not an unusually lovely face [...] It is her smile that has made her fortune through the centuries [...] What is she smiling at? The efforts of the musicians to entertain her? The leisurely diligence of an artist who paints her through a thousand days and never makes an end? Or is it not just Mona Lisa smiling, but woman, all women, saying to all men: "Poor impassioned lovers! A Nature blindly commanding continuance burns your nerves with an absurd hunger for our flesh, softens your brains with a quite unreasonable idealization of our charms, lifts you to lyrics that subside with consummation – all that you may be precipitated into

> parentage! Could anything be more ridiculous? But we too are snared; we women pay a heavier price than you for your infatuation. And yet, sweet fools, it is pleasant to be desired, and life is redeemed when we are loved."

"Sweet fools", she smiled. Yes, when we embrace the whole of Being, all so very human foibles are redeemed, enfolded within and so manifesting the whole. As with the Greek spirit of "play", so too the Renaissance placed its value on "all consuming laughter". But, as Kundera (1996) has pointed out, humor, play, laughter signify much more than mere mirth. Something deeper is being brought forth – a relation to the world in which dogmas are relativized, presuppositions called into question and self-importance deflated by implying alternative possibilities. "Laughter is the instrument of detachment; it breaks down the spiritual rigidity that seeks to clutch at its values as it they were so many coins hoarded by a miser" (Barrett, 1972, p. 204).

Interregnum. The Ascendancy of the Scientific Attitude: Excluded Knowledge

This Renaissance spirit spread north from Italy, through much of Europe. France, Holland, England were particularly imbued. We can recall Erasmus' quirky and brave *In Praise of Folly*, a mischievous satire against orthodoxy. Or Rembrandt's work, for example, his magnificent painting *The Night Watch*, to gather an illustration of the power of seeing people within their engaged world-relations. In contrast to previous group portraiture, wherein the people merely stood still, Rembrandt's painting captures them in the moment, in action, moving about the nighttime streets of the town, on duty. The effect was a startling revolution in vision.

But the Renaissance did not survive the violent reactions to the schism within Christendom that followed the Protestant Reformation. When a religious fanatic assassinated Henry IV, the humanist ruler of France who sought to institutionalize multi-denominational tolerance, the hopes of the Renaissance were eclipsed by a continent-wide plunge into sectarian religious warfare – the infamous Thirty Years War. It became a generation-long slaughter, ultimately decimating central Europe as effectively as had the Black Death of the plague. Positions hardened with the battle lines, orthodoxy was re-established, and the deviant were driven into silence. Sin and guilt became paramount once again, along with the compulsory darkened confessional box. Women covered themselves, and chastity once more replaced ecstasy. But the slaughter went on, and on, and on, as the Catholic and Protestant sides were relatively evenly matched. And so millions were massacred, in the name of religion. It finally ended when, under the cynical tutelage of Cardinal Richelieu, Catholic France switched sides, and fought with the Protestant faction to defeat the Catholic empire of Austria, to attain the pre-eminence of the major land power on the continent. All in the name of religion.

From that catastrophe, intellectuals recoiled in horror at the corruption of the authority of religion, and rushed to put together another basis for legitimation, an authority that could not be so cynically corrupted. Science, of course, was their alternative. And the next two generations, from Descartes to Newton, built an edifice of certainty based on Science as the legitimating authority (Toulmin, 1992).

But this Science derived its authority from an epistemology of dualism and a metaphysics of mechanistic causality. Newton's science of nature was not about the world of human experience but only of "brute" matter (Burtt, 1932). This approach, promising the desperately sought for certainty, was quickly adopted not only for physics, but also for all the human studies. For example, the British Empiricists saw the mind as likewise governed by "laws of association" and in the next century the search was on for the "elements" of consciousness, analogous to the periodic table of elements from chemistry. Modernity dawned, not as a continuation of the Renaissance (as is sometimes mistakenly assumed by postmodernists, e.g., Kvale, 1990), but as its repudiation.

The Third Wave. Contemporary Humanistic Psychology in the United States

For the next three hundred years this view of science dominated inquiry into human experience as well as into nature. And when, in the late nineteenth century, the various social sciences established themselves independently from philosophy, they very self-consciously pledged their allegiance to this standard of science. Indeed, as the recently converted so often do, they strove even to out-orthodox the orthodox. Hence the long sterility of modern psychology, locked into a dualistic conception of its own subject matter. But its long search for the "laws of mental life" proved barren, epitomized by the reign of behaviorism through the mid-twentieth century.

Finally, as part of a larger shift in the *Zeitgeist*, a reform movement emerged within European and American psychology. Inspired by previous developments in existential-phenomenological philosophy begun by Edmund Husserl (1934/1965, 1954/1970, 1911/1981), psychologists on both sides of the Atlantic began to revision the basic presuppositions of elementism and mechanism, and a new wave of broadly humanistic thought emerged. Key figures steeped in the phenomenological tradition included Ludwig Binswanger, Medard Boss, R. D. Laing and J. H. van den Berg from Europe, and, in the United States, Rollo May and Amedeo Giorgi. This was a very loosely emerging movement, with no sole leader, so there were many different lines of development (Aanstoos, 1987), eventually including an indigenously American humanistic movement, pioneered especially by Carl Rogers and Abraham Maslow and a transpersonal movement pioneered by Ken Wilber. It quickly grew and became a very multifarious movement, but guiding and pervading it was a sense of valuing the human as a whole. One of its early and most prominent advocates, Rollo May, even characterized it in 1958 as "the endeavor to understand man by cutting below the cleavage between subject and object which has bedeviled Western thought and science since shortly after the Renaissance" (May *et al*, 1958, p. 11). This depiction was entirely in line with the thrust of phenomenological philosophy, of which Merleau-Ponty wrote: "the chief gain from phenomenology is to have united extreme subjectivism and extreme objectivism in the notion of the world" (Merleau-Ponty, 1945/1962, p. xix). Likewise, Simone de Beauvoir (1946, p. 363) summarized this core insight with this extraordinary potency and succinctness:

> One of the immense merits of phenomenology consists in having restored to man the right to an authentic existence by abolishing the opposition between subject and object. It is impossible to define an object while cutting it off from the subject by which and for which it is an object. And the subject reveals itself only through the objects in which it engages itself. Such an affirmation merely makes explicit the content of our naive experience. But it is rich in consequences... Hence it is of extreme importance to establish solidly and to restore to man that child-like audacity which his years of verbal docility have deprived him: the audacity to say "Here I am".

The other chapters in this volume provide an exemplary variety of concrete illustrations that demonstrate this holistic taproot contributed by phenomenology to contemporary psychology. Rather than adding further to that, I would now like to emphasize how relevant and timely holism is as we move toward the future.

The Impact of a Holistic Vision

This claim of timeliness can be gleaned by considering some of the prospective benefits from a holistic vision. There are many areas in which we could demonstrate that claim, but here I can focus only briefly on four urgent crises in which this prospect is particularly evident: the medical, the social, the spiritual and the ecological.

Holistic Health

Despite enormous and ever-increasing expenditures, health care in this country is in a state of seemingly intractable crises. Immunities weaken while bacteria become resistant, fitness declines while obesity increases, cancer is epidemic while toxins proliferate, and the population consumes ever larger amounts of Prozac in the face of an epidemic of depression. And worldwide "rising incidence and prevalence of psychosomatic diseases, mental disorders, anxiety and neurosis" (Lambo, 2000, p. 114). The old "medical model" seems unable to comprehend or respond adequately to the new challenges we face, precisely because they do not conform to the old, mechanistic view of the body and disease.

In the past twenty years, however, humanistic psychologists such as Achterberg (1985), Borysenko (1988) and Criswell (2001) have been developing a "holistic" approach, in the sense of a "mind/body" holism. Such developments have already demonstrated many significant concrete results, such as the healing potential of imagery, counseling, meditation and yoga on life-threatening illnesses, from heart disease to cancer. The next step is to comprehend the even larger whole: beyond one's own mind/body is the wider relationship of person/world, most clearly manifest through the immune system, and approached through the emerging field of psycho-neuro-immunology. And the powerful impact of an even more comprehensively holistic vision on health is only now beginning, as we start to study nonlocal and transpersonal impacts on healing (Dossey, 1999).

Globalization and Its Discontents

As technology weaves its world wide web, the planet has become smaller than ever. And boundaries that once stood as impediments are now so permeable that popular commentaries now use the metaphor that "the world is flat" (e.g., Friedman, 2006). Transnational corporations now exercise tremendous power everywhere, as capital has become so incredibly mobile that a country's currency can be withered overnight. The resultant acceleration in the pace of economic development has disrupted indigenous economies and cultures, forcing upon them within a single generation the changes western cultures took the previous three centuries to transition.

The serious crises generated by rapid globalization have accrued because thinking and planning on this issue has tended to be too short term and too fragmented. The contextual inter-relationships woven within an indigenous culture (such a local farming techniques for this particular region, rather than a generic chemical-based agribusiness) have been ignored or simply over-looked (Diaz-LaPlante, 2007; Norbert-Hodge, 1991), leading to increasing divisiveness between young/old, urban/rural, and different ethnic and religious groups. These differences are not endemic, but have been exacerbated by economic tumult. It is the humanistic vision of holism that can redress this neglected awareness, and thus humanize this wrenching shift of globalization.

A Spiritual Emergence

Mainline religions become less meaningful and people drift increasingly toward fundamentalism, or substance abuse, driven by a spiritual hunger the modern era knows no way of satisfying. The loss of meaning, or anomie, has been the haunting side effect of the most materialistically abundant century in the history of humanity. Our culture now pays entertainers far more than thinkers, as distraction and escape become ever more paramount goals.

As the distinction between religion and spirituality is increasingly recognized by humanistic psychologists (e.g., Elkins, 1998), the value of a holistic vision of spirituality is now becoming more evident. Contemplative, meditative and mindfulness traditions are now being deployed in many arenas, from chronic pain (Kabat-Zinn, 1994) to psychotherapy (Epstein, 1995; Welwood, 2000) to living everyday life more fully (Kornfield, 2000; Walsh, 1999), while other scholars are striving to build a psychology fully integrative with spirituality (e.g., Wilber, 1995, 2000). Questions of meaning and the ultimate purpose of one's life simply cannot be drowned out by television and antidepressants. They must eventually be addressed by a holistic psychology uniquely positioned to serve the spiritual well-being of the next generation.

The Ecological Crisis

Daily we are now confronted by the evidence of looming ecological disasters: the polar ice caps are melting as we live through the hottest decade on record, penguins are washing up on shores a thousand miles off their traditional migratory path as even the ocean currents have been shifted to that extent, the accumulation of greenhouse gases has changed global climate and weather extremes become ever more commonplace, the air is poisonous smog, the rain is acid, the ozone is depleted, the land is deforested, the groundwater contaminated, and oxygen endangered, deserts are growing while topsoil is lost, and mountains of nuclear waste will remain radioactive until the sun burns out. No longer the purview merely of a counter-cultural perspective, the recognition of a serious ecological crisis has been widely acknowledged even by the most mainstream scholars (e.g., Gore, 2006; Friedman, 2008).

A "deep ecology" movement (e.g., Naess, 1986) has recently been coalescing around the basic vision of radical inter-connectedness. The utter compatibility of this movement with humanistic psychology's holistic vision is just now being comprehended, and an emerging subfield of ecopsychology is being born. Metzner (1999, p. 2) urges psychology to undergo a "fundamental [...] revision that would take the ecological context of human life into account". Pilisuk & Joy (2001, p. 107) note that ecological and humanistic thought converge in challenging the basic assumption of a mechanistic worldview. Roberts (1998) and Roszak, Gomes & Kanner (1995) provide that subfield with a variety of practices aimed at restoring the earth and healing the mind.

Conclusion

As can be seen from the peaks of these waves of holistic thinking in the west, this vision has a long history – co-terminus actually with the very history of western thought. In this light, we can see it is not merely a one-generation reform movement that will pass away with the ending of its late 20th century incarnation. Rather, though it may only peak at timely occasions, holism provides psychology with an enduring taproot, a vision of the meaning of being human more than twenty-five centuries in the making. As the heirs to this legacy, contemporary psychology has the opportunity, and responsibility, of bringing this vision of wholeness to fulfillment – precisely when it is most needed.

References

Aanstoos, C.M. (1987). A comparative survey of human science psychologies. *Methods, 1*(2), 1-36.

Aanstoos, C.M. (1996). Reflections and visions: An interview with Amedeo Giorgi. *The Humanistic Psychologist, 24*, 3-27.

Aanstoos, C.M. (2007). Holistic psychology: A history and statement of purpose. In M. Tarozzi (Ed.). *New frontiers of phenomenology: Proceedings of the International Human Science Research Conference*, University of Trento, Italy.

Aanstoos, C.M. (2009a). *The development of the human sciences: Holism in Renaissance humanism.* Paper presented to the International Human Science Research Conference, Molde, Norway, June.

Aanstoos, C.M. (2009b). *Foundations of humanistic psychology.* Lectures presented at University of West Georgia, Fall.

Aanstoos, C.M. (2009c). Holism and the human sciences. In M. Tarozzi (Ed). *Phenomenology and Human Science Today. Thoughts and Research.* Bucharest, Rumania : Zetabooks.

Achterberg, J. (1985). *Imagery in healing.* Boston: Shambhala.

Angyal, A. (1965). *Neurosis and treatment: A holistic theory.* New York : Wiley.

Barnes, H. (1937). *An intellectual and cultural history of the western world: Vol. 2: From the renaissance through the eighteenth century.* New York : Dover.

Barzun, J. (2000). *From dawn to decadence: 500 years of western cultural life.* New York: Harper Collins.

Borysenko, J. (1988). *Minding the body, mending the mind.* New York: Bantam.

Bullock, A. (1985). *The humanist tradition in the west* (pp. 11-47). New York: Norton.

Burtt, E. A. (1932). *The metaphysical foundations of modern science* (rev. ed.). New York: Anchor, pp. 15-35 and 303-325.

Cahill, T. (2003). *Sailing the wine dark sea: Why the Greeks matter.* New York: Doubleday.

Criswell, E. (2001). Humanistic psychology and mind/body medicine. In Schneider, K., Bugental, J. & Pierson, J. (Eds.). *The handbook of humanistic psychology* (pp. 581-591). London: Sage.

DeBeauvoir, S. (1946). Review of Merleau-Ponty's *Phenomenology of Perception. Les Temps Modernes, I,* p. 363.

Diaz-LaPlante, J. (2007). Humanistic psychology and social transformation: building the path toward a livable today and a just tomorrow. *Journal of Humanistic Psychology, 47,* 54-72.

Dillon, J. (2008). Reclaiming humanistic psychology from modernity: Problems and solutions. *Journal of Humanistic Psychology, 48,* 221-242.

Dossey, L. (1999). *Reinventing medicine : Beyond mind/body to a new era of healing.* New York: Harper-Collins.

Durant, W. (1939). *The life of Greece.* (*The story of civilization: Volume 2*). New York: Simon & Schuster.

Durant, W. (1953). *The Renaissance: A history of civilization in Italy from 1304-1576 A.D.* (*The story of civilization: Volume 5*). New York: Simon & Schuster.

Elkins, D. (1998). *Beyond religion: A personal program for building a spiritual life outside the walls of traditional religion.* Wheaton, IL: Quest.

Epstein, M. (1995). *Thoughts without a thinker: Psychotherapy from a Buddhist perspective.* New York: Basic Books.

Ficino, M. (2002). *De vita libri tres.* (Trans. as *Three books on life* by C. V. Kaske & J. R. Clarke). Tempe, AZ: The Renaissance Society of America. [Original work published 1489]

Ficino, M. (2006). *Theologia Platonica de immortalitate animae.* Cambridge, MA: Harvard University Press. [Original work published 1469-1474]

Fox, R.L. (2006). *The classical world.* New York: Basic Books.

Friedman, T. (2006). *The world is flat* (expanded ed.). New York: Farrar, Straus & Giroux.

Friedman, T. (2008). *Hot, flat and crowded.* New York: Farrar, Straus & Giroux.

Giorgi, A. (1970). *Psychology as a human science.* New York: Harper & Row.

Giorgi, A. (1976). Phenomenology and the foundations of psychology. In William Arnold (Ed.), 1975 *Nebraska symposium on motivation: Conceptual foundations of psychology* (pp. 281-348). Lincoln: University of Nebraska Press.

Giorgi, A. (1981). Humanistic psychology and metapsychology. In J. Royce & L. Mos (Eds.), *Humanistic psychology: Conceptual criticisms* (pp. 19-47). New York: Plenum Press.

Giorgi, A. (1984a). Toward a new paradigm for psychology. In C. M. Aanstoos, (Ed.), *Exploring the lived world: Readings in phenomenological psychology. West Georgia College Studies in the Social Sciences, 23* (pp. 9-28). Carrollton: Eidos.

Giorgi, A. (1984b). Toward a phenomenologically based unified paradigm for psychology. In D. Kruger (Ed.), *The changing reality of modern man: Essays in honor of J. H. van den Berg* ((pp. 20-34). Capetown, South Africa: Juta.

Giorgi, A. (Ed.). (1985). *Phenomenology and psychological research.* Pittsburgh: Duquesne University Press.

Giorgi, A. (1992). Whither humanistic psychology? *The Humanistic Psychologist, 20,* 422-438.

Giorgi, A. (1994) The idea of human science. In F.J. Wertz (Ed.). *The humanistic movement: Recovering the person in psychology* (pp. 89-104). Lake Worth, FL: Gardner.

Giorgi, A. (2006). The value of phenomenology for psychology In P. Ashworth & M. Chung (Eds.), *Phenomenology and psychological science: Historical and philosophical perspectives.* New York: Springer.

Giorgi, A. (2007). The contrasting approaches of postmodernity and phenomenology to the limits of the empirical paradigm in psychology. *Encyclopaideia, Anno XI, 22,* 31-52.

Giorgi, A. (2008). Phenomenological psychology. In C. Wiley & W. Stainton-Rogers (Eds.), *The Sage handbook of qualitative research in psychology.* London: Sage.

Giorgi, A. (2009). *Descriptive phenomenological method in psychology.* Pittsburgh: Duquesne University Press.

Goldstein, K. (1939). *The organism: A holistic approach to biology derived from pathological data in man.* New York: American Book Company.

Gore, A. (2006). *An inconvenient truth.* New York: Rodale.

Hale, J. (1994). *The civilization of Europe in the Renaissance.* New York: Knopf.

Hamilton, E. (1930). *The Greek way.* New York: Norton.Heidegger, M. (1971). The origin of the work of art In M. Heidegger, *Poetry, language, thought* (A. Hofstadter, Trans.). New York: Harper. (Original work published 1960)

Heidegger, M. (1975). *Early Greek thinking* (D. Krell & F. Capuzzi, Trans.). San Francisco: Harper. (Original works published 1950-1967)

Heidegger, M. (1977). Letter on humanism. In D. Krell (Ed. & Trans.), *Martin Heidegger: Basic writings.* New York: Harper & Row. (Original work published 1947)

Heidegger, M. (1992). *Parmenides* (A. Schuwer & R. Rojcewicz, Trans.). Bloomington: Indiana University Press. (Original work published 1982)

Heidegger, M. & Fink, E. (1979). *Heraclitus seminar* (C. Seibert, Trans.). Evanston: Northwestern University Press. (Original work published 1970)

Hickey, D. (2003). A house undivided: Andrea Palladio and the science of happiness. *Harpers*, April, 57-69.

Husserl, E. (1965). Philosophy and the crisis of European man. In E. Husserl, *Phenomenology and the crisis of philosophy* (pp. 149-192) (trans. by Q. Lauer). New York: Harper & Row. (Original work published in 1934)

Husserl, E. (1970). *The crisis of European sciences and transcendental phenomenology: An introduction to phenomenological philosophy* (David Carr, Trans.). Evanston: Northwestern University Press. (Original work published 1954)

Husserl, E. (1981). Philosophy as rigorous science (Quentin Lauer, Trans.). In P. McCormick & F. Ellison (Eds.). *Husserl: Shorter works* (pp. 166-197). Notre Dame, IN: University of Notre Dame Press. (Original work published 1911)

Kabat-Zinn, J. (1994). *Wherever you go, there you are.* New York: Hyperion.

Kornfield, J. (2000). *After the ecstasy, the laundry: How the heart grows wise on the spiritual path.* New York: Bantam.

Kristeller, P. O. (1964). *The philosophy of Marsilio Ficino.* Gloucester, MA: Peter Smith.

Kundera, M. (1996). *Book of Laughter and Forgetting.* New York: HarperPerrenial.

Kvale, S. (1990). Postmodern psychology: A contradicto in adjecto? *The Humanistic Psychologist, 18*, 35-54.

Lambo, A. (2000). Constraints on world medical and health progress. In Lanza (Ed.), *One world: the health and survival of the human species in the 21st century*. Santa Fe: Health Press.

Levin, D.M. (1985). *The body's recollection of being.* New York: Routledge.

MacGregor, M. (1959). *The story of Greece.* Edinburgh: Thomas Nelson.

Mahoney, E.P. (2006). Marsilio Ficino and Renaissance Platonism. In C. Celenza & K. Gouwens (Eds.), *Humanism and creativity in the Renaissance* (pp. 231-244). Boston: Brill.

May, R, Angel, E., & Ellenberger, H. (Eds.). (1958). *Existence: A new dimension in psychiatry and psychology* (pp. 3-36). New York: Basic Books.

Merleau-Ponty, M. (1962). *Phenomenology of perception* (trans. by C. Smith). New York: Humanities Press. (Original work published 1945)

Metzner, R. (1999). *Green psychology: Transforming our relationship to the earth.* Rochester, VT: Park Street.

Murray, E. L. (1975). *Lectures on Heidegger.* Duquesne University, Pittsburgh.

Naess, A. (1986). The deep ecology movement. *Philosophical Inquiry, 8*, 10-13.

Nauert, C. (1995). *Humanism and the culture of Renaissance Europe.* Cambridge, UK: Cambridge University Press.

Norbert-Hodge, H. (1991). *Ancient futures: Learning from Ladakh.* San Francisco: Sierra Club Books.

Pagels, E. (1979). *The gnostic gospels.* New York: Random House.

Pagels, E. & King, K. L. (2007). *Reading Judas: The gospel of Judas and the shaping of Christianity*. New York: Viking.

Pilisuk, M. & Joy, M. (2001). Humanistic psychology and ecology. . In K. Schneider, J. Bugental, & J. Pierson (Eds.), *The handbook of humanistic psychology* (pp. 101-114). London: Sage.

Rabil, A. (Ed.). (1988a). *Renaissance humanism: Foundations, forms and legacy*. (3 vols.). Philadelphia: University of Pennsylvania Press.

Rabil, A. (1988b). The significance of "civic humanism" in the interpretation of the Italian Renaissance. In A. Rabil (Ed.), *Renaissance humanism: Foundations, forms and legacy: Volume 1: Humanism in Italy* (pp. 141-174). Philadelphia: University of Pennsylvania Press.

Rice, E. F. (1988). The Renaissance idea of Christian antiquity: Humanist patristic scholarship. In A. Rabil (Ed.), *Renaissance humanism: Foundations, forms and legacy: Volume 1: Humanism in Italy* (pp. 17-28). Philadelphia: University of Pennsylvania Press.

Roberts, E. (Ed.) (1998). *Humanistic psychology and ecopsychology* (a special issue of *The Humanistic Psychologist, 26*, 1-3.

Robinson, J.M. (1968). *An introduction to early Greek philosophy*. New York: Houghton Mifflin.

Roszak, T., Gomes, M. & Kanner, A. (Eds.). (1995*). Ecopsychology*. San Francisco: Sierra Club Books.

Sallis, J. (1975). *Being and logos: The way of Platonic dialogue*. Pittsburgh: Duquesne University Press.

Scully, V. (1979). *The earth, the temple and the gods: Greek sacred architecture* (rev. ed.). New Haven: Yale University Press.

Seidel, G.J. (1964). *Martin Heidegger and the pre-Socratics*. Lincoln: University of Nebraska Press.

Stinger, C. (1988). Humanism in Florence. . In A. Rabil (Ed.), *Renaissance humanism: Foundations, forms and legacy: Volume 1: Humanism in Italy* (pp. 175-208). Philadelphia: University of Pennsylvania Press.

Tarnas, R. (1991). *The passion of the western mind*. New York: Ballantine.

Toulmin, S. (1992). *Cosmopolis: The hidden agenda of modernity*. Chicago: University of Chicago Press.

Trinkaus, C. (1960). A humanist's image of humanism: The inaugural orations of Bartolommeo della fonte. *Studies in the Renaissance, 7*, 90-147.

Valla, L. (1433). *De Voluptate [On pleasure]*. Translated reprint available at: http://www.humanistictexts.org/valla.htm

Von Hildebrand, A. (Ed.). (1966). *Greek culture: The adventure of the human spirit*. New York: Braziller.

Walsh, R. (1999). *Essential spirituality*. New York: Wiley

Welwood, J. (2000). *Toward a psychology of awakening: Buddhism, psychotherapy, and the path of personal and spiritual transformation*. Boston: Shambhala.

Wertz, F. J. & Aanstoos, C.M. (1999). Amedeo Giorgi and the project of a human science. In D. Moss (Ed.). *Humanistic and transpersonal psychology* (pp. 287-300). Westport, CT: Greenwood.

Wheelwright, P. (Ed.). (1966). *The presocratics.* Upper Saddle River, NJ: Prentice Hall.

Wilber, K. (1995). *Sex, ecology, spirituality.* Boston: Shambhala.

Wilber, K. (2000). *Integral psychology: Consciousness, spirit, psychology, therapy.* Boston: Shambhala.

Note

1 Of course I am aware that a variety of non-Western cultures also have a history of holistic thinking: native American (especially Amazonian), Arctic (especially Inuit, Suomi, and Siberian), Polynesian (especially Maori and Australian aboriginal), African (especially Fong, Kung and Xhosa), and south and east Asian (especially Vedic, Buddhist and Taoist). But, since the contemporary human science approach arose mainly from western roots that have only recently been deeply impacted by these nonwestern sources, I wanted to discover our own indigenous sources of holism.

BEYOND SCIENTISM AND RELATIVISM: AMEDEO GIORGI'S COMMITMENT TO HUMAN SCIENCE

Marc Applebaum, Ph.D.

Saybrook University
United States

Abstract

Amedeo Giorgi has sought to offer an alternative to the scientism of psychology conceived as positive science, on the one hand, and the relativism implicit in many of the research approaches based upon hermeneutic or postmodernist philosophy, on the other hand. Giorgi's body of work strives to articulate and defend a human scientific psychological research method that does justice to the human subject. Such an approach must demonstrate fidelity to psychological subjectivity as a lived phenomenon. Additionally, the approach must be methodical, teachable, and yield intersubjectively verifiable knowledge. In other words it must yield scientific knowledge. The phenomenological tradition, broadly defined, includes an important tension between descriptive or Husserlian perspectives and the interpretive (hermeneutic) perspectives articulated by Heidegger, Gadamer, and Ricoeur. I will argue that the meaning of the tension between Husserlian phenomenology and hermeneutics depends in large measure upon whether one's motivating interest is primarily scientific or philosophical. I will seek to describe Giorgi's contribution to psychology in terms of his insistence on the scientific status of phenomenological psychological research. I will seek to situate Giorgi's body of work vis-à-vis hermeneutic approaches in order to highlight the uniqueness of his contribution to the field.

> Although the genuine though never radically clarified idea of philosophy has by no means been completely sacrificed, the multiplicity of philosophies, which can hardly be comprehended any more, nevertheless has the result that it is no longer divided into scientific directions, such that they could still seriously work together, carry on a scientific dialogue through criticism and countercriticism, and still guide the common idea of one science toward the path of realization, in the manner of the directions within modern biology or mathematics and physics; rather, they are contrasted as societies of aesthetic style, so to speak, analogous to the "directions" and "currents" in the fine arts. Indeed, in the splintering of philosophies and their literature, is it still possible at all to study them seriously as works of one science, to make use of them critically and to uphold the unity of the work done?
>
> – Edmund Husserl, *The Crisis of European Sciences*

Why should the *scientific* status of human science research be a compelling issue for the next generation of qualitative researchers?[1] Today a current of epistemic relativism underlies many presentations of qualitative research, fed by an aestheticizing discourse which represents research in human science more as an artistic activity than a scientific one.[2] The result is a climate in which the pursuit of epistemological rigor is viewed skeptically, and the question "what makes human science scientific?" appears antiquated or irrelevant, the relic of a time before the so-called "death of epistemology".[3] Advocates of aestheticizing approaches to research are likely to place exclusive emphasis upon the "human" in human science – dwelling upon the multiplicity of meanings and issues of interpretation – while giving short shrift to the meaning of science for qualitative research, or the demands which science, properly understood, might place upon qualitative researchers. In other words, they will tend to advocate a kind of criterionlessness in which the researcher's freedom and individual expressivity is exalted above any intersubjective, epistemological requirements to which researchers work might be held accountable. Human science research might even be envisioned as aiming primarily at conveying the researcher's experience *of* research, rather than to yield knowledge intended to enrich a community of fellow researchers.

When such a conception of research holds sway, a seemingly absolute gulf opens up between the natural and human sciences, with the consequence that the idea of science *as such,* that is, a science of which the natural sciences are but one species and the human sciences another, is reduced to a nullity. Severed from any larger, encompassing notion of science, human science research is reduced to a species of aestheticism indistinguishable from the writing of fiction: an activity that aims solely at creativity, objectivity (however it might be understood in relation to human being) having been dispensed with. The point of departure for the following discussion is the premise that the fulfillment of psychology as a human science depends upon the development of psychological research approaches adequate to the study of the human person, and simultaneously able to argue their scientific status.

Amedeo Giorgi's career has been dedicated to establishing the psychology as a human science, retaining a strong sense of the scientific, which he seeks to articulate in relation to the human person. Giorgi envisions his work as a contribution to laying the foundation for a psychological science to come, one which clearly delineates its subject matter and is capable of rigorously arguing its human-scientific status. He has defined psychology broadly as "the study of subjectivity", and argued that psychology must seek to understand subjectivity "precisely as subjectivity expresses itself in the world" (unpublished lecture at University of Alberta, p. 1). Naturally, subjectivity is open to investigation in myriad ways: philosophy, literature and the arts all explore dimensions of lived subjectivity. Within these realms a multiplicity of motivating interests are possible other than a specifically *scientific, research interest.* Even within the domain of psychology, a clinical practitioner interest differs from a scientific interest to the extent that the aim of the clinician is to arrive at knowledge of an individual person in order to more adequately intervene with him or her. At stake in the following discussion are the precise meanings of "scientific" for the psychological investigation of subjectivity, from a human science standpoint. I will argue that when psychological research is shaped by an aesthetic interest, the resulting praxis and findings do not contribute to the founding of psychology as a human science, because the very criteria which would justify such a foundation are neglected. The resulting efforts, to the extent that they claim scientific status, serve to weaken rather than strengthen the case for human scientific psychology as an alternative to the dominant, empiricist paradigm.

According to the humanistic critique, psychological science in the main has been developed along empiricist lines "in dialogue with nature rather than humans" (Giorgi, 1992, 208-209). Hence mainstream psychology "never had to grapple with the meaning of human *as* human" (Giorgi, 1992, 208-209). Mimicking natural scientific praxis, psychology naturalized consciousness rather than allowing human phenomena to stand forth in their uniqueness. Such a limited empiricism continues to dominate contemporary psychological research, and as Kuhn (1996) observed, the only problems which a scientific community "will admit as scientific or encourage its members to undertake" are those that fit within its dominant paradigm (p. 37).

For Giorgi the empiricist paradigm when applied to psychical is a Procrustean bed, deforming the object it purports to investigate through the imposition of natural scientific categories upon human phenomena (1985). However, Giorgi's work is not an attack on empiricism per se. Instead Giorgi follows Husserl in arguing that psychical phenomena exceed the scope of *empiricist* methods (2006). Consequently empiricist psychology has failed to provide a unifying perspective capable of embracing the full range of psychical phenomena; neither has the psychological community as a whole come to relative consensus on core epistemological and anthropological assumptions (Giorgi, 1982). These fundamental gaps lead Giorgi to conclude that the precise meaning of psychology "is still not yet an historical achievement" (2008, p. 42).

Psychology, therefore, has yet to be properly founded as a science. In the attempt to contribute to this founding, Giorgi has devoted considerable attention to delineating what the psychical realm is, and what is required for a scientific approach to psyche. Giorgi has described the psychical as a "lower level of organization of subjectivity" which is "para-objective, para-rational, and para-normative" (unpublished lecture, June 17, 2005). "Para" indicates not that psychical phenomena *oppose* categories like rationality, but that the psychical arises alongside and goes beyond the objective, the rational, and the normative (Giorgi, 1993). In order to allow these phenomena to stand out to scientific reflection without theory-laden distortion, Giorgi turned to Husserl's phenomenological philosophical method, from which he developed a descriptive method for psychological research.

Husserl presented phenomenology as a method of philosophical inquiry whereby researchers "accept as given everything we encounter in perceiving awareness, as it confronts us, but also only within the limits within which it confronts us" (Kohák, 1978, p. 167). Giorgi drew upon Husserl and Merleau-Ponty's phenomenology in the attempt to develop a genuinely scientific approach to the study of subjectivity. Phenomenological psychology seeks to attain the mode of objectivity appropriate to human phenomena by "grasping subjectivity precisely as it presents itself" (Giorgi, personal communication, January 21, 2009).

Giorgi's commitment to the scientific status of psychological research is arguably the defining difference between his work and that of other qualitative researchers who invoke phenomenological and/or hermeneutic philosophy. Giorgi argues that the meaning of "science" as such must be articulated in such a manner as to embrace both empiricist and alternative approaches. He contends that whether quantitative or qualitative, a research approach must be methodical, critical, general, and systematic if it is to constitute science (Giorgi, personal communication, January 21, 2009). Like Husserl, Giorgi regards the scientific attitude as a consciously chosen attitude toward human phenomena, one which reflects a particular research interest (1970). Giorgi thus acknowledges that the world of science and the scientific object itself are co-constituted by the scientist (1969). Therefore the discoveries of science do not represent ahistorical, de-contextualized, "Platonic" truths, but truths *for* a community of researchers in a given context.

I will argue that in the absence of a motivating scientific interest – be it quantitative or qualitative – research and its fruits are limited to the realms of individualistic reflections upon philosophy, aesthetics, or clinical practice. If research is not shaped and sustained by a scientific interest – which implies participation in a community of co-researchers – and instead focuses exclusively on the personal meaning a phenomenon has for a given writer, the resulting findings, however suggestive, do not rise to the level of scientific knowledge. An attitude which privileges the research experience while denigrating method undermines the possibility of science.

In this paper van Manen's (1990, 2002) hermeneutic phenomenology will be criticized along the preceding lines. The aim of the critique will be to show that to the extent van Manen's approach yields knowledge, it does not rise to the level of science. My aim is not to argue that van Manen's approach fails to yield valuable reflections about subjectivity, but rather that those reflections are framed in a primarily aesthetic rather than scientific manner – an important limitation. This limitation may be irrelevant to van Manen's project; however, it is critical from a foundational perspective, because such an approach does not contribute to strengthening the scientific status of qualitative human science research as a rigorous alternative to the hegemonic, empiricist method.

Criteria for Science

Those psychologists guided by empiricism have the luxury of taking their underlying philosophical premises for granted as givens. Empiricist premises are so firmly established in mainstream practice that they are equated with science as such, a state of affairs exemplifying what Kuhn (1996) termed "normal science". Advocates of alternative scientific research approaches are obliged to repeatedly argue their premises because their work represents a challenge to the scientific community's "received beliefs" (Kuhn, 1996). Consequently researchers informed by the philosophical premises of non-empiricists such as Husserl, Heidegger, or Gadamer must make an explicit case for their guiding assumptions, spending significant time laying out the philosophical underpinnings of their work. In such cases the lines between philosophy and psychology is somewhat blurred of necessity. Nevertheless, if research is guided by a scientific interest, the philosophical discussion will be preparatory for, rather than in lieu of, a discussion of praxis. The transition Giorgi wants to make is from philosophy to science, since the two are not equivalent. A transformation is required.

Giorgi (1970) regards psychology as an as-yet unfounded science – unfounded in that the guiding assumptions and procedures of natural science were prematurely imposed upon psychology in the attempt to legitimize it. Overshadowed by these inadequately investigated empiricist assumptions, psychology has not yet articulated itself independently. As a consequence, psychology lacks disciplinary unity, since psychologists have not achieved broad consensus on the meaning of their object or upon "the methods, procedures, rules of interpretation" appropriate to the study of the psychical (1985, p. 45). Giorgi's work is directed toward a more comprehensive, shared disciplinary understanding that is not yet an historical achievement (1985).

In order to clarify the meaning of psychology as a human science, the meaning of "science" must be freed from the exclusively empiricist, positivist interpretation with which it has become popularly and institutionally identified. This effort requires that psychologists reflect upon the notion of science per se and identify unifying criteria required for knowledge to be considered scientific.

Having identified such criteria, which ought to be comprehensive enough to apply to both empiricist and other modes of scientific inquiry, it may then be asked how the criteria are to be applied when the object of inquiry is the human being. Giorgi (1997) argues that to constitute science, any quantitative or qualitative research approach must yield knowledge which is systematic, methodical, general, and critical (p. 249).

The Greek term *syst□ ma* implies an organized whole, or a body comprised of parts. Systematic knowledge means that a research approach is capable of producing interrelated findings that contribute to a picture of a whole. In psychology, this means that the knowledge produced would be interrelated and "regulated by laws, concepts, or meanings" (Giorgi, 1997, p. 249). Hence Giorgi understands "systematic" in terms broad enough to encompass natural scientific and human scientific research. So while a framework of laws might be applicable to research in chemistry, a network of interrelated meanings or concepts might be applicable in psychological, sociological, or anthropological research. A systematic approach to human science research is conducted in dialogue with existing understandings of the phenomenon under investigation, reflecting the view that "there are relations among aspects of knowledge that can be synthesized" (Giorgi, 1990, p. 113). Systematic psychological research communicates an anticipatory sense of psychology as an organized, holistic body of knowledge.

The Greek term *methodos* implies a reliable path of inquiry that has been confirmed over time and can be shared with fellow researchers. Science aims at enriching the community's shared understanding, not simply in yielding personal insight. Scientific discovery is never a private achievement, but always an implicitly communal one. To be scientific, knowledge must be arrived at through a praxis in which others can be instructed. If a research approach cannot be imparted to others and implemented independently by them, the accumulation of a body of knowledge would be impossible; discoveries would be limited to isolated insights lacking any necessary interrelationship. In contrast research methods achieve their results through the application of a focused, well-grounded, explicit, shared, and repeatable means of data gathering and analysis. An adequately precise and limited focus is a precondition of research, because, as Giorgi (2006) has noted, "the data will always be richer than the perspective brought to it but it is the latter that makes the analysis feasible" (p. 354). Repeatability in the context of human science does not imply a literal recapitulation of the lived experience of inquiry and discovery, which would be impossible. Instead repeatability refers to the straightforward fact that research steps are explicit and sequential and can therefore be performed again by multiple researchers in varied contexts.

A methodical research approach provides a collectively understood means of access to the phenomenon under investigation, and must be appropriate to the phenomenon being investigated, avoiding the use of "an *a priori* technique that may hinder access to or obscure the phenomenon because of reification or decontextualization" (Giorgi, 1990, p. 113). Method, *qua* method, lends itself to being taught to a community of fellow researchers. By this standard, a research approach which is incapable of methodical articulation, or whose advocates substitute an overly idiosyncratic, obscure, or artistic conception of their praxis for a methodical one cannot claim scientific status.

A research approach yields general knowledge if the findings have broad application rather than being limited to shedding light on the research participants themselves, or guiding interventions focused to specific individuals. If research is motivated by a scientific interest, its aims are disciplinary. Accordingly, a research approach which produces knowledge only of an individual or group of individuals, could yield insight without rising to the level of science. This guiding disciplinary interest does not imply a denial of the uniqueness of an individual case or diminish the meaningfulness of a participant's experience. However, if the researcher hopes to contribute to scientific community's understanding of the phenomena under investigation, he or she will seek to understand that experience upon a horizon inclusive of but more expansive than the life of any particular participant. Regarding validity in qualitative research, it ought to be noted that generalizability of research findings is not argued by means of statistics, but in terms of meaning.

Finally, a research approach is critical if practitioners invite and respond to critique by publishing procedures and findings for review by qualified members of the scientific community. This criterion could fail to be met if findings are expressed in either of two extreme forms: assertions of unquestionable truth, or assertions which are themselves unquestionable because their implicit relativism or positioning as artistic or poetic work undermines the very possibility of dialogue and critique. In either case, science has not been achieved.

Giorgi's four criteria are conservative in the sense that they are clearly based in the scientific tradition. Giorgi's intention, however, is to liberate psychological research from the constraints of empiricist philosophy while maintaining fidelity to science as such. Thus when empiricism is bracketed as merely one form of science and the preceding criteria are inquired into openly in the context of human science, the result is a radical re-envisioning of praxis. Giorgi has frequently written that human scientific psychology must discover what objectivity, reliability, and validity mean in the human science context, it being taken for granted that the significance of these concepts are different when the object of inquiry is subjectivity.

At the same time, the criteria make evident why research that is unsystematic or anti-methodical, which fails to yield general results or evades critical review may deepen understanding while nevertheless failing to rise to the level of science. In such a case, the approaches taken might be better characterized as philosophical or literary reflection, on the one hand, or practitioner-oriented reflections upon individual clinical cases, rather than as contributions to psychological science.

A variety of approaches to human science research in psychology invite critique from Giorgi's standpoint because they fail to meet the preceding criteria. Such critique is particularly important since psychology lacks internal coherence as a discipline. As Kuhn (1996) argued, once a viewpoint has become the paradigm for a discipline, "It is declared invalid only if an alternative candidate is available to take its place" (p. 77). Research which fails to pass muster as scientific – albeit a sense of "science" appropriate to the human subject, not one constrained by the empiricist worldview – cannot serve as an alternative to empiricist psychology. Thus debates between Giorgi's approach to psychological research and those of others such as van Manen (1990) are not parochial but reflect an effort to clarify the meaning of science per se, and serve as a reminder that approaches which bypass the question of their scientific status invite dismissal as unscientific.

Van Manen's Hermeneutic Phenomenology

Van Manen (1990) names his research approach "hermeneutic phenomenology" and presents it as founded in the human scientific tradition (*Geisteswissenschaften*).[4] I will focus primarily upon *Researching Lived Experience* (1990), his most extensive published presentation of his conception of hermeneutic phenomenology. I believe a strong case can be made that van Manen's hermeneutic phenomenology fails to fully satisfy any of the four criteria Giorgi proposes for science while neglecting to offer alternative criteria. The following discussion will concentrate almost exclusively upon Giorgi's first criterion, that scientific research must reflect a methodical praxis, examining the status of *method* and *methodical inquiry* in van Manen's hermeneutic phenomenology. My argument will be that hermeneutic phenomenology is conceptually anti-methodical. As a result of this limitation and van Manen's emphasis on the literary-aesthetic character of hermeneutic phenomenological writing, his approach is best characterized as a mode of aesthetic reflection, sensitive to the meanings of human phenomena, but one incapable of yielding rigorously scientific knowledge.

I propose that the foregoing limitation is a consequence of the fact that in van Manen's work the status of human science *as science* is not a central concern. Establishing hermeneutic phenomenology as scientific is therefore not a priority. On the contrary: van Manen wants to assert that his approach is human scientific without articulating criteria for the conduct of scientific research. Van Manen (1990, 2006) invokes the work of Heidegger, Gadamer, Derrida and Foucault in his presentations of hermeneutic phenomenology. Recently (2002) he made the claim, indebted to postmodernist discourse, that research is a form of creative writing akin to the production of literature.[5]

The philosophical premises cited by van Manen are not compatible with each other, making hermeneutic phenomenology's assumptive framework a moving target and hence difficult to critique. It is tempting to link this characteristic to van Manen's affinity for postmodernist discourse, which frequently prefers literary presentations to systematic argumentation.[6] But the central tension in the following critique of van Manen's hermeneutic phenomenology is that between on the one hand the need for a discovery of an human scientific alternative to the empiricist research paradigm, and the simultaneous need to elucidate public criteria for human science *quâ* science which can ensure rigor, reliability, and the validity of scientific findings.

In *Researching Lived Experience* (1990) van Manen attempts to appropriate Husserl's phenomenology while simultaneously deploying Heidegger and Gadamer's philosophy to advocate what is in essence an anti-methodical research approach. In more recent writing (2006) van Manen has continued to invoke Husserl while drawing upon Derrida's postmodern philosophy to advocate an anti-methodical and anti-disciplinary research approach. In these presentations van Manen severs Husserl's core praxis terms from their original, meaningful context in the phenomenological method, and mixes Husserl's descriptive-methodological terms with arguments drawn from incompatible philosophies such as Gadamer's philosophical hermeneutics or Derrida's deconstruction. In addition, van Manen (1990) equates method *per se* with mechanical technique, and makes the overly simplistic claim that research practice cannot be methodically articulated but can only be learned by doing. Van Manen's interpretation of hermeneutic phenomenology is beset by multiple internal contradictions in large part because epistemological clarity, disciplinary and methodological rigor, are framed as non-issues. Hence this type of hermeneutic phenomenology is anti-methodical for two chief reasons: because it argues explicitly against methodical praxis, and because it's underlying epistemological premises are contradictory and thus incapable of sustaining a methodical approach to research.

Anti-methodical Implication

Van Manen's standpoint vis-à-vis methodical research praxis in *Researching Lived Experience* (1990) is beset by internal contradictions. The text appears to provide guidelines for data gathering and analysis, making extensive use of the foundational terms with which Husserl described his practice of phenomenological inquiry.[7] Husserlian terms appropriated by van Manen (1990) include bracketing, free imaginative variation, description, explication and essence. These terms have technical meanings in Husserl's phenomenology, and van Manen's deployment of the foundational Husserlian terms strongly implies that they shape the practice of his hermeneutic phenomenology as well.[8] Van Manen's anti-methodical account of research praxis (1990), however, is incompatible with the indisputably methodical implications of the Husserlian terms he appropriates. Husserl's phenomenology is not a matter of abstract insights or theories, but rather a systematic and carefully delineated path of methodical inquiry. As Husserl's student and translator Dorion Cairns (1973) recognized, "the peculiar character of Husserlian phenomenology lies not in its content but in the way the latter is attained. Whatever its sense, an account is phenomenological in the Husserlian sense if, and only if, it is produced 'phenomenologically'" (p. 223). For this reason, Cairns noted, "one must also know Husserlian phenomenological method" (p. 223)[9].

In arguing that van Manen's hermeneutic phenomenology is anti-methodical in its approach to data gathering and analysis I must acknowledge that while characterizing methodical praxis in pejorative terms as a merely technical enterprise van Manen (1990) simultaneously claims to be following a "phenomenological method" (p. 111). While appropriating Husserl's technical terms, he misrepresents those terms in a manner which frequently renders Husserl's actual method incomprehensible and thus inaccessible to the reader. For example, van Manen (1990) mischaracterizes Husserl's well-known insistence that the researcher adopt an attitude of presuppositionlessness as "a methodology that tries to ward off any tendency toward constructing a predetermined set of fixed procedures, techniques, and concepts that would rule-govern the research project" (p. 29). But this is a distortion of Husserl.[10] As Kockelmans' (1994) overview of Husserl's phenomenology demonstrates, Husserl's methodical bracketing, phenomenological reductions, and free imaginative variation are all "procedures". Perhaps due to his desire to simultaneously follow Gadamer, van Manen, *contra* Husserl, poses an overly simplistic dichotomy between infinitely malleable, unfixed research practices (inscribed as humanistic and thus praiseworthy) and mechanical research techniques (inscribed as technocratic and thus blameworthy). He paradoxically characterizes the former alternative as constituting a "phenomenological method" and is thereby free to assert that his hermeneutic phenomenology is methodical.[11] In so doing van Manen confuses the openness of phenomenological research with a rejection of method and consistency. More recently van Manen (2006) has drawn upon Heidegger to argue that a genuinely phenomenological approach is a dynamic, creative endeavor that cannot be contained within a "preconceived method" (p. 720).

In addition van Manen (1990) privileges the researcher's individual freedom, making it absolute in a way, which renders methodical inquiry impossible. This consequence is evident in his claim that human science research cannot be constrained by a defined method because researchers must be free to engage in "choosing directions and exploring techniques, procedures, and sources that are not always foreseeable at the outset of a research project" (p. 162). While appearing to grant that "human science is a systematic study of human experience" (p. 168) van Manen (1990) claims that in the practice of hermeneutic phenomenology "there is no research design or blueprint to follow"– an obvious contradiction (p. 167). His presentation repeatedly implies a dichotomy – which is conceptually awkward and unnecessary from a Husserlian standpoint – between an idealized freedom and a mechanical, technique-driven "blueprint" for the conduct of research. On van Manen's account, method is misleadingly equated with robotic procedure. This misconstrual can be read as an attempt to turn Husserl's (1970) critique of the use of natural scientific methods for the study of consciousness against the methodical implications of Husserl's phenomenology.

A range of procedures for data-gathering and analysis are mentioned in *Researching Lived Experience* (1990), including prompting research participants to report their experiences in terms of the four "existentials" of spatiality, corporeality, temporality, and relationality (p. 101), meeting subsequently with participants to engage in "collaborative hermeneutic conversations" (p. 99), and adopting a "wholistic or sententious approach," a "selective or highlighting approach", or a "detailed or line-by-line approach" in the analysis of data (p. 92-93). However in the light of van Manen's pointed rejection of methodical praxis and research design, the practices he enumerates cannot be taken as comprising a unified or sequential research *method.* Given van Manen's presentation of hermeneutic phenomenology, the procedures he references cannot be understood as steps in a repeatable method – even steps to be implemented in a manner sensitive to the data. Rather, they must be understood as varied elements or alternate strategies to be drawn upon at the researcher's discretion in the course of a fundamentally spontaneous, unstructured (and in principle un-structurable) discovery process. To argue otherwise would be to read into hermeneutic phenomenology a consistent, repeatable research design – something van Manen explicitly rejects (1990).[12]

Epistemological Inconsistencies

It may be objected that the foregoing criticism is mere nitpicking and misses the point: namely, that van Manen's work seeks to encourage researchers to maintain an attitude of openness and adaptability. Nevertheless, if human science research aims at achieving scientific findings possessing disciplinary value, then a research approach must provide researchers with adequate guidance and conceptual clarity to conduct research. In this light, van Manen's hermeneutic phenomenology demonstrates epistemological confusion. Consider the following assertion regarding the practice of hermeneutic phenomenology:

> It is a descriptive (phenomenological) methodology because it wants to be attentive to how things appear, it wants to let things speak for themselves; it is an interpretive (hermeneutic) methodology because it claims that there are no such things as uninterpreted phenomena. (van Manen, 1990, p.180)

The former, descriptive assertion would appear to be an affirmation of Husserl's (1982) descriptive phenomenology. The latter, interpretive assertion is amplified in van Manen's claim that "understanding is always an interpretation" (p. 180). The two statements, taken as guidance for conducting research, are plainly contradictory.[13]

Obliged to acknowledge the "implied contradiction" in his argument (1990, p. 180), van Manen seeks to resolve the logical inconsistency by blurring the lines between description and interpretation.[14] But as Delius (1953) observed, descriptive and interpretive research approaches embody "a difference of attitude in which [...] research is undertaken", attitudes which are irreducible to each other (p. 306). Careful reading of hermeneutic phenomenology reveals multiple such attempts to blur important differences. For example the practice of hermeneutic phenomenological research is described as "a process of insightful invention, discovery or disclosure" (1990, p. 79). This combination of disparate terms presents a problem for the researcher, because "invention", "discovery", and "disclosure" are not equivalent and imply different attitudes on the researcher's part. As a researcher, "invention" suggests that in the course of research I create an idea whole-cloth through my own efforts; "discovery" suggests a state of affairs that is already present to me and which I make explicit through my own efforts; "disclosure" implies something given to me to understand, something I receive rather than creating. Clearly, these terms are not equivalent and imply different attitudes toward the research situation, the aim of data gathering, and the meaning of findings. These differences in attitude are suppressed in van Manen's (1990) presentation, but the conceptual inconsistencies remain, with the result that hermeneutic phenomenology does not cohere in an integral approach to research.

As has been noted, van Manen frequently invokes the core concepts and practices of Husserl's phenomenology such as bracketing, imaginative variation, essence, and the call to a "return to the things themselves" (e.g. 1990). However he mixes these references with arguments drawn from philosophical hermeneutics and postmodernism, and in so doing consistently obscures the fundamental differences between Husserl's phenomenology, Gadamer's philosophical hermeneutics, and Derrida's deconstruction. The latter two schools of thought –whatever their respective merits – are founded upon premises significantly different from and in some cases clearly incompatible with Husserl's work. Two examples illustrate these inconsistencies.

Van Manen asserts in *Researching Lived Experience* (1990, p. 180) that "understanding is always an interpretation", a paraphrase of Gadamer's (1986) remark in *Truth and Method* that "interpretation is not an occasional additional act subsequent to understanding, but rather understanding is always an interpretation" (p. 274). For van Manen, as for Gadamer, reflective understanding necessarily involves *adding* meaning *to* one's perceptions, rather than reflectively explicating meanings which are already present, though perhaps implicitly so.[15] Van Manen's assertion, while perhaps according with Gadamer's philosophy, contradicts a central tenet of Husserl's (1982) descriptive phenomenology, his "principle of all principles".

Husserl founded his approach to inquiry upon the assertion that in perception objects are immediately (intuitively) present to consciousness. Husserl's (1982) Principle of all Principles crystallizes his strong case that inquiry, to be rigorous, must limit itself to the given as it is given to the researchers within a chosen research attitude (p. 44). Husserl regarded meaningfulness as a constituent of perception, not an interpretive addition to perception. His descriptive phenomenological investigations aimed at rendering explicit those meanings that are already present, but implicitly so. Hence a descriptive approach aims at "achieving an adequate account of a certain given phenomenon", that is, a phenomenon which "presents itself to *direct* investigation" (Delius, 1953, p. 306). A premise of descriptive approaches is that a given phenomenon, recognized by a community of fellow-researchers, is capable of being investigated and research verified intersubjectively, because the phenomenon itself is *given to* researchers rather than being the interpretive *creation* of the researcher.[16] As a consequence, a researcher adopting a Husserlian approach seeks to explicate what is phenomenally given, while an interpretive researcher – for example, one following van Manen's (1990) approach – seeks to creatively invent a novel understanding, making use of the data, other artistic or literary materials, and self-consciously interpretive discussions with the research participants. These two approaches are mutually exclusive because they imply radically different attitudes toward the meaning of research as a lived-activity.

Indisputably, methodical inquiry – qualitative or quantitative – relies upon an orderly sequence of steps in gathering and analyzing data. Finally, van Manen's (2006) disavowal of "preconceived method" must be taken at face value (p. 720). A mode of inquiry which disallows "preconception" may yield spontaneous insight, but it cannot be responsibly termed methodical. Van Manen's opposition to "prescription" and "preconception" render his approach incapable of guiding methodical inquiry, since any research method must to some degree "prescribe" and "preconceive" how research is to be conducted. Van Manen (1990) draws his readers' attention to the etymological root of the word "method", the Greek *hodos,* which he translates as "way" (p. 28). But *hodos* means "way" in the sense of a path or a road, and phenomenologically we can say that *hodos,* like "method", is not a one-of-a-kind, idiosyncratic route which I take entirely on my own and without precedents. On the contrary, it is a well-beaten path: a *hodos* or method can be named a "path" or a "road" *precisely* because others may have traveled this way before me, others can travel this way with me, and others will travel this path after me.[17] A research path is always given in the mode "for us" – never is it merely "for me".

Appropriating Gadamer and Aestheticizing Research

This rejection of methodical praxis appears to flow from the fact that van Manen envisions research as aimed exclusively at the researcher's experience of "disclosure" and its aesthetic expression. As is well known, Heidegger and Gadamer describe the hermeneutic experience of understanding as an "event," a "disclosure of truth" (Palmer, 1969, p. 245). On my analysis, van Manen's (1990) framing of hermeneutic phenomenological research in aesthetic rather than scientific terms results in its incompatibility with methodical research procedures. Consistent research design is regarded as obstructing the unpredictable disclosure of truth, an event van Manen (1990) compares to the creation of artwork. Such assertions reflect van Manen's reliance upon philosophical hermeneutics, perhaps particularly upon Gadamer who he frequently cites (1990). Since Gadamer's philosophical hermeneutics is frequently called upon not only by van Manen but by other hermeneutically-influenced philosophers critical of Husserl, or psychologists critical of Giorgi's Husserlian research approach, a digression is in order.

Gadamer (1986) insisted that in *Truth and Method* he "did not remotely intend to deny the necessity of methodical work within the human sciences" (p. XVII).[18] He did, however, argue that the use of a given method of inquiry does not, in and of itself, guarantee truth – an observation fully compatible with Husserl's phenomenology (Amedeo Giorgi, personal communication, July 28, 2009).[19] Gadamer contended (2004) that the human sciences "have no method of their own", since a natural scientific method had been imposed upon the human sciences (p. 7). Moreover, he argued that a phenomenological account reveals that the lived-phenomenon of understanding is always richer and more complex than any method can account for – and in this particular philosophical sense, Gadamer was critical of method in the human sciences: the discovery process can never be fully subsumed within a method (J. N. Mohanty, personal communication, August 19, 2009).

Gadamer's work is relevant in the present discussion because van Manen (1990) appropriates it precisely *as* a guide for the conduct of research, despite Gadamer's (1986) protestations that he did not intend to offer "a methodology of the human sciences" or "to make prescriptions for the sciences" (p. XIII). As Gadamer wrote in his introduction to *Truth and Method* (1986) "My real concern was and is philosophic: not what we do or what we ought to do, but what happens to us over and above our wanting and doing. Hence the methods of the human sciences are not at issue here" (p. XVI). For this reason, seeking to shape hermeneutic phenomenological research along "Gadamerian" lines is arguably a misapplication of Gadamer's philosophy. Just as Giorgi seeks to appropriate Husserl's philosophy to guide and structure psychological research, van Manen seeks to appropriate Gadamer's philosophy (as well as that of Heidegger and Derrida) to guide pedagogical and other human scientific research.

The critical difference is that whereas Husserl intended his phenomenology as propaedeutic, preparing the ground for a more rigorous founding of the sciences, Gadamer's aim is radically different. He states explicitly that he is not seeking to guide the sciences but to reflect philosophically upon them as they present themselves. He states his aim in *Truth and Method* was "to understand what the human sciences are, beyond their methodological self-consciousness" (1986, p. XIII). Thus he explores the meaning of method while seeking to articulate a descriptive account of the experience of truth – Gadamer's primary interest. As Grondin (2003) observed, for Gadamer this experience of truth "is not really "knowledge", but power and a discovery which does not forget that it cannot discover everything, and that something of the truth essentially remains hidden" (p. 22). Gadamer argues philosophically that the truth "does not only, and perhaps not even primarily, rely upon what has an absolutely firm foundation, as scientific methodology insists" (Grondin, 2003, p.22). Furthermore, Gadamer's philosophical hermeneutics "is neither an art or method of providing accurate interpretations, nor a way of regulating interpretation" (Moran, 2000, p. 270). Instead as Habermas (1994) has written, it is "a critique – that is, it brings to consciousness in a reflective attitude experiences which we have of language in the exercise of our communicative competence" (p. 294). Therefore Gadamer's philosophical interest is far removed from that of a scientific researcher; his aim is neither to propose "better" research methods nor to advocate self-consciously anti-methodical research praxes in the sciences.

Gadamer (1986) does argue, however, that in Germany the "humanistic heritage" brings the human sciences "close to other, quite different, extra-scientific experiences, and especially those proper to art" (XVII).[20] By "science" Gadamer means the procrustean bed of the natural sciences, and here he has common ground with the larger phenomenological tradition including Husserl and of course Heidegger. But Gadamer's project is not to develop an alternative vision *for* science; for him, it would be hubris for a philosopher to deduce "from principles the way in which "science" must change in order to become philosophically legitimate" (p. XVII). Presumably, for Gadamer, science is driven by its own "immanent law of advance" (1986, p. XVII) and the arts, including the humaniora, are a different sort of human activity: the arts are creative whereas "science" is mechanical.[21]

This dichotomy raises a second feature of the difference between Giorgi and van Manen's approaches. Giorgi (1970) seeks to transcend the limits of empiricism by contributing the founding of psychology along qualitative, phenomenological lines – an approach, which implies an alternative, humanistic epistemology to guide human science. In contrast, van Manen (1990) seeks to transcend empiricism by classifying human science research as a fundamentally *aesthetic* activity, which enables him to largely dismiss epistemological and disciplinary questions as non-issues. For this reason the scientific status of hermeneutic phenomenological research is of little concern for van Manen and is consequently unaddressed.

Van Manen represents human scientific research as a form of literature "not unlike an artistic endeavor", rather than as a [potentially artful] articulation of distinctly scientific findings (1990, p. 39). On van Manen's (1990) account, the human science researcher is implicitly encouraged to envision his or her work in predominantly personal and literary-aesthetic terms.[22] In his more recent writing (2006) van Manen follows Derrida and other postmodernists in framing phenomenological research as primarily an experience of writing. This writing is for the sake of aesthetically expressing one's subjectivity, not in order to contribute to a disciplinary-communal body of knowledge. Thus "one does not write primarily for being understood; one writes for having understood being" (2006, p. 721).

The aesthetic and ontological dimensions of experience are privileged over the clarification of experience, which enables van Manen (2002) to dispense with questions of method or epistemological inconsistency as uninteresting and unimportant. Such issues are dismissed as largely mechanical, vestiges of a scientific worldview, which has been transcended. Hence van Manen (2002) states that research "methods, techniques, form, and style" are "mundane issues", whereas "questions of metaphysics [...] the limits of language [...] the enigmatic nature of words, text, interpretation, and truth" occur at a "more reflective level" (2002, p. I). He writes:

> Human science research as writing is an original activity. There is no systematic argument, no sequence of propositions that we must follow in order to arrive at a conclusion, a generalization, or a truth statement, because that would be to see writing itself as technical method. (1990, p. 173)

The researcher is engaged not in a methodical praxis but in "a free act of "seeing" meaning", and in this sense his or her activity is closer to the artist than the scientist (van Manen, 1990, p. 79). The assessment is the natural consequence of van Manen's adoption of artistic expression as his guiding paradigm. Research is framed more as a personal exercise in literary creativity than as participation in a disciplinary community. Research data and phenomenological writing is conceptualized as "texts" which must validate the researcher in a personal way, having an impact seemingly indistinguishable from that of literature such as poetry. Hence van Manen (2002) claims that:

> We experience an addressive moment when a text suddenly "speaks" to us in a manner that validates our experience, when it conveys a life understanding that stirs our sensibilities, when it pulls the strings of unity of our being [...] the reader must become possessed by the allusive power of the text – taken, touched, overcome by the addressive effect of its reflective engagement with lived experience. (p. 237-238)

In this move toward the artistic not only scientific criteria but disciplinary criteria are shed. Van Manen (2001) writes approvingly that qualitative researchers "have moved far beyond traditional discipline-based methodologies and methods" (p. 851). Viewed through the lens of Giorgi's approach, hermeneutic phenomenology does not rise to the level of a scientific research approach because the epistemological clarity required for methodical inquiry is lacking.

Giorgi: Human Science and the Context of Discovery

Giorgi (2009) views method in human science as requiring the articulation of understandable, sequential research procedures meant to guide the discovery process and insure rigor. Method is not envisioned as a mechanical exercise which, by virtue of its formal structure, guarantees valid research findings. Throughout his career (1970, 2009) he has consistently argued that rather than mimicking the methods of natural science, psychology must discover the unique meanings of methodical inquiry for human science. Early in his work Giorgi (1970) concluded that "in order to be faithful to the phenomenon of man, either a new type of science had to be invented or the meaning of science as it was understood had to be considerably broadened" (p. 53). From Giorgi's standpoint "technique" would be regarded critically if what is meant is a reductive, mechanical procedure – but this is arguably an impoverished conception of technique.[23] More broadly, Giorgi argues that science (human or natural) is unattainable in the absence of methodological rigor.

There is an important interplay of form and formlessness in Giorgi's articulation of phenomenological research, and this point is critical because Giorgi's phenomenology offers an alternative to the overly formless, criterionlessness of approaches such as van Manen's. For Giorgi, method is regarded as providing guidance and scaffolding, so to speak, within which the researcher may engage in an open-ended discovery process. This discovery process is understood in Husserl's terms as *intuitive*. Lacking a structure and coherence adequate to ensure that research is methodical, systematic, general, and critical, research will not yield knowledge that enriches the scientific community. Conversely, if a research method is overly theory-laden, the researcher will prejudge the phenomena to be encountered, precluding genuine discoveries.

For this reason Giorgi (1985) has emphasized that phenomenological research is conducted within a context of discovery rather than a context of verification, noting: "we are trying to systematize scientific activity within the context of discovery" (1985, p. 14). Consequently alongside or within the framework of his research method, "a certain open-endedness is also maintained so that genuine discoveries may ensue" (p. 13). Giorgi (1985) has described the phenomenological researcher's attitude using phrases such as "circumscribed indeterminateness," "empty determinateness", and "open expectancy". In these expressions Giorgi seeks to convey the lived experience of adopting a phenomenological attitude in research. This attitude is founded upon Husserl's phenomenological method of bracketing in order to behold the given *as* given. Giorgi, like Husserl, insists upon two simultaneous needs: that a methodical praxis frame inquiry, and that this method is adequately transparent to the "things themselves" so as to allow for genuine discovery.[24]

Consequently for Giorgi (1985) method is one of the primary means by which a discipline constitutes the research situation, within which disciplinary intuitions—perceptions framed by the shared interests of a disciplinary community of fellow researchers, a specifiable research question and approach to participants – may be fulfilled and intersubjectively verified. The psychological structures, which are intuitively (perceptually) present within such a research attitude, are not Platonic, universal, nor acontextual. Rather, they are situated within and given to a describable intersubjective research community.

Van Manen, as has been seen, emphasizes the "free act of "seeing" meaning", as central to research (1990, p. 79). Giorgi similarly emphasizes openness. Yet for Giorgi psychological research is a scientific activity, not an artistic one; science aims first and foremost at communal knowledge, not individual, creative expression – hence it demands shared criteria for knowledge. The meaning of openness in qualitative research depends upon whether research is envisioned as a scientific or an aesthetic endeavor.

Why should such a distinction matter for the next generation of qualitative researchers? Defining human science research as an artistic activity, freed from the constraints of science, is arguably the reflection of a much larger socio-historical trajectory in European and American history. Eagleton (1990) argues that in modernity the aesthetic has come to be regarded as "providing us with a kind of paradigm of what a non-alienated mode of cognition might look like" (p. 2). Amid the "progressively abstract, technical nature of modern European thought", he writes, "art would still appear to speak of the human and the concrete, providing us with a welcome respite from the alienating rigours of other more specialized discourses, and offering [...] a residual common world" (p. 2).

The aesthetic realm promises to reunite the fragmented discourses of ethics and truth by "swallowing up" these realms, with the result that "everything should now become aesthetic", and "truth, the cognitive, becomes that which satisfies the mind, or what helps us to move around the place rather more conveniently" (p. 368). In such a context "truth is no longer in fashion", having been supplanted by a postmodernist-inflected emphasis on "ambiguity, indeterminacy, [and] undecidability", a stance presented as "subversive strikes against an arrogantly monological certitude" (p. 379-380).[25] It is but a short step from this philosophical stance to van Manen's assertions that the qualitative researcher seeks elusiveness rather than clarity, writes not to be understood but "for having understood Being" (2006, p. 721), and "in a moment of transcendental bliss [...] may experience the privilege of the gaze of Orpheus" the archetype of the artist as inspired poet (2002, p. 244).

Arguably, redefining research as inspiring literature, discarding disciplinary constraints, and eschewing potentially turgid epistemological debates free practitioners to focus exclusively on conveying the lived meanings of human phenomena in the most compelling manner possible. However doing so also yields the field of science entirely to exponents of the positivist paradigm. If qualitative psychological researchers seek refuge in the arts and a postmodern equating of research with fiction, they invite the charge of subjectivism and the further marginalization of qualitative approaches as literary and hence irrelevant to science.[26]

Reducing method to mechanical technique unnecessarily impoverishes the conception of human science. Method is a means by which, as scientists, we constitute a shared world of inquiry within which insights can arise for a community of fellow researchers, to be interrogated and refined. Van Manen and others quite rightly argue that openness to human phenomena as they are lived is the essence of qualitative research. So too, such openness is rightly regarded as not being the mechanical byproduct of any series of rote procedural steps. From a philosophic perspective the essence of one's openness to another may indeed demonstrate a dimension of mystery and "unknowing". But at the same time, as researchers we need not *mystify* our openness: if qualitative research requires an attitude of open inquiry, does not this openness reflect a describable attitude which we learn over time in dialogue with mentors, with a framing method, with fellow-researchers, and within a shared humanistic tradition? It is this current in the human scientific tradition which Giorgi seeks to continue.

References

Bernet, R., Kern, I. & Marbach, E. (1993). *An introduction to Husserlian phenomenology.* Evanston: Northwestern University Press.

Cairns, D. (1973). An approach to Husserlian phenomenology. In *Phenomenology: Continuation and criticism: Essays in memory of Dorian Cairns* (pp. 223-239). New York: Springer.

Dancy, J. & Sosa, E. (Eds.). (1998). *A companion to epistemology.* Malden, MA: Blackwell Publishers, Inc.

Delius, H. (1953). Descriptive interpretation. *Philosophy and Phenomenological Research, 13*(3), 305-323.

Dodd, J. (1998). Attitude–facticity–philosophy. In N. Depraz & D. Zahavi (Eds.). *Alterity and facticity: New perspectives on Husserl.* Boston: Kluwer Academic Publishers.

Duvenage, P. (2003). *Habermas and aesthetics: The limits of communicative reason.* Malden, MA: Blackwell Publishing Inc.

Eagleton, T. (1990). *The ideology of the aesthetic.* Cambridge, MA: Basil Blackwell Inc.

Gadamer, H. G. (1986). *Truth and method.* G. Barden and J. Cumming (Trans.). New York: Crossroad.

Gadamer, H. G. (1994). Rhetoric, hermeneutics, and the critique of ideology: Metacritical comments on truth and method. In K. Mueller-Vollmer (Ed.). *The hermeneutics reader* (pp. 274-292). New York: Continuum.

Gadamer, H. G. (1996). *The enigma of health: The art of healing in a scientific age* (J. Gaiger and N. Walker, Trans.). Palo Alto, CA: Stanford University Press.

Gadamer, H. G. (2004). *Truth and method.* (2nd Ed.). J. Weinsheimer and D. G. Marshall (Trans.). New York: Continuum.

Giorgi, A. (1970). *Psychology as a human science: A phenomenologically based approach.* New York: Harper & Row, Publishers.

Giorgi, A. (1985). Sketch of a psychological phenomenological method. In A. Giorgi (Ed.). *Phenomenology and psychological research* (pp. 8-22). Pittsburgh: Duquesne University Press.

Giorgi, A. (1993). Psychology as the science of the paralogical. *Journal of Phenomenological Psychology, 24*, 63-77.

Giorgi, A. (1997). The theory, practice, and evaluation of the phenomenological method as a qualitative research procedure. *Journal of Phenomenological Psychology, 28*(2), 235-260.

Giorgi, A. (2006). Difficulties encountered in the application of the phenomenological method in the social sciences. *Análise Psicológica* 3:XXIV 353-361.

Giorgi, A. (2009). *The descriptive phenomenological method in psychology: A modified Husserlian approach.* Pittsburgh: Duquesne University Press.

Grondin, J. (2003). *The philosophy of Gadamer* (K. Plant, Trans.). Montreal, Quebec: McGill-Queen's University Press.

Habermas, J. (1994). On hermeneutics' claim to universality. In K. Mueller-Vollmer (Ed.). *The hermeneutics reader: Texts of the German tradition from the enlightenment to the present*, New York: Continuum.

Himmelfarb, G. (1997). Tellingt it as you like it: Postmodernist history and the flight from fact. In K. Jenkins (Ed.). *The postmodern history reader* (pp. 158-174). New York: Routledge.

Husserl, E. (1970). *The crisis of European sciences and transcendental phenomenology: An introduction to transcendental phenomenology* (D. Carr, Trans.). Evanston: Northwestern University Press.

Husserl, E. (1982). *Ideas pertaining to a pure phenomenology and to a phenomenological philosophy: First book: General introduction to a pure phenomenology* (F. Kersten, Trans.). Boston: Kluwer Academic Publishers.

Ihde, D. (1980). *Hermeneutic phenomenology: The philosophy of Paul Ricoeur.* Evanston: Northwestern University Press.

Kockelmans, J. J. (1993). *Ideas for a hermeneutic phenomenology of the natural sciences, Volume 1.* Norwell, MA: Kluwer Academic Publishers.

Kockelmans, J. J. (1994). *Edmund Husserl's phenomenology.* West Lafayette, IN: Purdue University Press.

Kohák, E. (1978). *Idea & experience: Edmund Husserl's project of phenomenology in ideas I.* Chicago: University of Chicago Press.

Kompridis, N. (1999). Heidegger's challenge and the future of critical theory. In P. Dews (Ed.). *Habermas: A critical reader* (pp. 118-152). Malden, MA: Blackwell Publishers.

Kuhn, T. S. (1996). *The Structure of Scientific Revolutions (3rd Ed.).* Chicago: University of Chicago Press.

Maraldo, J. C. (2003). Rethinking God: Heidegger in the light of absolute nothing, Nishida in the shadow of onto-theology. In J. Bloechi (Ed.). *Religious experience and the end of metaphysics*, Bloomington: Indiana University Press.

Moran, D. (2000). *Introduction to phenomenology.* New York: Routledge.

Palmer, R. E. (1969). *Hermeneutics: Interpretation theory in Schleiermacher, Dilthey, Heidegger, and Gadamer.* Evanston: Northwestern University Press.

Ransom, J. S. (1997). *Foucault's discipline: The politics of subjectivity.* Durham, NC: Duke University Press.

Spiegelberg, H. (1965).*The phenomenological movement: A historical introduction, Volume one (2nd Ed.).* The Hague: Martinus Nijhoff.

The Holy Bible: New Revised Standard Version. (1977). New York: Oxford University Press.

Van Manen, M. (1990). *Researching lived experience: Human science for an action sensitive pedagogy.* Albany: SUNY Press.

Van Manen, M. (2001). Transdisciplinarity and the new production of knowledge. *Qualitative Health Research, 11*(6), 850-852.

Van Manen, M. (2002). Writing in the dark. In M. van Manen (Ed.). *Writing in the dark: Phenomenological studies in interpretive inquiry*, London, Ontario: The Althouse Press.

Van Manen, M. (2006). Writing qualitatively, or the demands of writings. *Qualitative Health Research, 16*(5), 713-722.

Notes

1 I want to express my gratitude to Amedeo Giorgi and J. N. Mohanty for their willingness to dialogue with me during the writing of this article.

2 The terms "aesthetic", "aestheticizing", and "artistic" are used in this article not to refer to the philosophy of art or the activity of creating artwork, but rather to designate a style of thought and argumentation that has been critiqued by both Eagleton (1990) and Habermas (1996), one which in Habermas' view "would collapse the difference between logic and rhetoric, between normal and "poetic" language, between problem solving and meaning creation" (Kompridis, 1999, p. 137).

3 This position is associated with philosophers such as Rorty (see Dancy & Sosa, 1998, pp. 88-91).

4 Of course the term "hermeneutic phenomenology" refers to a rich tradition of philosophical inquiry including Heidegger and Ricoeur (see Spiegelberg, 1965, p. 323; Kockelmans, 1993, and Ihde, 1980). In the present discussion the term is used solely in reference to van Manen's research approach.

5 Commenting on his historical work *The History of Madness,* Foucault wrote "it is necessary that what it asserts is somehow "true", in terms of historically verifiable truths. But what is essential is not found in a series of historically

verifiable proofs; it lies rather in the experience which the book permits us to have. And an experience is neither true nor false: it is always a fiction" (cited in Ransom, 1997, p. 57).

6 Himmelfarb (1997) contends that postmodern scholarship rejects "normal standards of discourse", renounces "all pretence of rational, logical, "enlightened" discourse", and abandons "the conventions regarding the presentation and documentation of evidence" (p. 172). Her analysis is made in the context of historiography, but is applicable to other disciplines.

7 For Husserl's emphasis on method, see Bernet, Kern & Malbach (1993), Chapter 2.

8 For example, he writes that "insight into the essence of a phenomenon" is accomplished by "making explicit the structure of meaning of the lived experience" (1990, p. 77); similarly, "*In determining the universal or essential quality of a theme our concern is to discover aspects or qualities that make a phenomenon what it is and without which the phenomenon could not be what it is.* To this end the phenomenologist uses the method of free imaginative variation in order to verify whether a theme belongs to a phenomenon essentially" (p. 107). Such statements initially appear to be paraphrases of Husserl.

9 As Dodd (1998) observed, "Philosophy, for Husserl, is not a perspective that we can switch to at will (though it flows from our freedom); it must be isolated, rebuilt and fortified. As such it is approachable only if reflection adopts a certain rigor; for method is the space within which philosophy emerges as philosophy, and in doing so it merges with the method itself, giving it, the method, a concrete meaning, relevance" (p. 67).

10 Similarly van Manen's (1990) assertion that "the method of phenomenology is that there is no method" and yet there somehow remains a "methodological ground" (p. 30) is fallacious, unless van Manen means to exclude Husserl and Husserlian thought from the phenomenological tradition!

11 The same unfortunate dichotomizing is evident in van Manen's (1990) claim that hermeneutic phenomenology "is decidedly unmethodological in a purely prescriptive or technocratic sense", with its curious equation of "prescription" with "technocracy" (p.3).

12 Likewise, maintaining that Husserl's phenomenology rejects well-articulated techniques and procedures is unsupportable, as it would require omitting the epoché, bracketing, and imaginative variation (all of which are methodical praxes) from one's account, something which would render Husserl's phenomenology unrecognizable. The rejection of methodical research praxes cannot itself constitute a method of inquiry.

13 The argument is circular: if all phenomena are mediated by interpretation, then phenomena are in principle *never* immediately present to a researcher (or any experiencer). In that case, description as such is impossible – all that remains is interpretation. But if there is no presence to be interpreted, then there is no given: in which case, how does the subject have access to an object

of interpretation? When the presence of the given is ruled out of order, it is difficult to see how interpretation would be possible. The attempt to resolve the epistemological inconsistency by incorporating description as a subset of interpretation fails logically.

14 He expands thusly: "invention (my interpretive product), discovery (the interpretive product of my dialogue with the text of life), disclosure of meaning (the interpretive product "given" to me by the text of life itself)" (p. 88). Labeling everything interpretation does not resolve the problem – rather, it conceals the implicit contradictions.

15 Warnke (1987) noted that for Gadamer, "all understanding involves projecting a meaning upon one's perceptions that is not strictly contained in the perceptions themselves" (p. 75).

16 Of course, this givenness has a context of research interest, language, culture, et cetera.

17 Hence the use of *hodos* in Matthew, Chapter 7 verse 14: "the gate is narrow and the road [*hodos*] is hard that leads to life, and there are few who find it" (1977). Hermeneutic phenomenology privileges the researcher's unique subjectivity above intersubjectivity – but paths and research methods are intrinsically intersubjective.

18 As Palmer (1969) noted, Gadamer states that "he is doing ontology, not methodology" (p. 47).

19 This is so because the fulfillment of intuition, in Husserl's terms, is not the mechanical outcome of implementing fixed procedures. This includes disciplinary intuitions, i.e. intuitions arrived at in the context of a given field of inquiry such as psychology or anthropology. When it occurs, the fulfillment of an intuition takes place within a context, and in scientific inquiry the context includes multiple givens which can be specified, such as the defining of a research question. Of course an intuition may remain unfulfilled: from a Husserlian perspective, there is no guarantee that a given presentational process will result in intuitive fulfillment (Amedeo Giorgi, personal communication, July 28, 2009).

20 Gadamer appears to equate science as such with the modern natural sciences. This is important in order to properly understand why Gadamer asserts that the experience of understanding in the human sciences is closer to the arts. In a collection of essays published in 1996 he writes "the term "art" seems to belong to that domain in which someone's skills and abilities enable them to construct something, to "make" something [...] this is not the typical way of modern science, which has learnt to erect constructive models on the basis of experience, experiment, and correct quantitative calculation" (p. 95). He writes, "Our science is based not on the experience of life but on that making and producing [...] this science is essentially [...] a kind of mechanics: it is *mechane*, that is, the artificial production of effects which would not come about simply of themselves" (1996, p. 38).

21 For Giorgi, in contrast, the humanities and the human sciences ought not to be collapsed together.

22 Van Manen (1990) asserts that "just as the poet or the novelist attempts to grasp the essence of some experience in literary form, so the phenomenologist attempts to grasp the essence of some experience in a phenomenological description [...] the artist recreates experiences by transcending them" (p. 96-97).

23 The Greek term *tekhne* has much broader connotations including art, skill, craft, method, and system.

24 Were one to address this situation in ontological terms, the question might be framed thusly: how can method simultaneously be full as a delimiting and constituting of the research situation, and empty as a transparency to the given as given? This simultaneity of seeming opposites is expressed in the philosophy of Kyoto School philosophers Nishida Kitaro and Nishitani Keiji using the Japanese term *soku.* (see Maraldo, 2003)

25 Arguably, many of the chief theorists of postmodernism such as Derrida, Lyotard, and Foucault critiqued Husserl in precisely this manner.

26 As Duvenage (2003) notes, Habermas has argued "it is possible to apply non-objectivist modes of inquiry [...] in science, but this should not violate science's primary orientation toward truth" (p. 60).

ART AND FLESH: A PSYCHOLOGY OF ART BY WAY OF MERLEAU-PONTY

Thomas F. Cloonan, Ph.D.

Marymount College of Fordham University (Emeritus)
United States

Abstract

Artistic experiences and aesthetic experiences may instigate changes in the psychological character of existence by way of ontological re-structurings of the person. This conclusion arises from the study of Merleau-Ponty's writings on art and his last work posthumously published, The Visible and the invisible (1964/1968). The essay presented here progresses from a discussion of Merleau-Ponty's ontological concepts of flesh and the visible and invisible and their relationship to art, to the nature and role of consciousness for ontology and a psychology of art, and finally to the parts played by imagination and physiognomy in a psychology of art. Artistic experiences and aesthetic experiences are agencies of change in the ontology and psychology of human beings.

Artistic and aesthetic experiences are not to be confused, much less conflated, with "art appreciation". The latter term involves cognitive assessment and value judgment of works of art. Art appreciation is employed in the domain of education. An application of it is found in the commercial enterprises of for-profit art galleries and of art auctions. [Etymologically, "to appreciate" derives from *ad* + *pretium*; that is, "to, towards, or for price".] Museum acquisitions involve both educational and purchase meanings.

Art appreciation is a term generic in its definitional direction and it is nonspecific with respect to the intensity and depth prepotencies that issue from the ontological dimension of the work of art. These prepotencies burgeon in artistic and aesthetic experiences. While art appreciation is informational in character, artistic and aesthetic experiences touch upon and are touched by the ontology of works of art. Those contacts institute psychological consequences. The focus of this essay is on the experiences of the visual arts of painting, drawing, and print-making which may not be *pars pro toto* for all of the arts, but which do have a kindred significance for the other fine arts of sculpture and architecture and, in less direct ways, for the performing arts such as music, dance, theatre, and, in subtle ways, for literary art.

"Artistic experiences" are on the part of the makers of the work of art. Documents by artists such as correspondence and journals, research and journalistic interviews of artists, and their autobiographies and biographies include accounts of artistic experiences. "Aesthetic experiences", which are had with the perceptual response to completed works of art, are equally available to the inquiries of investigators and to programs of research. The ontological dimension is to be engaged existentially, not solely on the level of philosophical conceptualizations. Ontology is the deepest stratum of genuine works of art. It is to that place that this essay seeks to go.

Maurice Merleau-Ponty's writings are outstanding in this regard. He plumbs the art of Cézanne in "Cézanne's Doubt" (1993a), considers the art of language and the language of painting in "Indirect Language" and the "Voices of Silence" (1993c), and addresses the visual experience in "Eye and Mind" (1993b). These three essays, especially "Eye and Mind", are preamble to Merleau-Ponty's (1964/1968) *The visible and the invisible*, which is the primary text of reference for this essay and which is explicit in its discussion of the ontological character of what Merleau-Ponty calls "flesh" and the "visible and invisible" that intertwine in visual art.

Johnson (1993) points out that, "Eye and Mind" was first published in January 1961. It was the last work Merleau-Ponty published prior to his sudden, premature death on 3 May 1961, at the age of fifty-three (p. 36). The terribly untimely close to Merleau-Ponty's life, in addition, intervened in the completion of what would have been Merleau-Ponty's further work, *The visible and the invisible.* Claude Lefort was the assembler and organizer of that work's material for posthumous publication (1964/1968). However much its character as a work-in-progress (especially the "Working Notes" part of it), *The visible and the invisible* is the most developed edge of Merleau-Ponty's thoughts on ontology.

The Merleau-Ponty aesthetics reader is a solid resource volume in which the editor, Galen A. Johnson (1993), has gathered together the three essays by Merleau-Ponty mentioned above, a number of authoritative essays on Merleau-Ponty's aesthetics, and his own perspicacious commentaries on Merleau-Ponty's essays. They are all within the realm of philosophy. Recourse, here, is had to this volume. Reference is also made to Edward Casey's (1976) philosophical discussion of imagination in relation to artistic and aesthetic experiences.

From the perspective of phenomenological psychology, the work of Amedeo P. Giorgi (1985, 1987, 2009) is a crucial part of the caravan that this essay musters in a phenomenological psychological understanding of the making of art and of aesthetic experiences. The "mission of art", which is the redirection of ordinary quotidian perception (Ó Cluanáin, 1979), and imagination's role (Ó Cluanáin, 1987) and physiognomy's assignment in these experiences (Cloonan, 2005), in addition, are core to them. The Gestalt psychologists Rudolf Arnheim and Wolfgang Metzger's works deserve recognition from phenomenologists. Arnheim (1966) is an agent for clarification of the interaction between perception and imagination and that is acknowledged in this essay. The less well known but no less important Metzger (1936/2006) has conducted investigations on the psychology of perception that at least at one point arguably verge on Merleau-Ponty's ontological "visible and invisible" – with all the reservations that one must have toward the presence of naturalist assumptions in those investigations. In the presentations of this essay, all these references intercalate with the primary Merleau-Ponty documents that are above mentioned.

The thesis of this essay is that Merleau-Ponty's presentation of "flesh and the visible and invisible" is the clearest ontological explication of the context within which artistic and aesthetic experiences take place. The essay progresses from the discussion of these terms for the sake of a phenomenological psychology with its existential program for a re-directed living through both making art and aesthetically experiencing it, to the position of consciousness in the psychology of art, and finally to imagination and physiognomy's roles in artistic and aesthetic experiences.

Flesh and the Visible and Invisible

Merleau-Ponty's ontology lexicon is a stumbling block to the writers and readers of mainstream psychological literature. The subtlety of language in Merleau-Ponty's "Eye and Mind" that continues and flourishes in his *The Visible and the invisible*, quite manifestly in its "Working Notes", may dissuade psychologist readers from expectation that Merleau-Ponty's writings have accessible relevance to the psychology of art. I refer here particularly to Merleau-Ponty's vocabulary of "flesh and the visible and invisible".

The positivist nature of American psychological glossary is the major contributor to that difficulty. Johnson says, "We need a new philosophical language that would not ignore the strangeness of the world, even if it would of necessity speak indirectly and in half-silence" (1993, p. 37). More so, psychologists need to appreciate the inadequacy of conventional psychological language for discourse on ontology and its relationship to psychology in general and to the psychology of art and aesthetics specifically. Let us attend, therefore, to Merleau-Ponty's "flesh and the visible and invisible".

Flesh

"Flesh" is provocative. Its provocation lies in the various denoted and connoted meanings of it that range from the raw and freshly butchered meat of the slaughterhouse, to the naked body in erotic situations, and then to the religious and shocking, "whoever eats my flesh and drinks my blood will live in me and I in him" (John 6:56). Why is a word with such combustive qualities used in the presentation of ontological conceptualizations?

Merleau-Ponty's employment of the word "flesh" is neither sensationalist nor arbitrary. The antecedents of it go back to Husserl's description of the "touching and being-touched" phenomenon (1952/1989, pp. 152-159). Husserl's discussion of touching and being touched and his incorporation of the perceptible within the perceiver (grasped "in the flesh") are part of his legacy to Merleau-Ponty. A propos of this legacy, Merleau-Ponty (1960/1964) in his essay, "The philosopher and his shadow" in *Signs*, says,

> When my right hand touches my left, I am aware of it as a "physical thing". But at the same moment, if I wish, an extraordinary event takes place: here is my left hand as well starting to perceive my right, *es wird Leib, es empfindet* [it becomes Body (flesh), it senses (feels)]. The physical becomes animate. Or, more precisely, it remains what it was (the event does not enrich it), but an exploratory power comes to rest upon or dwell in it. [...] it ("this description") results in an ontological rehabilitation of the sensible. [...] When we say that the perceived thing is grasped "in person" or "in the flesh" (*leibhaft*), this is to be taken literally: the flesh of what is perceived [...] reflect(s) my own incarnation and [is] its counterpart. (pp. 166-167)

The German wording, "*Es wird Leib, es empfindet*" ["it becomes body (flesh), it senses (feels)"], is straight from Husserl (in German, 1952, p. 145; in English translation, 1989, p. 152). In "The intertwining" – The "chiasm" section of *The Visible and the invisible* (1964/1968, pp. 130-155), Merleau-Ponty makes a number of references to the touching and being-touched phenomenon, references that occasion his discussion of flesh and the visible and invisible. There is a *segue* of development from Husserl's thoughts on the cogent phenomenon of touch, therefore, to Merleau-Ponty's new ontology of flesh and the visible and invisible.

The word "chiasm" is a key for understanding Merleau-Ponty's articulation of his new ontology of flesh and the visible and invisible. He says, "the idea of *chiasm*, that is: every relation with being is *simultaneously* a taking and a being taken, the hold is held, it is *inscribed* and inscribed in the same being that it takes hold of" (1964/1968, p. 266). Merriam-Webster's 11th Collegiate Dictionary defines "chiasma" ("chiasm") as, "an anatomical intersection or decussation". Reference to the etymology of the word, from the same source, brings us to a more generic level of the meaning of the word, at which level Merleau-Ponty's usage of it may become clearer; "chiasma": New Latin, X-shaped configuration, from Greek, crosspiece, from *chiazein* to mark with a chi, from *chi* (X)".

The essence of chiasm is intersection such as the intersection of a cross. Decussation is "the action of crossing". Merleau-Ponty's use of the word chiasm is for the "crossing" of the referents in whatever contexts his book's passages are presenting (e.g., the crossing of "touching" and "being touched"; the crossing of the "visible" and "invisible"). Chiasm functions as a metaphor in the service of "a fundamental identity-and-difference" of ontology. It is among other metaphors (such as dehiscence, fission, divergence [*écart*], and intertwining) that Merleau-Ponty employs for this purpose, as Dillon (1988) points out. With respect to this fundamental identity-and-difference and these metaphors for it, Dillon says, "there is here no "monism of the phenomenon", but there is no dualism, either. There is, instead, flesh [...]" (1988, p. 157).

Perceptual psychologists are familiar with the word "chiasm" in the physiology of the eye. In optic chiasm, "the nerve fibers from the nasal half of each retina cross, so that each hemisphere of the brain receives input from both eyes" (VandenBos, 2007, p. 651). This partial crossing, the definition continues, is called a partial decussation. The decussation of optic chiasm is in reference to a neural, structural intersection in which there is a "crossing" of neural fibers for the purpose of crosslateral transmission of neural messaging to terminal visual cortical centers in both hemispheres. Through the neural operations afforded by the optic chiasm, the visual experience is a more integrated and fuller reality. At the cortical level, binocular depth perception is enhanced over and beyond the overlapping of visual fields that register from the neural messaging coming solely from just, respectively, the left and right eyes.

The understanding of chiasm's decussation in the physiology of visual experience may facilitate the perceptual psychologist's appreciation of Merleau-Ponty's employment of chiasm, for example, in the experience of touch, the dynamics of flesh (e.g., "flesh coils upon flesh"), and rather pertinently in the experience of the visible and invisible. Using the word "chiasm", Merleau-Ponty adheres to the etymological and generic meaning of chiasm's decussation, the "intersecting or crossing". For perceptual psychologists, the optic chiasm is available as an analogy for the chiasmic bonding of "touching" and "being touched" in tactile activity whose non-anatomical decussation is simply the instant of "touching-touched". It becomes an analogy for the chiasmic bonding of the "visible" and "invisible". The decussation or crossing of the visible and invisible, Merleau-Ponty tells us, is effected in the painterly action of the visual artist.

Barbaras (1991/2004) comments on the antecedence of Husserl's thought on "touch" for its significance for Merleau-Ponty (pp. 153-161), and he specifies "intertwining and chiasm".

> Such is the meaning, then, of the intertwining and of the chiasm: the duality of subject and object, which merges at the level of the one perceiving because the one perceiving makes himself world, merges thereby at the level of the perceived; the perceived is "on my side", it is set into my flesh, in agreement with visibility [...]. Ultimately, it is a matter of taking literally Husserl's formula according to which the thing is grasped "in person", "in the flesh (*Leibhaft*) [...]". (pp. 158-159)

Merleau-Ponty thus extends the legacy of Husserl's presentation of the phenomenon of touch to the use of the term flesh in *The visible and the invisible.* Merleau-Ponty formulates ontological implications of touch in his presentation of flesh. His new ontology presents a radicality that distinguishes it from the ontology of Husserl's philosophy. Along with it, he proscribes any assumed derivation of flesh from a duality of body and spirit. Merleau-Ponty (1964/1968) declares, "we must think it (flesh), as we said, as an element, as the concrete emblem of a general manner of being" (p. 147). He continues later on:

> The flesh of the world is not explained by the flesh of the body, nor the flesh of the body by the [...] self (cf. spirit) that inhabits it [...]. The flesh of the world is not *self-sensing* (*se sentir*) as is my flesh – it is sensible and not sentient – I call it flesh, nonetheless [...] (p. 250)

The non-dualist difference between the flesh of the world and the flesh of the body (body understood as embodied subjectivity, Merleau-Ponty's *le corps propre*) is a difference of differentiating distinction. It is not a difference between metaphysical realities in exclusion of each other. With continuing emphasis, Merleau-Ponty states, "flesh [...] is the sensible in the twofold sense of what one senses (the sensible) and what senses (the sentient)" (p. 259).

For some, an immediate misunderstanding of flesh in Merleau-Ponty's presentation is that it is an expression of philosophical monism. Their number is perhaps greater. Merleau-Ponty is declarative on the non-monistic nature of flesh. "The flesh of the world is not *self-sensing* (*se sentir*) as is my flesh – It is sensible and not sentient" (p. 250). As Dillon (1988) puts it in his reading of Merleau-Ponty, "[Merleau-Ponty] repeatedly rejects the monistic resolution: that an apparent difference between visible and invisible can be resolved by a real identity" (p. 157).

The subtlety of the distinction between flesh as sensible and flesh as sentient is lost to philosophical monist analyses just as it is lost to the mutual exclusivity of dualist thinking. Dillon (1988) expatiates on Merleau-Ponty's position:

> Trees and mountains do not see; they are blind witnesses to my own visibility. The body as exemplar sensible does not function as an example of sensibility in inanimate things. The human body is that particular kind of flesh that allows the flesh of the world to double back on itself and be seen. (p.169)

With finality, Merleau-Ponty says toward the end of *The visible and the invisible*, "a world that is neither *one* nor two in the objective sense – which is pre-individual, generality" (p. 262). Merleau-Ponty then says, "start from this: there is not identity, nor non-identity, or non-coincidence, there is inside and outside turning about one another" (p. 264).

Merleau-Ponty, finally, references flesh to Being.

> The flesh of the world is of the Being-seen, i.e. is a Being that is *eminently percipi* [to be perceived], and it is by it that we can understand the *percipere* [to perceive]: [...] all this is finally possible and means something only because *there is* Being [...]. (1964/1968, p. 250)

Merleau-Ponty refers to the "amorphous" perceptual world in relation to painting as, "at bottom Being in Heidegger's sense [...] which, apprehended by philosophy in its universality, appears as containing everything that will ever be said, and yet leaving us to create it [...]" (1964/1968, p. 170). If the word "flesh" is provocation for some empiricist psychologists, perhaps the word "Being" with its philosophical provenance is scandal to them. For its justification, beyond the way in which Merleau-Ponty refers to it, readers may refer to the work of the Swiss phenomenological psychiatrists Ludwig Binswanger and Medard Boss and to the work of the American existentialist psychologist Rollo May and others.

The Visible and Invisible

The distinction between visible and invisible in Merleau-Ponty's ontology is not a dichotomy. The invisible inheres in the visible. Chiasm effects the context of the intertwining of the visible and invisible as it does the context of the intertwining of touching and being touched, which is – see above – the antecedent of Merleau-Ponty's discussion of flesh.

The "otherness" of the invisible to the visible cannot suggest alterity, a state of being alien to the visible. The invisible abides in and is complement to the visible. Merleau-Ponty says, "Meaning is *invisible*, but the invisible is not the contradictory of the visible: the visible itself has an invisible inner framework (*membrure*), and the in-visible is the secret counterpart of the visible, it appears only within it [...]" (1964/1968, p. 215).

Merleau-Ponty, moreover, declares of the "invisible" that, "it is the invisible *of* this world", and that it is "that which inhabits this world, sustains it, and renders it visible, its own and interior possibility, the Being of this being" (p. 151). The invisible here in Merleau-Ponty is not some arcanum. It is not some idealized repository of realities that is esoteric in character and philosophically Platonic in derivation. It is *of* this world.

The Gestalt psychologist Wolfgang Metzger (1936/2006) discusses "visible and invisible forms" from the perceptual point of view. The discussion stimulates considerations of the visible and invisible in visual fields, the locus of Metzger's investigations, in such manner that the one who is read in Merleau-Ponty cannot help but consider possibilities of an ontological dimension to it. Reference to contexts of naturalistic assumptions, of course, is obligatory. One of Metzger's graphic illustrations for points on "visible and invisible forms" is the "ambiguous figure" so familiar to psychologists. In that phenomenon of figure-rivalry, the alternative potential figure dwells in a "formless intermediate space" until there is a required suppression of the incumbent figure that allows the alternative to "figure" in the visual field. Metzger's descriptions and language at the perceptual level here tease speculation on correlations with Merleau-Ponty's visible and invisible – again, with respect for differences of philosophical assumptions.

They also suggest a bridging of Merleau-Ponty's ontological conceptions to the praxis of painters in their studios standing before the challenge of the easel – the challenge of the invisible. The study of a connection here requires respect for the distinctions between that which is perceptual and that which is ontological – at the same time that one awaits the occasioning of the ontological through perceptual experiencing.

Flesh and the Visible and Invisible in Relationship to Art

Merleau-Ponty says, "to the flesh – the invisible structure can be understood only through its relation to logos, speech – the invisible meaning is the inner framework of speech [...]" (1964/1968, p. 224). The invisible becomes present to flesh through the vehicle of "logos, speech". Merleau-Ponty also refers to a "Logos of lines" (1993b, p. 142). One may say that Merleau-Ponty acknowledges art as a logos – at least as a kind of speech. He says, "[...] painting speaks in its own way" (1993c, p. 84). In further advocacy of painting, Merleau-Ponty declares, "writers must not underestimate the painter's labor and study, that effort which is so like an effort of thought and which allows us to speak of a language of painting" (p. 92). Merleau-Ponty, moreover, refers to the legitimacy of treating painting as a language (p. 112). In a sense, "the privilege language enjoys over painting or the practices of life remains relative" (p. 115). In sum, the art of painting participates in the revelation of the meaning of the invisible to flesh.

Artists testify to the invisible and the visible. They do so sometimes with startlingly explicitness. Odilon Redon (1945) has declared, "my whole originality, therefore, consists in having made improbable beings live humanly according to the laws of the probable, by as far as possible putting the logic of the visible *at the service of the invisible* [italics added]" (p. 361).

Paul Klee (1945), an artist among the ones to whom Merleau-Ponty refers in "Eye and Mind" (1993b), has said, "one learns to look behind the façade, to grasp the root of things. One learns to recognize the undercurrents, the antecedents of the visible. One learns to dig down, to uncover, to find the cause, to analyze" (p. 444). To recognize *the antecedents of the visible*, the antecedents that are the invisible inherent in the visible. The artists Redon, Klee, and others through their art arrive at the invisible that has always been there. One may say that they have "created" it, but they have not created it *ex nihilo*. Priest (2003) says:

> Painting is revelatory of being because it is a depiction of the visible which makes an awareness of the invisible possible. By construing painting as a kind of language addressed to being Merleau-Ponty is drawing attention not only to the fact that paintings are not painted *ex nihilo*, but also to his claim that the visible presupposes the invisible and the invisible presupposes the visible. (p. 219)

Redon and Klee's testimony to the visible and the invisible undergoes specification in the considerations of line and its phenomenality in the visual arts. Merleau-Ponty (1964/1968) offers us a starting point for these considerations. The invisible, he says, "is *in the line* of the visible, it is its virtual focus, it is inscribed within it (in filigree) [...]" (p. 215). The line that the artist draws manifests the invisible's meaning in its "coiling over on flesh". The presentation of the invisible through its presence-ing to the visible is achieved by the artist who depicts, limns, and renders explicit the invisible in visible lines. The artist's line participates in "a system of equivalences, a Logos of lines, of lighting, of colors, of reliefs, of masses – a nonconceptual presentation of universal Being" (Merleau-Ponty, 1993b, p. 142). The Logos of the artist's line discloses Being graphically just as the Logos of speech communicates Being notionally. Merleau-Ponty a bit further on says eloquently:

> Whether it be representational or nonrepresentational, the line is no longer a thing or an imitation of a thing. It is a certain disequilibrium contrived within the indifference of the white paper; it is a certain hollow opened up within the in-itself, a certain constitutive emptiness – an emptiness which, as Moore's statues show decisively, sustains the supposed positivity of things. (1993b, p. 144)

Consciousness in the Psychology of Art

The default understanding of consciousness in our culture is cartesian. It is pervasive and laggard to philosophical history's development from the time of Immanuel Kant. As phenomenologists point out, the cartesian sense communicates a "consciousness" that is container to variously filling thoughts, perceptions, images, memories, etc. This customary employment of the word "consciousness" is that consciousness is a subjectivity onto-itself, and that of which it is conscious is considered as reflecting an other-than-self objectivity. Phenomenologists' understanding of the word "consciousness" differs from this.

Phenomenological philosophers and psychologists consider consciousness as an instance of "intentionality". Intentionality, a "tending toward", always assumes a "that" toward which there is the intending. Intentionality is relational. In his comments on intentionality for psychologists, Giorgi says (2009):

> This being directed to other than itself on the part of subjectivity is what intentionality means, although reflectively, subjectivity can make aspects of itself an object of such directed activity. [...] The intentional relation is the basis of meaning and so phenomenological psychological analyses seek a type of meaning as the basis for understanding psychological reality. This is in contrast to natural scientific psychology, which interprets psychological reality in terms of cause-effect relations. (p.184)

In the above quotation, Giorgi situates for modern psychology the significance of intentionality and consciousness as phenomenologically understood. Consciousness, manifestation of intentionality and agent for meaning, is in a roster of philosophical thinking that is fundamentally different from that of cartesian thinking. Phenomenological psychologists who are familiar with the literature of Edmund Husserl and with Merleau-Ponty's earlier *Phénoménologie de la perception* (1945) are conversant, of course, with "intentionality".

Some among them who are unread in *The visible and the invisible*, nevertheless, may be puzzled (although they should not be puzzled) by Merleau-Ponty's statement in his "Working Notes" of *The visible and the invisible*, "there is no longer consciousness – projections – In itself or object" (1964/1968, p. 227). The puzzlement intensifies with Claude Lefort's (1964/1968) statement that in *The visible and the invisible* Merleau-Ponty revisits his early analyses:

> [...] in order to show that they acquire their full meaning only outside of a psychological interpretation, when they are enveloped in a new ontology. It alone can now ground their legitimacy [...] by disclosing the impossibility of further maintaining the point of view of consciousness. (p. XXI)

Merleau-Ponty's "move" of analyses from out of psychological interpretation to the new ontology of *The visible and the invisible* that involves the seeming retirement of consciousness raises questions such as, "Where is intentionality in this ontology, and how does intentionality thereby enact in the lifeworld?"

Lingis (1986) ratchets up the radicalism of Merleau-Ponty's understanding of intentionality in his ontology of flesh. Lingis says that Merleau-Ponty, "transposed the format of intentionality into the essence of corporeity; intentional analysis now [...] [operates] within a philosophy of nature where consciousness itself is produced by an "overlapping" of nature [cf. flesh] upon itself". "Intentionality", Lingis continues, "which for Husserl was a transcending of the sensible [...] Merleau-Ponty reformulates as a power of the sensible" (p. 31).

Has there been, indeed, the retirement of consciousness? Merleau-Ponty says that his new ontology discloses how, "it was meaningless to thus realize the consciousness before the consciousness" (1964/1968, pp. 250-251). That is, it is meaningless to posit a consciousness and that of which it is conscious (cf. psychology) before a foundational consciousness or intentionality that is primordial to and embracing of transcendent positings (cf. ontology). *Foundational* consciousness is not retired. Intentionality for Merleau-Ponty, as Lingis says, is reformed as "a power of the sensible". Merleau-Ponty has repurposed the designations of intentionality and consciousness in a thematically and more explicitly ontological direction.

Barbaras (2004) points out that,

> Merleau-Ponty's ontology proceeds entirely from the decision to reconceive intentionality as an originary "reality", to recognize the irreducible and in some way unrendable character of the intentional fabric. [...] Intentionality rejects a type of analysis that tries to undo it in order to reconstruct it, to rediscover in it a unity starting from a prior duality. In other words, for Merleau-Ponty the issue is one of understanding *intentionality as being* through the notion of flesh. (p. 170)

Flesh as understood by Merleau-Ponty surmounts the intentionality of consciousness that Husserl had tried to reconstitute from the "duality of matter and form" (Barbaras, 2004, p. 170).

The re-presentation of intentionality as the intentional fabric of flesh in *The visible and the invisible* does not bespeak a rupture in the conceptual development of Merleau-Ponty's thought from *Phénoménologie de la perception* (1945) to *The visible and the invisible* (1964/1968). Merleau-Ponty declares a commonality of thread between the ontology of *The visible and the invisible* and that before it:

> I must show that what one might consider to be "psychology" (*Phenomenology of Perception*) is in fact ontology. Do so by showing that the being of science [which includes, of course, the science of psychology] can neither be nor be thought as *selbständig*. (1964/1968, p. 76)

Merleau-Ponty declares here that psychology has, at the very least, an intimate relationship to ontology that is both subtle and complicated. Psychology then, in this context, is the study of the Being of the human being. Merleau-Ponty says further, "results of *Ph.P.* [*Phénoménologie de la perception*] – Necessity of bringing them to ontological explicitation" (1964/1968, p. 183). Dillon addresses this continuing thread in Merleau-Ponty's work.

> [...] the thesis of the primacy of phenomena which grounds the implicit ontology of the *Phenomenology* [*of Perception*] culminates in the doctrine of the element of flesh wherein the term "flesh" occupies in the explicit ontology of *The Visible and the Invisible* the same conceptual space as the term "phenomenon" (or "Gestalt") occupied in the earlier work. "Phenomenon", "Gestalt", and "flesh" name the same fundamental reality: the always presupposed foundation of all rationality, all value and all existence (p. 174).

For Dillon, flesh has been implicitly present in *Phenomenology of Perception's* reference to "phenomenon" ("Gestalt") and it is articulated explicitly in *The visible and the invisible.* Intentionality (and the operations of consciousness) is now ontologically presented as the "power of the sensible", as Lingis says. It inheres in sentient flesh. Consciousness is not repudiated. Merleau-Ponty professes Being as the place of consciousness in ontology. "Being is the "place" where the "modes of consciousness" are inscribed as structurations of Being [...] and where the structurations of Being are modes of consciousness" (1964/1968, p. 253).

It is the argument of this essay from all of this that what is occurring at the psychological level of consciousness and its discourse is at that moment an occurrence at the ontological level as it is presented in *The visible and the invisible.* Reflection on this concurrence suggests that the making and the aesthetic experiencing of art encompass ontological simultaneities. Some may impute to the above thoughts a conflation of the psychological and the ontological. The differentiation between the two rests in their levels of discourse. The experiencing of art is both psychologically addressable and ontologically referable.

In all of this, three lines of development have so far been presented. The first is that of Merleau-Ponty's development of an explicitly ontological significance to touch that he terms flesh from the antecedent of Husserl's discussion of the phenomenon of touch. The second line of development is within the chronology of Merleau-Ponty's own work as outlined by Dillon above: from the implicit ontology of phenomenon (or Gestalt) in *Phénoménologie de la perception* to its explicit ontological characterization as flesh in *The visible and the invisible.* The third line of development is Merleau-Ponty's repurposing of the designation of consciousness from Husserl's phenomenology of it to an understanding of its modes as "structurations of Being" and the intentionality of consciousness as the intentional fabric of flesh.

For the phenomenological psychologist of art informed by Merleau-Ponty's ontology, transfigurations of Being in the ontological dimensions of flesh and its visible and invisible that are effected by artistic and aesthetic experiences signify psychological consequences. Just as these transfigurations of Being are the purpose of art in its ontological articulation, the purpose of art in its psychological expression is "the mission of art" that is defined by Ó Cluanáin (1979) as:

> [...] the propaedeutics of perception for a more authentic living of life. That is to say, the perceptual experience of art returns the viewer or listener to a *Lebenswelt* which is now perceptually experienced as illuminated with significances formerly inapparent or obscure – and this "return" motivates the person toward a more authentic living. (p. 245)

Imagination and Physiognomy in the Psychology of Art

With Merleau-Ponty's repurposing of the designations of intentionality and consciousness, what are the dynamics of the artistic experiences and aesthetic experiences at the psychological level in its mission of art that may resonate at the ontological level for re-structurings of Being? Philosophical reflections and psychological investigations disclose that imagination is a key player here. It is proposed, furthermore, that physiognomy is its theatre of activity.

Imagination

Imagination is the executive partner with perception in making art and in experiencing art. It empowers perception to reach beyond its limits. In the spirit of Merleau-Ponty's languaging, imagination enables vision to fathom the invisible that is inherent in the visible.

Imagination, Kearney (1991) says, is dialogical in character. It is not a "free agent"; it is not autonomous in agency. One does not "just imagine". Kearney says:

> The imagination addresses an invisible meaning in the visible world and the world responds only because both participate in a common core of Being. It is precisely because of this cognate genesis that imagination may serve as an agent of creative dialogue rather than monologue [...] imagination is dialogical. (p. 115)

The dialogue is concrete and it may be difficult. Anyone who makes art is working with a material medium; e.g.; canvas and pigments, stone and sculpting tool, musical sound and its instrumentation, or word sounds and representations with their combinations. The medium resists the "making" done to it by the artist. Imagination has to deal with that perceptually experienced resistance. Imagination's efforts may be frustrated, fulfilled, or "in process". Imagination never, however, lofts independently from perception into an artistic activity that seeks to exact a total obedience from the medium's materiality. It is in dialogue with the visibility of its medium and with that medium's material resistance. Tacitly, the goal is to focus on arriving at the invisible.

Amedeo Giorgi (1987) in his discussion of the psychology of imagination presents participant experiential reports with respect to the imaginational process. Giorgi analyzed those descriptive reports of the participant artist according to the phenomenological psychological method that he has developed over the years since the latter part of the 1960's (e.g., 1985, 2009). He quotes an artist participant in his study, whose goal was to depict the "ideal cat".

> I have to kind of sit back and let the ideas, the images, the figures, kind of flow out. Like I said, it's like giving myself over to it. I have to get out of the way [...] new images [...] just sort of come if I'm looking at the paper in the right way [...] all else just kind of falls to the wayside. I'm just there. It's a great feeling, you know. (p. 31)

Giorgi comments, "it seems that the role of imagination is to bring to presence in consciousness whatever is not directly perceivable or actually given in any other way. [...] for the creative type [the artist], the various images he gets helps him to become clearer about his guiding idea". He adds, "the succession of presences helps the painter to achieve an artistic object" (1987, p. 38). Giorgi continues:

> [...] it is the meaningful relationship between present reality and the imagined events that helps us to understand the specifics of the imagined events. The reality lacks are fulfilled by the irreal presences of the imagination, and these presences are psychologically meaningfully related to the gaps in reality. (p. 41)

"Various images" and "the succession of presences" are the configurations drawn from the artistic media and their respective material resistances. "Present reality" is the point of departure for the dialogue between imagination and its perceptually experienced medium. "Reality lacks are fulfilled by the irreal presences of the imagination." In the ontology of Merleau-Ponty, one would say that lacks within the visible are fulfilled by the inherent invisible that is elicited by the artistic activity with the assistance of the imagination. The dynamic of dialogue is explicit here.

Introductory to his phenomenological psychological analysis of the results obtained in his investigation, Giorgi had presented a phenomenological philosophical context for his position that "the key to understanding the phenomenological approach to imagination is to understand that the image is a modality of consciousness" (p. 23). The philosophers to whom he referred in his investigation were Jean-Paul Sartre, Edmund Husserl, and Edward Casey. Giorgi did not refer to Merleau-Ponty in his 1987 investigation. The essay being presented here extends the psychology of imagination as Giorgi has studied it to relationship with Merleau-Ponty's thoughts on flesh and the visible and the invisible. The writer of this essay believes that the extension is consonant to Giorgi's 1987 study.

In the discussion of the results of his study of the psychology of imagination, Giorgi says, "overall, it seems that the role of imagination is to bring to presence in consciousness whatever is not directly perceivable or actually given in any other way […]" (1987, p. 38). In the context of Merleau-Ponty's new ontology, "whatever is not directly perceivable or actually given in any other way is candidate for the visible's invisible". The artist initiates the artistic process through commitment to it. The implementation of the commitment, however, takes on "a life of its own". The artist does not control the situation. "[The artist] was responding to a noematic discovery; he was not in control" (Giorgi, 1987, p. 42).

The art-making forays of the artist are at the psychological level. The artist with learned skills engages the material and its resistances. Imagination associates with the involved perceptual processes. Perception by itself, no matter how focused on art-making, is inadequate to the task. Imagination in relationship to perception is neither simplistically a "tag on" nor is it, within a reductionist perspective, some kind of "gesture" exercised by perception. Imagination, with perception, is the enabler of artistic activity and of aesthetic concurrence. At the philosophical ontological level, then, the artist's efforts importune the invisible to disclose itself through the medium in which the artist is working.

With respect to aesthetic imagination, it is guided by the artistic imagination that has been accomplished in the work of art. The clearest evocation of this is reported by Giorgi (1987) from one of the participants in his study:

> When I say "caught", I kind of mean, something helped me imagine this scene, to think about it. Something about the picture called me to imagine, something about the season, and the possibilities of winter called me, kind of spoke to me, like prompting me to imagine. They like helped stimulate my imagination, would be another way of saying it. (p. 34)

In this case, the photographer's caught image of the participant and his wife skiing, not necessarily artistic but available as example of a finished exercise of imagination (through composition, control of lighting, angle, etc.) and suggestive of artistic image, has called to the participant's imagination. In aesthetic experience, the imagination of the experiencer responds to this call and it is in *perceptual* tandem to the artistic imagination that has been enacted in the completed work of art. Ó Cluanáin (1987) points out, "imagination [that is aesthetic] is subsequent to and contingent upon the perception of the work of art" (p. 86). With attention to Rudolf Arnheim's (1966) careful and rigorous treatment of the perceptual character of the aesthetic experience, Ó Cluanáin (1987) says that in the aesthetic experience, "imagination is directed and fulfilled through the structure(s) of the perceived work of art" (p. 97). Imagination that wanders from that structure(s) is withdrawing from the aesthetic experience. *Subsequent to* the aesthetic experience, imagination stirred by the aesthetic experience may range wherever it will. In the case of the participant in Giorgi's study, his imagination then wandered after having been caught by the photograph. He "began to imagine the coming ski season" (1987, p. 34).

This is an important point. Casey seems to suggest that in the aesthetic experience of art, especially in theatre, we have an extension of aesthetic experience, "from its initial perceptual basis [...] onto an imaginative plane" (1976, p. 140). This is a compromise of the primacy and authority of the work of art. As it has been said above, "the imagination of the experiencer is in tandem to the artistic imagination that has been enacted in the completed work of art". This is within the perceptual experience of the work of art. Experience of a work of art exits from aesthetic experience proper when the experiencer's imagination exceeds the boundaries of the artistically enacted imagination in the work of art. "The receptivity of aesthetic imagination [...] requires a "hold" on the ordinary imagination" (Ó Cluanáin, p. 106). Post-aesthetic imagination, despite its own authority and validity, is adventitious to aesthetic imagination.

Physiognomy

Earlier in this essay it was said that,

> The non-dualist difference between the flesh of the world and the flesh of the body (body understood as embodied subjectivity, Merleau-Ponty's *le corps propre*), however, is a difference of differentiating distinction and not the difference between metaphysical realities in exclusion of each other.

A concept facilitative of the appreciation of Merleau-Ponty's distinction between "flesh of the world" and "flesh of the body" is that of physiognomy. Physiognomy interfaces embodied subjectivity and nature with each other; it interfaces flesh of the body and flesh of the world with each other. It is a kind of pellicle utterly porous and transparent through which embodied subjectivity and nature open to each other and intertwine. It is with risk that the word pellicle is offered here – positivist reifications could subvert the metaphoric character of the word as it is offered in this understanding of physiognomy. I define physiognomy as (2005):

> [...] the specification of expression. It is the structural specification of the phenomenon in its expressiveness. Another way of saying it is that expressiveness characterizes all of nature both human and physical, and that physiognomy reflects the structural differentiation of expressiveness in the instantiations of nature. In this context, "expression" [or "expressiveness"] [...] is a general character of all

> phenomenal reality. This position emerges from reflection both on the thoughts of Merleau-Ponty in his phenomenological review of expressiveness and physiognomy, and also on the thoughts of Arnheim in his Gestaltist understanding of visual experience. (p. 220)

Further on, I say, "one can appreciate that analysis of works of art progresses through experience of the physiognomy [of them] and that that experience is not had by way of pieces, by way of visually sectioning the work. It is direct and immediate" (p. 233). Recognition of the "look", of the physiognomy, of whatever is before us is the recognition of kinship. Flesh coils over flesh. Embodied subjectivity, *le corps propre*, and Nature are reconciled to each other through interfacing physiognomy. The artist experiences this in the making of art. Reciprocally, the experiencer of the completed work of art is experiencing the reconciliation. Within that aesthetic experience, as I (1987) say, "perceptual embrace of the work of art [...] [is] the embrace that both contours itself totally to the physiognomy of the art in order to be informed by it, and also stands as the sufficient basis of the aesthetic experience" (p. 86). Specifically, in the "physiognomy" of the art there resides the enacted artistic imagination to which fits the experiencer's imagination.

Conclusion

The thesis of this essay has been, "that Merleau-Ponty's presentation of "flesh and the visible and invisible" is the clearest ontological explication of the context within which artistic and aesthetic experiences take place". The achievement of that understanding of art's ontology immediately distinguishes artistic and aesthetic experiences of art from the educational and assessment purposes of art appreciation. It is the position of this essay that Merleau-Ponty's thoughts on art's ontology within a psychology of art clarify how genuine experiences of art institute psychological consequences for experiencers.

To understand how art instigates psychological – and ontological – consequences, there has to be consideration of Merleau-Ponty's repurposing of the designations of intentionality and consciousness. This essay suggests that the engagement of the two levels of psychological discourse and ontological discourse clarifies the reciprocity and simultaneity between the psychological and ontological dimensions of artistic and aesthetic experiences. The experiencing of art is both psychologically addressable and ontologically referable. Lastly, imagination and physiognomy are constitutive of artistic and aesthetic experiences. All the above serve the "mission of the psychology of art": the re-direction of everyday living to more authentic living.

References

Arnheim, R. (1966). *Toward a psychology of art.* Berkeley, CA: University of California Press.

Barbaras, R. (2004). *The being of the phenomenon: Merleau-Ponty's ontology* (T. Toadvine & L. Lawlor, Trans.). Bloomington, IN: Indiana University Press. (Original work published 1991)

Casey, E. (1976). *Imagining: a phenomenological study.* Bloomington, IN: Indiana University Press.

Cloonan, T. F. (2005). Face value: The phenomenology of physiognomy. *Journal of Phenomenological Psychology, 36*(2), 219-245.

Dillon, M. C. (1988). *Merleau-Ponty's ontology.* Bloomington, IN: Indiana University Press.

Giorgi, A. (Ed.). (1985). *Phenomenology and psychological research.* Pittsburgh, PA: Duquesne University Press.

Giorgi, A. (1987). Phenomenology and the research tradition in the psychology of the imagination. In E. L. Murray (Ed.). *Imagination and phenomenological psychology* (pp. 1-47). Pittsburgh, PA: Duquesne University Press.

Giorgi, A. (2009). *The descriptive phenomenological method in psychology: A modified Husserlian approach.* Pittsburgh, PA: Duquesne University Press.

Husserl, E. (1952). *Ideen zu einer reinen phänomenologie und phänomenologischen philosophie. Zweites Buch.* (M. Biemel, Ed.). Dordrecht: Kluwer.

Husserl, E. (1989). *Ideas pertaining to a pure phenomenology and to a phenomenological philosophy: Second book* (R. Rojcewicz & A. Schuwer, Trans.). Dordrecht, The Netherlands: Kluwer Academic Publishers. (Original work published 1952)

Johnson, G. A. (Ed.). (1993). *The Merleau-Ponty aesthetics reader.* Evanston, IL: Northwestern University Press.

Kearney, R. (1991). *Poetics of imagining: From Husserl to Lyotard.* London: HarperCollins *Academic.*

Klee, P. (1945). Notes from his diary. In R. Goldwater & M. Treves (Eds.). *Artists on art* (pp. 441-444). New York: Random/Pantheon.

Lefort, C. (1968). Editorial Note. In M. Merleau-Ponty, *The visible and the invisible* (A. Lingis, Trans.), pp. xxxiv-xxxix. Evanston, IL: Northwestern University Press. (Original work published 1964)

Lingis, A. (1986). *Phenomenological explanations.* Dordrecht: Martinus Nijhoff Publishers.

Merleau-Ponty, M. (1945). *Phénoménologie de la perception.* Paris: Gallimard.

Merleau-Ponty, M. (1964). *Signs* (R. C. McCleary, Trans.). Evanston, IL: Northwestern University Press. (Original work published 1960)

Merleau-Ponty, M. (1968). *The visible and the invisible* (A. Lingis, Trans.). Evanston, IL: Northwestern University Press. (Original work published 1964)

Merleau-Ponty, M. (1993a). Cézanne's doubt. In G. A. Johnson (Ed.). *The Merleau-Ponty aesthetics reader* (pp. 59-75). Evanston, IL: Northwestern University Press.

Merleau-Ponty, M. (1993b). Eye and mind. In G. A. Johnson (Ed.). *The Merleau-Ponty aesthetics reader* (pp. 121-149). Evanston, IL: Northwestern University Press.

Merleau-Ponty, M. (1993c). Indirect language and the voices of silence. In G. A. Johnson (Ed.). *The Merleau-Ponty aesthetics reader* (pp. 76-120). Evanston, IL: Northwestern University Press.

Metzger, W. (2006). *Laws of seeing* (L. Spillmann, S. Lehar, M. Stromeyer, & M. Wertheimer, Trans.). Cambridge, MA: MIT Press. (Original work published 1936)

Ó Cluanáin, T. P. (1979). Phenomenological psychological reflections on the mission of art. In A. Giorgi, R. Knowles, & D. L. Smith (Eds.). *Duquesne studies in phenomenological psychology: III* (pp. 245-277). Pittsburgh, PA: Duquesne University Press.

Ó Cluanáin, T. P. (1987). Towards a psychology of imagination in art and in esthetics. In E. L. Murray (Ed.). *Imagination and phenomenological psychology* (pp. 78-108). Pittsburgh, PA: Duquesne University Press.

Priest, S. (2003). *Merleau-Ponty*. London: Routledge.

Redon, O. (1945). From his journal and letters. In R. Goldwater & M. Treves (Eds.). *Artists on art* (pp. 358-361). New York: Random/Pantheon.

Rojcewicz, R. (n.d.). Translation of *Phénoménologie de la perception* (Merleau-Ponty, 1945). Unpublished.

Van Den Bos, G. R. (Ed.) (2007) *APA dictionary of psychology*. Washington, DC: American Psychological Association.

THE VALUE OF TRANSCENDENTAL PHENOMENOLOGY FOR PSYCHOLOGY: THE CASE OF PSYCHOSIS

Larry Davidson, Ph.D. & Lesley Anne Solomon[27]

Yale University
United States

Abstract

Conventional wisdom suggests that transcendental phenomenology holds little relevance for psychology, as psychology is presumed not to require performance of Husserl's "transcendental reduction". As an empirical science, psychology is thought to assume the existence of the natural world and to remain in this way transcendentally naïve. This chapter begins with a brief review and critique of this position and makes the argument – drawing both from Husserl's mature works and from concrete clinical examples – that for psychology to be grounded in phenomenology it must constitute a return to naïve positivity from the transcendental rather than stop short of taking the transcendental turn. The example of psychosis is used to demonstrate the difference which makes a difference when psychologists pursue a transcendental attitude prior to taking up their properly psychological subject matter, allowing history and culture to inform the context for their individualistic focus on everyday life.

Two roads diverged in a wood, and I –
I took the one less traveled by,
And that has made all the difference.

– Robert Frost, *The Road Less Traveled.*
(chosen in homage to Father Edward Murray)

In a 1927 letter to Roman Ingarden, Husserl complained that he was allowing himself to become depressed by the fact that his better students "overlook the depth dimension that I point to and instead of finishing what I started, time and again prefer to go their own way". He noted that this was particularly true, and particularly problematic, of a young Martin Heidegger, he described as a "natural power of a genius" and whom, he bemoaned, "carries all the youth away with him" (cited in Caputo, 1977, p. 86). These insights could be described as prescient if one agrees that the *approximately* 80 year history of phenomenology since 1927 has been populated primarily by Heidegger, his existentialist contemporaries, and their students – the vast majority of whom *have* followed Heidegger's lead of stopping short of the transcendental turn in their phenomenological explorations. But what if there was a "depth dimension" to Husserl's perspective which was overlooked in the process? How might phenomenology have looked different, and produced different results, especially for psychology, had Husserl's students, and their students after them, taken "the road less traveled"?

Amedeo Giorgi is one of the few students of Husserl's students who has grappled with this depth dimension and who has tried to see what lay down the alternative path to the one taken by Heidegger and his followers. Although heavily influenced by Merleau-Ponty earlier in his career, Giorgi has remained interested in the transcendental problematic posed by Husserl and has continued the work Husserl began of trying to develop a *pure* phenomenology by pursuing his investigations to their own inevitable conclusions. This has meant running up against the boundaries of the transcendental, considering the possibility of the transcendental reduction, and wondering *whether* there are implications for psychology deriving from this otherwise (and properly) philosophical domain – all of which pertain to the "depth dimension" of which Husserl wrote above. Appearing never to fear standing apart, and at times alone, Giorgi has continued from the time of his first major work, *Psychology as a Human Science: A Phenomenologically-Based Approach* (1970), to hold out the most stringent of expectations for a phenomenologically-based psychology; one that does not sacrifice its foundation in consciousness in order to retain a respectable vestige of naturalism (i.e., making it more readily accessible and understandable to fellow psychologists).

In the following chapter, we consider this dimension of Giorgi's legacy. We argue for and describe the less traveled road of a human science of psychology based in Husserl's transcendental phenomenology. We appreciate that the conventional wisdom has suggested that transcendental phenomenology holds little relevance for psychology and that psychology is presumed not to require performance of Husserl's "transcendental reduction". As an empirical science, psychology is thought to assume the existence of the natural world and to remain in this way transcendentally naïve. But we suggest that this view has overlooked the "depth dimension" to which Husserl pointed, and which we find to have significant implications even for an empirical science of psychology.

The chapter makes the argument, drawing from Husserl's mature works, that for psychology to be based in phenomenology it must constitute a *return* to naïve positivity *from* the transcendental rather than stop short of taking the transcendental turn. The example of psychosis is then used to demonstrate the difference which makes a difference when psychologists pursue a transcendental attitude prior to taking up their properly psychological subject matter. In Husserlian terms, this difference is no less than that between pursuing a "science of life" as opposed to a "science of death" (1970), or, in the terms suggested by the Husserl scholar J. N. Mohanty (1985), a phenomenology "of respect" as opposed to a phenomenology "of suspicion" (Davidson, Staeheli, Stayner, & Sells, 2004). Given the tragic history of psychosis within clinical psychology and psychiatry, we suggest that this offers an especially useful illustration of taking the road less traveled in phenomenology.

The Transcendental

> With the break with *naïveté* brought about by the transcendental-phenomenological reorientation there occurs a significant transformation, significant for psychology itself [...] In fact, for a genuine psychology, and for the exactness that belongs essentially to it, transcendental philosophy plays the role of the *a priori* science to which it must have recourse in all its actually psychological knowledge, the science whose *a priori* structural concepts it must utilize in its mundane inquiry. (Husserl, 1970, p. 210)

The relationship between phenomenology and psychology is admittedly complex, with Husserl's own views on the nature of this relationship evolving over the course of his career (Kockelmans, 1967). In previous articles (Davidson, 1988, 1994; Davidson & Cosgrove, 1991, 2002; Davidson, Staeheli, Stayner, & Sells, 2004), we have tracked this evolution through its various twists and turns and have argued at length for the necessity of the transcendental turn for the development of a phenomenologically-based psychology. We will not repeat those arguments here. Rather, we will assume as our primary point of departure what we take to be Husserl's mature position as reflected in his final, unfinished, work, *The Crisis of European Science and Transcendental Phenomenology* (1970; hereafter referred to as *The Crisis*), and will consider the implications of the transcendental phenomenology outlined there for the science of psychology. Psychology being the first and most crucial of the "European sciences" which Husserl considers to be in a "crisis", we will explore the nature of this crisis and the way in which the turn to the transcendental offers a way out of it.

So what, after all, is the depth dimension of the "transcendental" to which Husserl refers? In his earlier works, Husserl tended to define the transcendental *via negativa*; that is, in terms of what it was not. The transcendental was *not* constituted, was *not* worldly or mundane, was *not* the psychological, the anthropological, the historical, etc. It was what remained when all of these layers of naivety were bracketed through the phenomenological reduction, described variously as the transcendental ego, transcendental subjectivity, or transcendental intersubjectivity. As an epistemological absolute, such a concept was essential to Husserl's overcoming of psychologism and grounding knowledge in universal truths. As solely an epistemological concept, however, there was little to appeal to Heidegger or other phenomenologists interested in the intentional relation between the person and the life-world. It came across as bloodless and empty, and, apparently, was easily dismissed.

We cannot be contented with such a negative characterization of the transcendental. In order both to demonstrate the importance of the depth dimension of Husserl's work and to distill the implications of the transcendental turn for psychology, we are challenged to characterize the transcendental in positive terms as well. Erazim Kohak, another Husserl scholar, understood the nature of this challenge also, suggesting that Husserl's "recognition of the transcendental dimension of subjectivity may be his greatest challenge to his successors". Kohak describes this challenge as one of transforming the "transcendental dimension from an epistemological vanishing point to a conception of the Person as a transcendental presence" (1978, pp. 182, 175). While mindful of the magnitude of the task undertaken, and straining thus against the appearance of hubris, we shall, nevertheless, take a stab at a positive definition which we hope will allow us then to consider its implications for psychology.

We know that words such as consciousness, intentionality, subjectivity, and experience refer to the transcendental. We also know, however, that these words may be used in a parallel psychological as well as transcendental sense. They may be used to refer to worldly or objective realities as well as to the constitutive source of these realities. What may not be considered to have parallel psychological significance is the act of constituting itself. Our challenge is to come to an understanding of this act that does not objectify it; that does not falsely psychologize it. As Fink wrote in his commentary on *The Crisis*, the transcendental reduction "*deobjectifies* transcendental life" (1970, p. 133). We thus need to be able to characterize the transcendental in a positive fashion in other than objective terms; in a way that preserves its non-objective status. We need to come to an understanding of constituting subjectivity or consciousness as different from the psychological, historical, social, etc. How are we to understand this difference?

We know all of these objective realities to be constituted in nature. They are constituted by lived experience as the particular worldly appearances which may be taken on by lived experience. Experience may *appear*, that is, as psychic, as historical, as social, etc. in nature, even while it remains fundamentally transcendental. Each of these perspectives thus refers back to, or is an interpretation of, the transcendental. Each is constituted as a self-objectification of the non-objective transcendental. Perhaps, then, we can appreciate the nature of the transcendental as transcendental by viewing experience without the assistance of any of these worldly appearances or interpretations; by viewing it, in Mohanty's words, "freed from its mundaneity" (1985, p. 208). What would experience look like, we could ask, if it were seen as neither psychological nor historical, etc., in nature?

Kohak makes such an attempt in his discussion of the transcendental. Rather than asking what experience might look like *without* any of these self-interpretations, however, he simply defines the transcendental as being subjectivity *prior* to its taking any of them on. Building upon the "personalism" which Husserl offered especially in *Ideas II* (1952), Kohak equates the transcendental subject with the Person as constituting ego. He understands "Person", however, as the fundamental ontological entity, rather than as a psychological or anthropological being. It is the Person who may become the worldly focus of psychology or anthropology – or, for that matter, of biology or anatomy – but the Person itself exists prior to taking on any of these objective characteristics. Writes Kohak: "The Person is precisely the transcendental I in its full density but prior to the peculiarities of a culture or a personality" (1978, p. 185). In this sense, the transcendental is that which becomes (self-objectified as) the psychic or the historical, etc. It is that which takes on a worldly appearance, that which becomes objective. Considered in its own right, prior to the act of self-objectification, it is quite simply the "Person" as subject.

But how does such an approach, we might wonder, not make of the "Person" merely a blank slate upon which we then write any number of objective characteristics? How does it avoid making of the transcendental an epistemological "ideal limit"? Defining it solely as the "Person" prior to culture or personality would appear to be just another way of defining it negatively, in terms of what it is not (yet). Kohak himself realizes that: "The I which I am and am aware of being is emphatically not an epistemological vanishing point" (1978, p. 186). Yet how else are we to understand this "I"?

Husserl offers the following solution. He argues that the pure or transcendental I of lived experience (Kohak's Person) is not to be equated or identified with the experience itself. The subject of experience is not a real moment or part of the experiencing act. It is to be considered to be apart from, or different from, both the objects of these experiences and the experiences themselves as objectively interpreted. In his lectures on *Phenomenological Psychology*, Husserl writes:

> *From everything which is given directly as an object, reflection leads not only to constituting lived experiences in which the object is constituted as a pole, but at any*

> *time a reflection directed toward the identical I is possible: and this I is the subject of all lived experiences and the subject for all its objects as a pole of unity of its intentionalities; but it is not itself a lived experience. (1977, pp. 158-159)*

We must separate the subject of experience even from experiences of reflection upon experience. When we reflect upon our own experiences we thereby constitute, or objectify, as objects ourselves as subjects. This is required by the nature of intentionality and reflection. We should not thereby, however, mistake the constituted object of reflection to be the subject reflected on. "Of course every reflection which I relate to myself", writes Husserl, "is itself a lived experience and makes me objective – objective for me." Yet in the very fact that I am objectified for myself there is evidence of an I for whom I have become objective. There is still the I as subject functioning behind this reflection and allowing it to be a reflection *for me*. "I am as subject of the reflecting a functioning I"; and "even unreflectedly", he adds, "I am constantly a pole of identity in relation to which everything else is *objective*" (1977, p. 159).

It is this I functioning behind all lived experiences as their subject that Husserl equates with the transcendental. We therefore cannot understand the process of this I reflecting on, and thus objectifying, it as that of a psychological subject reflecting on him/herself. Psychological reflection takes place in the natural attitude, and we are speaking here of the transcendental perspective. To consider the pure subject to be a human being would be to lapse back into the natural attitude. While the objectified subject may become the object of history, of psychology, or of biology (etc.), the functioning I, the Person, remains neither psychological, nor historical, nor biological in nature. It remains a pole of identity in relation to which each of these objects may be considered to be objective. It is the "I" *for whom* I appear to be a psychic being; for whom my being a psychic being is "on hand".

Before criticizing Husserl's notion of the "pure I" for simply constituting more of the same empty talk of ideal limits and vanishing points, we should note that Husserl was clear to point out that this "pure I" is *not* to be considered merely "a dead pole of identity". It is not only an epistemological concept. It is not a generic, abstract, or unreachable Ego. Rather, he writes:

> It is the I of affections and actions, the I which has its life in the stream of lived experiences only because it on the one hand exercises intentions in them as intentional lived experiences, toward and busied with their intentional objects, and because on the other hand it is stimulated by these objects, in feeling is touched by them, is attracted to them, is motivated by them to actions […] The I is constantly there

> [...] not as an empty word, but as a directly exhibitable center, as a pole. (1977, pp. 159-160)

The pure I may be considered to represent more than a dead pole of identity or an empty word precisely because it is fully *alive*. It is not an ideal polar point, but an I who performs activities. It is a vital and vibrant I who touches and is touched in its living by the objects of its experiences. It is the primordial actor whose actions bring to life and enrich its surrounding world of objects as both constituted by previous actions and affecting and motivating future actions. This is the I of both the passive and active genesis of meaning: the I that is passively moved by a pre-given world of significance, but who also actively generates on this basis a new and original world of significance. Originality is possible, Husserl writes, "as a result of an active doing of the I on the basis of something or other given passively beforehand" (1977, pp. 160-161).

This makes of our pure I more of a substantive concept than a mere vanishing point or empty ideal polar point. In the recognition of the I's *living*, in the recognition of its being both affected and active, it does perhaps make more sense to use Kohak's term of the "Person". This carries with it the connotation of vitality and affect that Husserl here attributes to the I. In doing so, however, we must keep in mind that we are speaking of a transcendental concept. We must remember that this Person is not the psychological ego or human being *per se*, but is a Person equally present in its self-interpretations as psychological, historical, biological, etc. It is a Person equally as social as it is individual, equally as temporal and historical as it is spatial and material-physical. But it is also a Person whose life is not exhausted by the sum total of these varying perspectives on it. It is the living Person who takes on this number of varying modes of objective appearance, who provides the conditions for the very possibility of appearing in these ways, but who also is preserved as the source of constituting, of life, itself. It is, perhaps most accurately stated, the *life* of the Person who lives in certain objectively definable ways.

This last point might give us some cause to be dissatisfied with Kohak's formulation of the transcendental I as Person. To the extent that the I is pure subjectivity, pure life, we should acknowledge that it does not stand alone, it is not ontologically self-sufficient. Use of the term Person, no matter how de-objectified or de-anthropologized we may intend, would appear to imply an absolutizing of the individualized subject, an autonomy of the individual actor. Husserl, however, makes it clear that the transcendental is an intersubjective domain and that the pure I does not represent a self-contained or solipsistic world. Subjectivity is not "fragmentary" and split off into personally relative spheres; it is not autonomous and arbitrary, not relative to the whimsy of individual subjects, but is universally structured as teleological (1970, pp. 269-299).

We may thus only continue to refer to the transcendental as the Person if we are willing to consider the Person in its activity as relative to or subordinate to absolute subjectivity. Such a view would entail humility with respect to the Person's activity in the face of a more overarching domain of subjective life. This kind of humility is no different in principle, however, from the operative sense of humility presently entailed in naturalism: the humility we experience that is, in the face of Nature (e.g., in natural disasters and medicine, as well as in the awe of a beautiful landscape). As it is apparently acceptable to view the human body as subordinate to the over-arching causal nexus of Nature, of which it is but a part, Giorgi has suggested that there is no obvious reason to reject a parallel subordination of the Person as individual subject to an overarching motivational nexus of transcendental subjectivity of which it is also but a member (A. Giorgi, personal communication, 1988). Transcendental subjectivity may be considered as universally structured within phenomenology as is nature within naturalism. The basis of this structure is, of course, different, in that subjectivity has as its fundamental law, motivation, or teleology rather than naturalistic causality. Still, it would appear to be just as arguable that a subjective realm of motivation and teleology is the necessarily given context for individual Persons as it is that a natural world of causality is the necessarily given context for individual bodies.

With this understanding of the transcendental, we are now in a position to appreciate more fully Husserl's rejection of all forms of ism's, including particularly Dilthey's historicism. Any position that sought to elevate a constituted region of reality to the role of (transcendental) source or origin for reality would necessarily overlook the truly crucial and all-important role of *living*, affected and active, subjectivity in the constitution of this and all other worldly regions. It would replace the life of the subject with a lifeless region of constituted sense which, deprived of its life-giving relation to subjectivity, would be converted into a meaningless accumulation of facts. Kohak illustrates this point with respect to the example of sociologism, but it would apply equally well to all forms of psychologism as well; he writes:

> When sociologists explain delinquent behavior as a product of underprivileged environment, they leave society helpless in dealing with the delinquent. What we need is not to explain what "made" him do it but rather to understand what, as he understood his own acts, he *chose to do*. In our terminology, we need to understand what kind of [...] world he constituted about himself so that his behavior appeared appropriate to him. We have to understand his choice. Assigning human

> acts to material causes is a dubious procedure, since objects function as motives not qua material entities but as presented in consciousness [...] It is also not overtly helpful, for it leaves society no recourse other than behavioral conditioning, which may assure tranquility but contributes little to the growth of free moral persons. (1978, p. 137)

This example demonstrates clearly how an explanation of subjective activity grounded in deterministic understandings of history, sociology, psychology, etc., would miss the fundamental role of intentionality. It is the foundational importance of the life of the Person, the constituting activity of consciousness, which must be preserved in psychology and all forms of science. We have had to inquire back to the transcendental source of the horizons of our subject's experience and the experience itself in order to reach this dimension explicitly. Our account of our subject's experience will have to be situated explicitly upon its ground.

Kohak's phrasing, as well as his example in general, raises a problematic issue, however. He speaks of his young "delinquent" as "choosing" and as constituting his world. Are these not psychologistic appeals to constitution? Is this not precisely the view of behavior and experience that Husserl rejected under the label of "transcendental psychologism"? Such an example raises the question of how we are to get back to our psychological subject now that we have acquired our transcendental context. Now that we have situated experience within its varying horizons, what is left for us, as psychologists, to do? How do we understand the nature of the psychic within our newly won transcendental framework? What sense of the psychic remains following the turn to the transcendental? How do we return from this philosophical excursion to our task and interest as psychologists?

The Return

> Pure psychology is and can be nothing other than what was sought earlier from the philosophical point of view as absolutely grounded philosophy, which can fulfill itself only as phenomenological transcendental philosophy. But I as a pure psychologist or transcendental philosopher have not thereby ceased being a human being; no more has the actual being of the world and of all men and other beings in the world changed in the least. And I have also not ceased having this particular worldly interest which bears the title: universal science of human beings in respect to their psychic being, both individual-psychic and social; I thus return to the natural attitude, changing my vocation: I take up my work as a psychologist on the ground of the world. (Husserl, 1970, pp.259-260)

We have reached behind the appearance of psychological subjects to their constituting source of the transcendental I or Person. How are we now to get back to concrete psychological presence in the life-world? What light does this newly gained transcendental knowledge shed on the particular experiences of psychological subjects who are the product of a process of self-objectification? How does a psychology which comes after the transcendental reduction differ from one conducted before it?

Husserl referred to this issue as "the problem of *flowing in*" (1970, p. 208). Prior to the performance of the transcendental reduction the psychic was either understood as a material property of the human organism (in naturalism) or as a transcendental function of the human being (in transcendental psychologism). Following the performance of the transcendental reduction the psychic is now understood to be a self-objectification of transcendental intersubjectivity. The problem is one of how the transcendental "flows into" this self-objectification and "becomes apperceived as its newly revealed intentional background of constitutive accomplishments" (1970, p. 210). How does viewing the psychic in this way, in its relation to the transcendental, change our understanding of it? And, other than by becoming formally the first discipline to be taken up within transcendental phenomenological philosophy, how does the science of psychology differ as a result of it as well? What is the significance of this "flowing in" for our work as psychologists?

Viewing the psychic as a self-objectification of subjectivity means viewing it, along with the world in which it is situated, as a transcendental achievement. The psychic is no longer to be understood as a given, but rather as a region of sense constituted, and in the process of continuing to be constituted, by subjectivity. It is the correlate of certain experience-patterns, of the coherence of specific and definite structures of experiencing life. Paci writes concerning this transcendental understanding of the psychic:

> Mundane psychological life is now characterized in a particular way whereby the transcendental ego operates in it [...] Psychological life is revealed in its structure and thus allows for psychology as the science of a special region of transcendental life. The vast transcendental horizon comes to be determined as psychological life and thus constitutes psychology as a science to the extent that it establishes the essential region of those essential typical operations of transcendental consciousness which we can call psychological. (1972, p.147)

The psychic is taken to refer to one region of transcendental life, the study of which constitutes one regional ontology. As a region unto itself, the psychic has its own particular, definable character, its own "internal structure"

(Paci, 1972, p. 147). We are to describe and investigate a person's experiences as one instance of the typical way in which life comes to be internally structured as psychological. Were we historians rather than psychologists, we would find ourselves interested analogously in a different regional ontology: in describing and investigating the typical way in which life comes to be internally structured as historical. We have, then, but to characterize what is essential to the psychic as a region of constituted sense, as one typical way in which life comes to be internally structured.

We know that for Husserl psychology in all of its forms situates the psychic upon the pre-given ground of the life-world. Regardless of whether we view the life-world as an objective given or as an achievement of transcendental constitution, the psychic is given as existing within its horizon. This insight sheds initial light on the essence of the psychological. The life-world is pre-given to the psychic, and the psychic is experienced as taking in this reality existing outside of and independently of itself. The psychic is constituted, then, as a worldly and mundane reality that is essentially passively receptive in the face of the life-world. As described by Fink: "Psychology moves from the start within the self-explication of human experience as being only receptive and impotent" (Fink, 1970, pp. 118-9; cf., also, de Boer, 1978, p.168). The psychic is constituted as that region of sense characterized by a passive receptiveness and impotence in the face of the larger world in which it is situated and of which it is but a part.

Before one objects that people can experience themselves as active and potent in the face of the world as well as passive and impotent we must stress that this insight applies to the level of the ontological, not to the level of the ontic, in defining the essence of the psychic. The ways in which consciousness is passive, receptive, and impotent in the face of the world have to do, that is, with the transcendental constitution *of* the world in the first place, and not with specific responses to a specific world as experienced by a specific person. Phenomenology has taught us that there are both passively and actively generated strata of sense involved in any act of constitution. Transcendental subjectivity objectifies itself as embodied psychological subjectivity by objectifying its pre-given strata of passively generated sense as the defining characteristic of psychic being. The condition for the possibility of my having psychic being is the presence of the realm of passively generated sense pre-given to me in my active constituting life. Were the transcendental not to involve the passive generation of meaning, then it could not take on a worldly and mundane appearance. Were the sedimentation of previously generated sense as passively pre-given not possible, then neither would be self-objectification of the transcendental as psychic. It is thus the possibility and nature of this appearance, the possibility and content of the horizons of sedimented meaning, which constitute the psychic. Psychic being is determined on the basis of the characteristics of this (transcendentally) pre-given sense. I do not experience myself as free to "choose" to constitute any kind of world I wish to live in, but rather experience myself as having been born into a particular world that existed prior to me and as finding myself within particular concrete conditions not of my own making. How I then experience and am motivated by that particular context is the stuff of a psychological science.

We now are in a position to understand how the psychological ego parallels for Husserl the transcendental ego. The psychological ego is the manner in which the transcendental is able to appear in the world as a mundane reality. It is the Person, but now *as* constituted by all of the particularities of culture, history, personality, etc. It is the particular individuated and embodied way in which subjective life has come to exist here in this space and at this time. Psychic being thus includes all of the various horizons of sedimented meaning that have gone into constituting me to be the particular Person that I am right here and now. It includes all that I am passively receptive to and impotent in the face of, all that is pre-given to me as the ground upon which my activity may take place. As Paci writes: "The specific field of psychology is the field of conditionings, of what conditions me in relations with others, my motivations, and my projects" (1972, p. 186). It is the field of constituted sense in which the Person has objectified itself to be situated in order to become a part of the life-world. It is for Husserl thus the "first" self-objectification of the transcendental, the first appearance of subjectivity in, and as part of, the life-world (1970, p. 262). Other social sciences will build precisely upon this base.

Before proceeding on, it may be useful to point out that it is this parallelism between the transcendental and the psychological which is, according to Husserl, misunderstood in the case of a "phenomenological psychology", resulting in transcendental psychologism. The problem with phenomenological psychology was its (mis)understanding of the essential nature of the passivity and impotence described above. Rather than accepting an ontological sense of passivity and impotence in the face of the world as pre-given as a fundamental aspect of the transcendental constitution (self-objectification) of itself as psychological, phenomenological psychology is left to struggle with an ontic sense of passivity and impotence which it then mistakenly attributes to the psychological subject as the product of an act of "self-deception". Instead of acknowledging that we simply do not experience ourselves as constituting the world in which we live (in which, more accurately, we find ourselves), phenomenological psychologists insisted that psychological subjects did in fact constitute their personal worlds but then deceived themselves about this very act of constitution. The passivity and impotence which are, in fact, essential aspects of any act of transcendental constitution became personal fictions of which (certain) psychological subjects tried to convince themselves, but only as acts of pathological self-deception. In reality, however, neither convincing nor self-deception are required. What is required, we argue here, is understanding that constitution remains a transcendental act and that the psychological is but one self-objectification of the transcendental as a worldly being.

In a previous report, we used the example of a young woman with anorexia to illustrate this misattribution of transcendental subjectivity to psychological subjects in phenomenological psychology (Davidson & Cosgrove, 2002). We argued that from the perspective of phenomenological psychology, this woman would be described as viewing herself as a passive victim of the meanings she had herself constituted and as having constituted herself as powerless in the face of them. The structures of passivity and impotence were thus prominent in this proposed psychological understanding of her experience and world. In the view of phenomenological psychology, however, this was the result of our young woman deceiving herself about the origins of the meanings in terms of which she was living her life. She was deceiving herself about the fact that she had actually chosen these meanings, deceiving herself about the fact that she was the one actively constituting herself and the others around her to have the meanings that they did.

Having taken the transcendental turn, we now know, however, that our young woman did not constitute these meanings as a psychological subject, nor did she choose in any sense to have them pre-given to her. She did not choose, for example, to be born into a society in which women are valued for their physical attractiveness, and in which being physically attractive requires being thin. Nor would it make sense to say that as a teenager she knew "ontologically" that possibilities other than these really existed in the world; that she need not have taken for granted these implicit and sedimented meanings as valid for her as well. She did not choose nor did she actively generate the passively generated meanings which were pre-given to her. Having taken the transcendental turn, we now know that there are ways in which even transcendental subjectivity is passive and ways in which meanings are given to consciousness prior to and as the precondition for its own activity. Phenomenological psychology was psychologistic in attributing what were for our subject passively generated meanings to her personal psychological activity. In returning from the transcendental to the psychological we will not want to repeat this mistake. We will not want to hold psychological subjects responsible for the pre-given horizons in which they themselves come to be constituted as such.

How do we understand these pre-given horizons differently? We understand these pre-given horizons, along with the psychological subject him or herself, to be factical achievements of transcendental constitution. It is important that we not return to a pre-transcendental *naïveté* and attribute these structures to Nature nor to our psychological subject him or herself. However, it is not therefore necessary for us to become historians or political scientists rather than psychologists. As psychologists we are interested specifically in the ways these constituted structures have passively contributed to the constitution of this particular Person's experiences. Our focus is on the impact of these pre-given structures on individuals' experiences, not on the pre-givenness of the structures themselves. We may limit ourselves therefore to what we shall call the "motivational horizon" of our subject's experience: to that immediate environment of pre-given sense that directly informs his or her experience (Davidson, 1988). We pursue the transcendental origins of these structures to the extent necessary to come to an understanding of how this subject's experience has been structured by them. We return from the transcendental once we have a grasp on the character of the particular horizon in which this experience has arisen. While the psychic may be the first self-objectification of the transcendental, it is not the only one. The other forms of objectification may, however, be left to other disciplines to explore.

Psychology as a Science of Life

> Today, psychologists have a favorite word, and that word is maladjusted. I tell you today that there are some things in our social system to which I am proud to be maladjusted. I shall never be adjusted to lynch mobs, segregation, economic inequalities, "the madness of militarism", and self-defeating physical violence. The salvation of the world lies in the maladjusted [...]. (Martin Luther King, 1981, p. 23)

We remember that, in our return from the transcendental to positivity, we are not to return thereby to our pre-transcendental *naïveté.* As we are not to forget what we have learned transcendentally, we thus remain aware that subjective life is the only absolute given; that all else, including the psychic, derives its sense from this sole life-giving source. We therefore cannot consider the transcendental act of constitution to be one property of the psychological subject. Rather, we recognize that the psychic is only one (constituted) aspect of the transcendental Person. This Person we know to be as much historical, political, ethical, economic, etc., as it is psychological.

Psychology is the study of the ways in which individual subjects may be motivated to act. A significant portion of its subject matter consists of the meaningful ways in which prior acts of a subject motivate his or her future activity. But these acts themselves, the active generation of what later will become a part of the actor's motivational horizon as pre-given meaning, cannot be captured within psychology. Psychology can only study these acts retrospectively, as having played a role in the constitution of the subject's present motivational horizon (cf. Paci, 1972, p. 146). It can only study a constituted region of sense, not the acts of constitution themselves. The acts themselves transcend the boundaries of psychology, just as they transcend the boundaries of the psychological ego. They do not lie within the scope of the psychologist.

In restricting psychology to the study of the motivational horizon *for* individual activity we have therefore, however, limited significantly its competence as well as its scope. The implications of such a limitation for our new science may be considered fairly profound. It is obvious, for instance, that a transcendentally grounded psychology could not consider itself to be predictive in nature. It could not presume to explain in a deterministic manner each new action of the Person as simply being an effect of the operation of previous experiences acting as causes. While it would be able to delineate clearly the horizon for a given action, including its pre-existing possibilities, it would not be able to guarantee that this action would actualize any of the already given possibilities as opposed to creating a new one. Nor would it be able to explain how the creation of a new possibility came about, nor why it came about in this instance as opposed to that one, etc. While able, perhaps, to delineate "typical" patterns of experiencing (cf. Giorgi, 1979), it would not be able to know *in advance* how a given subject will act in a given situation.

Further, while the origins of our motivational horizon may not themselves be the proper object of study for the psychologist, they remain important for psychology nonetheless. Their impact on its subject matter cannot be overlooked, as they essentially constitute it to be what it is. They are present in the passive generation of the motivational horizon in which we do take an explicit interest. As we are no longer transcendentally naive, we may no longer allow ourselves the false comfort of naturalism or psychologism, in which the horizon of experience is viewed as an objective given. Rather than being an objective given, we understand the horizon to be the product of historical, political, social, cultural, and economic forces. All of these aspects we also know to contribute directly to the constitution of the psychic as psychic. In limiting the scope of psychology explicitly to this circumscribed segment of the whole, we thus also acknowledge explicitly the importance of the remainder of the landscape that we have left to our colleagues in other disciplines to explore. We recognize that we require the assistance of these disciplines in shedding light on the other aspects of the phenomena we take to be of psychological interest.

Following the return to positivity, the psychic, even within psychology, thus comes to be seen as only one segment of a much larger landscape. As Scanlon eloquently suggested:

> One gets the impression that even the most astute psychological description and analysis amounts, relatively speaking, to a brilliant flash of lightning which illumines momentarily a small segment of a vast landscape shrouded in darkness and extending to unknown depths. (1982, p. 198)

Psychology as a science becomes only a small part of a much larger interdisciplinary whole. It becomes situated as only one well-circumscribed avenue of access to the Person in his or her transcendental identity. But we remember that the Person is not to be exhausted by the sum total of these worldly perspectives either. It is not merely the psychological taken together with the historical, political, ethical, social, etc. that is to be appreciated. Rather, it is to be understood as a whole which is *more* than the sum of parts. It is the very presence of life which provides the condition for their possibility. In this sense, psychology is not one discipline that can simply be added to other disciplines to create an aggregate all-encompassing science. The sense of interdisciplinary used here is not that of independent sciences coming together externally. Rather, psychology, like all other positive sciences, is to be subordinated to the transcendental perspective in which it is situated. Each discipline is taken to be only one beam of light shone on what is to be considered an essentially trans-perspectival subject matter. It is the transcendental presence of the Person that always remains primary; the presence of the Person as non-psychological of which psychology only provides one glimpse.

Lastly, and perhaps most importantly for our present purposes, this subordination of the psychic to the transcendental implies that it is activity itself that is primary and passivity and receptivity secondary, even within psychology itself. While psychology is to be the study of passivity, it is to view passivity as only one moment of an active process. It is to be the study of the role of the motivational horizon in the on-going life of the subject, as opposed to the study of the motivational horizon as the cause or source of this life. Rather than being given as a motivational horizon which then causes or brings about the subject's activity, it is the activity of the subject him or herself, the intentional life of the Person, which brings to life the motivational horizon as that which motivated the activity to take on the particular form that it did.

To appreciate the far-reaching implications of this point one must in essence reverse one's ordinary ("natural") way of thinking. For Husserl, all meaning is to be understood only as playing a role in the intentional life of the Person, whether as product or as pre-given horizon. This constitutes, however, a Copernican reversal of the natural attitude view, in which the life of the Person is attributed to some constituted region of sense, whether it be that of the psychic, the biological, etc. According to Paci: "the meaning of the problem of the reabsorption" of the transcendental – what we have called the problem of "flowing in" – is captured in the development whereby "all the sciences become sciences of life" (1972, p. 155). The result of the transcendental's flowing into the psychic is that passivity, while remaining an essential moment of experiencing life, comes to be seen as playing a role *in the service of* activity, rather than as its source. Sciences thus become sciences of the on-going life of subjectivity, rather than remaining sciences of the constituted (lifeless) products of this life. They also move from being passive, receptive, and impotent, to being active, creative, and powerful (Paci, 1972, p. 152).

With this step we have stumbled onto what Husserl was referring to in the title of *The Crisis* as being the crisis of European sciences in the 1920's and 1930's. From the perspective of a German intellectual of Jewish heritage, Husserl was witnessing what he considered to be a tragic misuse of science, in which the methods and presumed results of science were being placed in the service of fascism. "Science" was being used to promote and justify the ascendancy, even fetishization, of one constituted region of sense over all others. Science was passive, receptive, and impotent in the face of political authority, and ceded its epistemological autonomy too readily in the service of promoting and preserving an emerging status quo. Furthermore, this emerging status quo was oriented to the destruction and death of any signs of life which diverged from its own fetishized ideal. For science not to be complicit with such meaningless destruction of life, it would have to be fundamentally transformed, re-oriented to a meaningful affirmation of life instead. This, according with Husserl, could be achieved through an appeal to transcendental phenomenology.

The transcendental turn has placed passivity and receptivity in the service of activity and creativity, constituted regions of sense in the service of the act of transcendental constitution. As applied to science, this means that the world can no longer be understood as an objective and independent reality which provides the source and foundation for the emergence of life. Rather, from a transcendental perspective this objective, independent world is to be understood as a pre-given constituted correlate of subjective activity. It is what *it* is only as a particular instance of the passive generation of meaning pre-given to active constitution. As such, it is simply the product of previous acts of constitution and the precondition for further such acts. It might be thought of as one frame abstracted from the movie that is the on-going process of the constituting of the world by subjectivity. The world is thus not itself the source of life, not itself an objective given. Rather, it is the ever changing and life-less product of transcendental subjective life. It is a realm of previously constituted, and now "dead", sense. It is only the realm of subjectivity itself which is absolute; the world follows after as *its* intentional achievement.

From this perspective, it makes little sense for science, or any other human pursuit, to insist on adapting a Person's activity to the world as it currently is. Of what value could it possibly be to adjust a Person's actions to a previously constituted stratum of sense? What would be the point of actively accepting that this realm of meaning has been passively generated to be pre-given to me, rather than using this realm of meaning as the point of departure for further active constitution? Life is to be found in the creation of the possible rather than in capitulation to the previous. It is only when science views subjectivity as arising out of, owing its origins to, a certain objectively existing state of affairs that it values adaptation to the status quo. It thus places activity and life in the service of what is in actuality a passively generated stratum of sense, a dead layer of previously constituted meaning. Given the nature of the world to which science was attempting to adapt people in the 1920's and 1930's, one can well appreciate Husserl's fear and distrust of this kind of science. One can understand his proclamation that not only society but its science as well was in a state of crisis.

What alternative is there? The transcendentally-grounded alternative is not to view the world as an objective given, as a complete and independent reality that is unchanging in the face of subjective life. It is rather to view the passivity, receptivity, and impotence characteristic of the psychic as playing a secondary, if nonetheless essential, role in the on-going and creative life of transcendental subjectivity. Psychology transcendentally-grounded would thus not view the Person as subject as solely passive and impotent in the face of the world, as it would also not view the world as given in advance. Rather, it would know the world to be contingent upon the activity of Persons and ever-changing as a result of this activity. It would view the world as playing a passive role as the stage upon which the teleological movement of subjective life takes place. The psychic *per se* would be one segment of the backdrop for this drama. Subjective life, however, would be elsewhere – it would be in the temporal unfolding *of* the drama itself.

Husserl writes that for the world as an intentional accomplishment of subjectivity its "being-in-advance is an absurdity" (1970, p. 265). Viewing the world as constantly in the process of being constituted, and thus constantly changing, our psychology has no objective world at its disposal to which it might attempt to adapt or adjust its patients. Any thought that there might be an objective world to which one might try to adapt would be the result of a psychologistic attribution of necessity to what is actually a contingent structure. As long as we remain within a transcendental framework there is no world that might be passively accepted by our subject or against which her or his experience might be compared and judged deficient. As a result of the transcendental turn, writes Husserl: "there now arises a humanistic science which does not have the world in advance and does not constantly hold onto the world" (1970, p. 326).

Rather than holding onto the world as the source of life and as that to which life must be adapted, transcendental phenomenology views the world only as that which has been constituted thus far. While existential phenomenology might have appeared to agree in principle with this sense of the world as "incomplete", it also seemed to view this incompleteness as something that one was passively to accept. The incompleteness of the world is not so much something one may accept, however, as it is something that one may confirm as it were by accident in the active process of the generation of new meanings. The incompleteness of the world is proven each time a new and different world is created. Transcendentally, we may thus view the world as providing the Person only with the precondition for the active generation of new meanings, with the tools or building blocks for further activity and further change. Transcendentally, the world is to be seen as a resource for life's on-going teleological activity, as part of its equipment, rather than as its source or origin.

Also, rather than viewing the subject as deficient and therefore needing to be chang*ed* by treatment, transcendental phenomenology views the subject as chang-*er* (cf. Kohak, 1978). It views the Person as a socio-cultural, historico-political, psychological, ethical, biological, etc., *actor* (cf. Paci, 1972) whose activity brings about substantive and meaningful changes in the world as constituted correlate of this activity. The function of psychology thus becomes to help patients as Persons understand the myriad ways in which their lives have been previously constituted, previously conditioned, in order to enable them to utilize this passively pre-given sense in their own activity. Psychology joins with the Person's on-going teleological life by viewing the world in which the Person lives as providing him or her with the tools or resources for further activity and change. It is thus not the *Person* who is seen as deficient. The Person is seen instead as having been inadequately *equipped* – whether through impoverishment, poor parenting or education, "bad" genes, etc. – for his or her present life tasks. It is by viewing the psychic in this way as a more or less adequate tool for life that psychology preserves its transcendental grounding even as it returns to positivity. It is in this way that it preserves the primacy of activity and life over passivity and death.

Transcendental phenomenology promotes a basic conviction in the responsibility of subjectivity for the nature of the world in which it situates itself. As one transcendentally grounded science, psychology provides some knowledge of how this on-going process has been conducted thus far. In providing Persons with a self-understanding of the ways in which their activity has been passively constituted, in providing them with an understanding of the ways in which the world has been pre-given to them, it calls them to participate actively and responsibly in the further constituting and changing of both themselves *and* their world (Husserl, 1970, pp. 340-341, 400). Husserl sees the resolution of the cultural crisis of his day to reside in the active pursuit of this kind of transformative science; a science that encourages Persons to take active responsibility for themselves and the world in which they live. Viewing the world simply as an accumulation of meaningless and dead facts, already determined in advance, leaves one powerless to change it. Viewing it as meaningful and contingent upon one's intentional constitution motivates one to be responsible for it and to take an active role in trying to change it. Grounding psychology in a transcendental framework thus not only brings value and meaning back into science (through the re-appropriation of the life-world), but, just as importantly, brings science back into the on-going life of the culture.

The Case of Psychosis

> In psychology the natural, *naïve* attitude has the result that the human self-objectifications of transcendental intersubjectivity, which belong with essential necessity to the makeup of the constituted world regimen to me and to us, inevitably have a horizon of transcendentally functioning intentionalities which are not accessible to reflection, not even psychological-scientific reflection. "I, this man", and likewise "other men" – these signify, respectively, a self-apperception and apperception of others which are transcendental acquisitions involving everything psychic that belongs to them, acquisitions which flowingly change in their particularity through transcendental functions which are hidden from the naïve attitude. We can inquire back into the transcendental historical dimension, from which the meaning and validity accomplishment of these apperceptions ultimately stems, only by breaking with *naïveté* through the method of transcendental reduction. (Husserl, 1970, pp.208-209)

So our job as psychologists is not to help persons with psychosis to adapt or adjust to the world as it currently is, but rather to help prepare them and/or assist them in taking an active role in further constituting and changing both themselves and the world. They, like everyone else who functions in the natural or naïve attitude, will not necessarily be aware of the role of their own subjectivity in constituting the constituted world; these transcendental functions may very well be "hidden", as Husserl suggests above. And it is not our job as psychologists to insist that people seeking help take the transcendental turn, as we ourselves had to do. It does appear to be our job, though, to come to understand and to identify for them the constituted horizon of pre-given meanings within which they live and which motivates them to act. It will then be up to them, to the degree to which they function as autonomous Persons within the motivational nexus of transcendental intersubjective life, to decide how they want to move forward in creating new meanings and a new world.

But *are we not* talking about people with psychotic disorders? *Are we not* talking about people whose very capacities for understanding and making informed decisions are lacking? Only if viewed from the perspective of a science of passivity and death. Viewing people as lacking in anything only makes sense when people are viewed as objects, when they are viewed against the backdrop of some constituted stratum of (dead) sense, in comparison to some static sense of "normality" to which everyone is presumed to aspire. And once we accept the view that they are lacking in some substance without which they cannot be whole, then our options for intervention are limited: either we attempt to fill them up from the outside with whatever they are presumed to be lacking (whether it be neurotransmitters or social skills) or we consign them to an empty or less-than-human life (whether it be in distant state hospitals or in under-funded and segregated community programs).

But what if what is most important is the action of constituting meaning (i.e., life) rather than any particular meaning that has been constituted (i.e., death)? From such a life-affirming perspective, persons with psychosis are viewed as already making decisions everyday and as making these decisions based on their own understandings of the circumstances and their roles within those circumstances. While well-meaning others might heartily disagree with some of those decisions, and the understandings upon which they are based, they would be hard-pressed to deny that the person continues to make such decisions, even if, in the Sartrean style, he or she decides not to decide (Sartre, 1956). Psychosis, in this sense, is not a disturbed or alternative mode of being-in-the-world, as suggested by the early phenomenological psychopathologists; it does not result in a fundamental distortion of the person's being or nature (Davidson, Staeheli, Stayner, & Sells, 2004). The person with psychosis, in Kohak's terms, is no less a Person.

What then is psychosis? Early phenomenological psychopathologists, as well as some contemporary theorists (e.g., Stanghellini, 2004), suggest that people with psychosis have lost or lack "common sense". As a technical term, "common sense" was used to refer "to the implicit assumptions, attitudes, and activities which underlie the person's experiences of a shared social world" and was purported "to account for their difficulty in establishing and maintaining social relationships" and otherwise participating in a consensual social reality (Davidson, 2007). For whatever reason, people with psychosis did not share the same sedimented stratum of sense that was pre-given to others in their social environment. They also appeared to lack the capacity to acquire it in the future. Finally, as insight into or awareness of the illness was thought to be an inherent part of the illness itself (part of what makes psychosis seem so alien), people were also assumed not to be aware of their own lack of common sense. Not only did they lack common sense, but they also lacked the common sense to know that what they lacked was common sense. No wonder psychosis was thought to be so intractable to intervention.

Fortunately, this has not been our experience. Not only do many, if not most, people with psychosis recover over time – with or without treatment – but we also have found people with psychosis to be the most knowledgeable reporters of their own experiences, needs, and interests (Davidson, 2003a; Davidson, Hoge, Godleski, Rakfeldt, & Griffith, 1996; Davidson, Stayner, Lambert, Smith, & Sledge, 1997; Flanagan, Davidson, & Strauss, 2007). They have insight not only into their own subjective life and processes, but also are acutely aware of how others perceive them as well. This awareness has had dire consequences, as people have believed the pronouncements of mental health professionals that they would never work again, never marry or have children, never live independently, etc., and have internalized the social stigma that has been associated with psychosis for the last several hundred years. For many people over many years, a major aspect of their pre-given horizon of meaning involved extremely negative, at times non-human, stereotypes of "psycho killers", "maniacs", and "mental patients". Acutely aware that others viewed, or may view, them in these terms, many people have withdrawn from society, refused to acknowledge having a mental illness, or otherwise rebelled against this destiny. The sciences of clinical psychology and psychiatry have done little to help them overcome this fate.

Much of this has been changing over the last thirty or so years, with the emergence of the "mental health recovery movement". This movement emerged in the gap created by de-institutionalization, when hundreds of thousands of people with serious mental illnesses were discharged from state institutions to communities where they were very few services or other resources for them. As a result, they began to band together to help each other out and to advocate for changes to mental health policies and programs, arguing that they maintained their civil rights and responsibilities and should be treated accordingly. This mental health consumer/survivor movement converged with longitudinal clinical research that showed that people living outside of hospitals often improved over time, and the mental health recovery movement was born.

We have learned many things from this recovery movement in mental health, despite the fact that it is still in its infancy. Of the many things we have learned, the most relevant to the present discussion is the fact that while people with psychosis may appear to have lost "common sense" –just as they may appear to have lost a sense of self and their *élan vital* (two additional important insights generated from phenomenological investigation) – they also are capable of re-acquiring these capacities or aspects of "normal" everyday life. Any such losses should be considered partial and temporary rather than absolute and permanent. We will describe how this is so in the remaining portion of this chapter, beginning with the issue of common sense. That this is so, however, is a reflection of the value of the transcendental for psychology. Common sense, a functional sense of self as an agent, and a sense of vital energy are all constituted products of transcendental intersubjectivity. They are products of experience rather than its source. As such, they can be lost but also found; they can be compromised or deteriorate but also be promoted or regenerated. Until the Person dies, however, they should never be denied.

To return to the concept of common sense, for example, we noted above that people with psychosis were thought to lack the common sense required to realize that what they were lacking (among other things) was common sense. This also has not been our experience. In fact, the following passage from a narrative-phenomenological interview with a person diagnosed with schizophrenia represents precisely the opposite position, which we have found consistently in the hundreds of interviews we have conducted over the past twenty years. Seth, a participant in one of our earlier studies, described to the interviewer how: "*People take for granted that you just do things.* A person with mental illness, it's sometimes hard [...] it's like you're distracted, you can't get involved because you're not sort of all there" (quoted in Davidson, Haglund, Stayner, Rakfeldt, Chinman & Tebes, 2001, p. 282).

With this one passage, Seth has offered us an alternative explanation of the issue of common sense in psychosis. It is not that people with psychosis lack common sense, and therefore are doomed to a life of disability and dependence. Rather, it is that they have difficulty participating in the mundane, trivial, and everyday activities that others are fortunate to be able to take for granted – and this because they are distracted by other aspects of their experience. What is "common sense" if it is not precisely that domain of the "taken for granted" in everyday life? People appear to lack common sense when they do not take for granted the same things that others do. This does not mean, however, that they cannot take these things for granted; *it is* just that they do not *do so*. Their attention, and perhaps effort, lies elsewhere. As Seth explains, having a serious mental illness may *sometimes* be experienced as posing distractions that make it difficult for the person to be "all there". Wherever else he or she may be, others – who are expecting the person to be attending to the same things they are – are likely to view the person as missing, as vacant or empty, or, as the clinical language suggests, as responding to internal stimulation.

But people with psychosis are not always "not all there". And many people have learned ways to manage these internal distractions so that they can "be there" more often than not over time. Granted, these successes may at first be achieved at a fairly concrete level, such as the woman we have called Betty who described how for her learning that she could regulate her own radio represented a turning point in her eventual recovery. As she said:

> It is being active, and I take pride and I'm independent to a certain extent [...] like in my jazz music, like *I'll* turn on my jazz radio, and *I'll* love it [...] it's *my* interest. *I* turn the radio on myself, no one had it going to nourish *them*-selves, to entertain *them*selves, like parents would at a house. *I* turn it on, *I'm* responsible, *I* enjoy the music, *I* make notes and draw while I'm hearing it [...] Then I turn it off, then I have some evidence, *I've* got something done, *I've* been productive, *I* have the drawings to look at [...] It was for me and by me, my own nurturing. So I'm proud of this effort (quoted in Davidson & Strauss, 1992, p. 138; emphasis in the original).

Most people take for granted that they can turn on and off a radio, and then listen to the channel of their choosing. But for Betty, who had been a promising music student before the onset of schizophrenia, this represented an accomplishment, and perhaps a hard won one as well. This is an interesting finding and worthy of further exploration. As it turns out, what was particularly difficult for Betty, as she described elsewhere in her interview, was first regaining a sense that she was a person at all; that she was an agent in her own life who could make decisions and act on those decisions on her own behalf. This is why she accentuated the words "I", "me", and "them" in the quote above. The achievement was not realizing that the radio could be turned on and off, or that it could be turned to the jazz station. "Parents" do it all the time. The achievement was that it was Betty herself who could do so, and do so for herself. For people disabled to this degree, this apparently is a formidable first achievement – but it is a possible achievement nonetheless.

In addition to rebuilding a sense of self that they can then eventually take for granted – just as everyone else does – people with psychosis have described becoming re-grounded in the present as another important challenge that contributes to their gradual re-acquisition of common sense. Minkowski (1970) and other phenomenological psychopathologists described what they saw as a loss of the *élan vital* in individuals with serious mental illnesses, considering the appearance of the person being not "all there" as an indication of his or her fundamental loss of vital energy. What they apparently did not consider as much was that people might be able to regain the vital contact with life that they had (temporarily) lost (Davidson, 2003b). Vital contact with life is another thing that we ordinarily take for granted in our everyday lives; it also is something that people with psychosis may need to work hard to regain. In terms very similar to those used above by Betty, Erica, a participant from Sweden, described this as follows:

> Before [...] everything was in the long term [...] Instead, having to hang on, to find strength, I live small moments more intensely. Now we're here, you and I, and my whole life is all here, only here. It doesn't matter what else happens [...] This moment here is more important than anything that might happen tomorrow [...] This was definitely decisive for me, this fact of living intensely what I'm doing instead of worrying about the future or other things was a real support, a cornerstone for everything [...] a very difficult awareness, a difficult position to take, but living intensely whatever I'm doing, being very concentrated, for me personally [...] I did this and no one told me to do it. I did it on my own and it works. (quoted in Davidson, 2007)

In order to take this position, people have to achieve some degree of awareness of or mastery over the more distracting symptoms of the illness; what we have described as "taming" the illness (adopting this use of the term from *Le Petit Prince* by Saint-Exupery, 1943). But perhaps equally important, they also have to experience a sense of interest, pleasure, or success in what they are doing or it will remain externally imposed and of no use in re-building their sense of self or reconnecting them vitally to life. Once people begin to appreciate these rich and personal experiences (i.e., experiences which are not yet taken for granted) and their positive repercussions, and once they begin to have a sense of self as agent, they can begin to plan for and pursue such experiences more intentionally. As Annica, another Swedish participant, described:

> My way is to simply see to it that I have something to do, to take a walk, light a cigarette, drink a cup of coffee, eat an apple, watch TV and be on the go. Like, I can't just sit around or lie down and sleep all day, I can't do that. It's just not something I can do [...] I feel well enough now that I want to do something, I want to be active, creative, have some company around me. I want to make something positive of the day, meet people,

> I want to talk. I'm pretty keen on having company and I don't just lie in bed and sleep all day [...] I can't understand how you could waste your days when you only have one life. And so you have to make something of it. (quoted in Marin, Mezzina, Borg, Topor, Lawless, Sells, & Davidson, 2005, p 228)

We are not suggesting that these experiences and accomplishments cure psychosis. What we are suggesting is that these experiences and accomplishments begin to lay the foundations for the person to take on active role in combating the illness and eventually either learning how to live effectively with it or, in many cases, to overcome it. There is a tremendous amount of diversity in what those roles look like and the ways that people find to do battle with the illness. Under-girding all of these efforts, though, appears to be a gradual process of relearning how to manage life, and oneself, on a day-to-day basis, the illness and its symptoms being only one of the many aspects of life that one has to manage. To appreciate the intricate and subtle steps that a person takes in order to lay this foundation, one might need to imagine what life would be like on a day-to-day basis if one could no longer take many of the basic givens of everyday life for granted. Erica, the Swedish participant we quoted from above, described the incremental nature of this process in the following passage:

> So I take it step by step. I have learned to hurry slowly and do it in stages and set partial goals when I have discovered that it makes sense [...] doing it by partial goals and making it manageable, then you get positive feedback that it's going okay and then you don't hit the wall. That's my strategy, the strategy for success: partial goals and sensible goals and attainable goals, and that's something I've learned to do in order to achieve things. When I have been able to deal with something that's been a struggle and feel secure, I move on. Step by step, put things behind me. (Marin, Mezzina, Borg, et al., 2005, p. 236)

Conclusion

Erica described the process above as "hurry[ing] slowly" both because it addresses an immediate and urgent need, without which one cannot function effectively (thus the need to hurry), and also because it requires painstakingly small steps, taken repetitively, over time (and thus the need to go slowly). It is as if a person did not feel confident that the floor below him or her was solid and would not give way each time he or she took a step forward. In this case, it would be understandable that each step would be taken slowly, cautiously, and with care so that the person would be able to spring back to the solid ground that was still there in case the floor in front of him or her were to dissolve before his or her eyes (as it does in some cartoons and video games). This is the challenge the person with psychosis faces in reconstructing his or her sense of self, reconnecting vitally to the world, and regaining a useful body of "common sense" – all objects being constituted products of transcendental intersubjectivity. They must, as it were, be constituted anew in the wake of the illness, incorporating what the person has come to learn about the illness, its effects, and his or her most effective ways of dealing with it. The more people do so, and the more visible role models of the possibility of recovery become through the mental health recovery movement, the more people with psychosis will contribute not only to recreating themselves but also to recreating the world. They will contribute to the creation of a world in which serious mental illness is no longer considered a death sentence, in which it is no longer shameful to be diagnosed with *it* or *to* seek help for a mental illness, and a world in which the pursuit of a *normal* life in the community is truly rendered possible for all.

References

Caputo, J. (1977). The question of Being and transcendental phenomenology: Reflections on Heidegger's relationship to Husserl. *Research in Phenomenology*, 7, 84-105.

Davidson, L. (1988). Husserl's refutation of psychologism and the possibility of a phenomenological psychology. *Journal of Phenomenological Psychology*, 19, 1-17.

Davidson, L. (1994). Phenomenological research in schizophrenia: From philosophical anthropology to empirical science. *Journal of Phenomenological Psychology*, 25, 104-130.

Davidson, L. (2003a). *Living outside mental illness: Qualitative studies of recovery in schizophrenia.* New York: New York University Press.

Davidson, L. (2003b). The restoration of vital contact with reality: Minkowski, Sartre, and *Joie de Vivre* as a basis for recovery. In Granger, B. & Charbonneau, G. (Eds.). *Phénoménologie des Sentiments Corporels.* Paris: Association Le Cercle Herméneutique, pp. 195-207.

Davidson, L. (2007). Habits and other anchors of everyday life people with psychiatric disabilities may not take for granted. *Journal of Occupational Therapy Research,* 27(S), 1-9.

Davidson, L. & Cosgrove, L. (1991). Psychologism and phenomenological psychology revisited, Part I: The liberation from naturalism. *Journal of Phenomenological Psychology,* 22, 87-108.

Davidson, L. & Cosgrove, L.A. (2002). Psychologism and phenomenological psychology revisited, Part II: The return to positivity. *Journal of Phenomenological Psychology*, 33(2), 141-177.

Davidson, L., Haglund, K.E., Stayner, D.A., Rakfeldt, J., Chinman, M.J., & Kraemer Tebes, J. (2001). "It was just realizing [...] that life isn't one big horror": A qualitative study of supported socialization. *Psychiatric Rehabilitation Journal*, 24, 275-292.

Davidson, L., Hoge, M.A., Godleski, L., Rakfeldt, J., & Griffith, E.E.H. (1996). Hospital or community living? Examining consumer perspectives on deinstitutionalization. *Psychiatric Rehabilitation Journal*, 19, 49-58.

Davidson, L., Staeheli, M.R., Stayner, D.A., & Sells, D. (2004). Language, suffering, and the question of immanence: Toward a respectful phenomenological psychopathology. *Journal of Phenomenological Psychology*, 35(2), 197-232.

Davidson, L., Stayner, D.A., Lambert, S., Smith, P., & Sledge, W.H. (1997). Phenomenological and participatory research on schizophrenia: Recovering the person in theory and practice. *Journal of Social Issues*, 53, 767-784.

Davidson, L. & Strauss, J.S. (1992). Sense of self in recovery from severe mental illness. *British Journal of Medical Psychology*, 65, 131-145.

De Boer, T. (1978). *The development of Husserl's thought.* (T. Plantinga, Trans.). The Hague: Martinus Nijhoff.

Flanagan, E., Davidson, L., & Strauss, J.S. (2007). Incorporating patients' subjective experiences into the *DSM-V*. *American Journal of Psychiatry*, 164(3), 391-392.

Frost, R. (1920). *Mountain interval.* New York: Henry Holt and Company.

Giorgi, A. (1970). *Psychology as a human science: A phenomenologically-based approach.* New York: Harper & Row.

Husserl, E. (1952). *Phanomenologische untersuchungen zur konstitution. Ideen zu einer reinen phanomenologie und phanomenologischen philosophie. Zweites buch* (M. Biemel, Ed.). The Hague: Martinus Nijhoff.

Husserl, E. (1970). *The crisis of European science and transcendental phenomenology* (D. Carr, Trans.). Evanston, IL: Northwestern University Press.

Husserl, E. (1977). *Phenomenological psychology* (J. Scanlon, Trans.). The Hague: Martinus Nijhoff.

King Jr., M. L. (1981). *Strength to love.* Philadelphia: Fortress Press.

Kockelmans, J. (1967). Husserl's original view of phenomenological psychology. In J. Kockelmans (Ed.). *Phenomenology: The philosophy of Edmund Husserl and its interpretations* (pp. 418-449). New York: Doubleday and Company.

Kohak, E. (1978). *Idea & experience: Edmund Husserl's project of phenomenology in Ideas I.* Chicago: University of Chicago Press.

Marin, I., Mezzina, R., Borg, M., Topor, A., Lawless, M.S., Sells, D., & Davidson, L. (2005). *The person's role in recovery.* American Journal of Psychiatric Rehabilitation, *8(3), 223-242.*

Minkowski, E. (1970). *Lived time: Phenomenological and psychopathological studies* (N. Metzel, Trans.). Evanston, IL: Northwestern University Press.

Mohanty, J.N. (1985). *The possibility of transcendental philosophy.* Boston: Martinus Nijhoff.

Paci, E. (1972). *The function of the sciences and the meaning of Man* (P. Piccone & J. Hansen, Trans.). Evanston, IL: Northwestern University Press.

Saint-Exupery, A.de. (1943). *The Little Prince* (K. Woods, Trans.). New York, NY: Reynal & Hitchcock.

Sartre, J.P. (1956). *Being and nothingness* (H. Barnes, Trans.). New York: Washington Square Press.

Scanlon, J. (1982). Empirico-criticism, descriptive psychology, and the experiential world. In J. Sallis (Ed.). *Philosophy and archaic experience* (pp. 185-198). Pittsburgh: Duquesne University Press.

Stanghellini, G. (2004). *Disembodied spirits and deanimated bodies: The psychopathology of common sense*. Oxford: Oxford University Press.

Note

1 Lesley Anne Solomon is a student who is in the process of formulating her graduate studies program in psychology.

SUBJECTIVITY, MEMORY, AND HUMAN SCIENCE

Magnus Englander, Ph.D.

Malmö University
Sweden

Abstract

Natural scientific psychology still fails to address the issue of subjectivity in a meaningful way. Amedeo Giorgi's descriptive phenomenological psychological method enables human scientific researchers to approach the realms of subjectivity while still meeting the rigorous criteria of science. The purpose of this essay is to highlight the notion of subjectivity in Giorgi's method as it applies to human science, and to do so by using the phenomenon of memory as an example. Recent efforts to place the phenomenon of memory in a biological and/or cognitive scientific model are critically examined from a phenomenological perspective. By utilizing Giorgi's qualitative method one is able to capture essential subjective, psychological aspects of lived memory. Some examples of descriptions of memory are provided with earlier human scientific results on memory, and they are integrated with the overall phenomenological dialogue on the intricate relationship between the phenomena of the body, memory, and self.

> Memory requires more than dating of a fact in the past. It must be dated in my past. In other words, I must think that I directly experienced its occurrence. It must have that "warmth and intimacy" [...] as characterizing all experiences "appropriated" by the thinker as his own.
>
> – William James, *Principles of psychology.*

Amedeo Giorgi, who established the descriptive phenomenological psychological method (Giorgi, 1975, 1985, 1997) as applied to human science research, has made it possible for researchers to access the qualitative aspects of human phenomena without sacrificing the rigorous criteria of modern science. In other words, what makes Giorgi's method so appealing to the human scientist is that it provides an option for scientifically describing the meaning of a phenomenon as lived by human subjects. Giorgi's qualitative method lets the researcher access the subjective realm in which lived meanings are pre-reflectively constituted and also allows for the possibility (through the use of the phenomenological psychological reduction, critical reflection, and the use of imaginative variations) of a discovery of a general, human scientific psychological structure about a human phenomenon of their interest. Hence, researchers in, for example, the fields of psychology and nursing science that are particularly interested in human meaning, as it is lived by subjects, find Giorgi's method to be a legitimate alternative to mainstream research methods that, more often than not, uncritically adopt a natural scientific approach in researching human phenomena. Human scientists that utilize Giorgi's method seem interested in the meaning of the phenomenon as it is lived by human subjects. The motivation for using a descriptive qualitative method has for its obvious reason that researchers, such as psychologists and nurses, in their actual work setting frequently encounter the subjectivity of a human being. For that reason alone they have a genuine interest of being true to the lived aspects of phenomena when they are conducting their scientific research. To further one's understanding of the meanings of phenomena that are experienced by one's clients or patients can evidently be helpful in therapeutic or caring situations in which connecting to a sense of inter-subjectivity is necessary.

In other words, these human scientists do not find it useful to give up certain qualitative aspects of the phenomenon present in the subjective realm in order to remain faithful to a traditional, natural scientific agenda. To use Sokolowski's (2008) recent expression, the *veracity* of these human scientists is in harmony with what they are looking for and thus they maintain a sense of responsibility in regard to the search for human knowledge. This does not imply that, for instance, psychologists or nursing scientists using natural scientific, research methods are not conducting legitimate science; however, it only suggests that there are qualitative methods that can, at times, be more appropriate in regard to certain research questions and purposes of a study.

The main purpose of this essay is to point out the necessity of staying with subjectivity in order to capture human scientific meaning as opposed to objectifying subjectivity for the sake of the natural scientific position. The phenomenon of memory will be used as an exemplar throughout the text of this essay. First, a critical examination of the cognitive and biological approaches to the phenomenon of memory is undertaken, especially in order to emphasize how such approaches can lead to misrepresentations of subjectivity. Second, a human scientific understanding of memory is considered, highlighting phenomenological themes such as the pre-reflective and reflective self. The argument here is that Giorgi's (1985, 1997) method can provide for the discovery of the meaning of the phenomenon of memory and thus re-direct the psychology of the phenomenon to the subjective realm. Such effort can aid in establishing more fruitful interdisciplinary labors in our quest for knowledge of human memory.

Since this essay's theme is the interrelation of subjectivity, memory, and Giorgi's (1985, 1997) human scientific method, it is essential at this point to clarify the term subjectivity before going any further. My intention here is to use the term subjectivity in the same sense as Giorgi (2004, p. 2) has done, that is, "[...] as a generic term to speak about persons, consciousness, experience, psyche, agency, the lived body, ego, self and all other such terms that refer to our source of life and awareness". This generic term, subjectivity, implies a commonality that Giorgi (2004, p. 2) claims to be a concept that is at the "center of all of the human sciences". Giorgi (2004, p. 2) also states, "Coming to grips with subjectivity is one of the key problems in the human sciences and this task was not approached properly by the natural science psychologist". I will not explicitly go into all the difficulties surrounding the "noun subjectivity and the adjective subjective" nor the "pejorative term *subjectivism*" since this has already been done by Giorgi (2004, pp. 3-5) elsewhere. However, there is what Giorgi (2004, p. 5) states a "key problem" in regards to subjectivity and human science that I think will be essential to set the stage for our present discussion. Giorgi (2004, p. 5) states:

> The key problem, therefore, is to try to understand how an experienced object necessarily requires subjectivity and yet can be known in such a way that one can claim that it is known unbiasedly. That is the central issue that is responsible for all of the vulnerabilities surrounding the effort to get knowledge of subjectivity. Science seeks knowledge that is objective. In the natural sciences that task means that scientists try to apprehend things and processes as they really are and subjectivity does not pose an insurmountable problem there. In the human sciences, however, an objective understanding usually means apprehending human activity including subjective expression. The paradox seems to be that human beings who are scientists must efface their own subjective biases in order to apprehend objectively the subjective expressions of others. This is the seemingly paradoxical task that the human sciences must face [...].

The solution offered by Giorgi (2004) is for human scientists to find a more balanced view on subjectivity. In other words, it is more rigorous to take subjectivity into serious consideration than to ignore it or misrepresent it (Giorgi, 1997).

A Phenomenological Critique of Biological and Cognitive Scientific Attitudes and Approaches Towards the Phenomenon of Memory

In a time and age of computer technology we use the term memory as a metonymy for both intelligence and efficiency. Memory has simply become an "abstract commodity" which we depend on at work and in everyday life. The term is also the main focus in the neurobiologist's laboratory in which a search for the underlying cellular and molecular mechanisms is of high priority on today's natural scientific agenda (Kandel, 1996). And, of course, memory has always had its privileged place in psychoanalytic theory (Freud, 1989/1899).

Other popular, contemporary, clinical theories such as, for example, eye movement desensitization reprocessing (EMDR) has memory at the core of their theory (Shapiro, 1995). In general, the phenomenon has become to the 21st century cognitive psychologist what learning was (and still is) to the behaviorist. However, the main direction of all the above mentioned attempts still looks at memory through the eyes of the natural scientific paradigm highlighting such issues as causality, trace, speed, and storage capacity in relation to biology and cognitive schemas. Not to mention the false memory debate that has amounted to almost nothing but the quest for the factual aspects of memory (Brown, 1996). Although some cognitively-oriented psychologists have tried to address autobiographical memories (e.g., Howe, 2000), its mode of inquiry is still limited to a pre-established cognitive scientific model. Nevertheless, memory has also always been at the heart of phenomenological theory and Husserl (1991/1893-1917) knew that he had to be able to account for temporality, and thus memory, in order to clarify his philosophical studies on consciousness.

Consequently, phenomenological psychologists have always shown a special interest in the phenomenon of memory and have throughout the 20th century launched heavy critiques against mainstream, natural scientific, psychological research efforts. Perhaps most notable is Straus' (1966) critique of psychologists' search for the memory trace and Giorgi's (1989) phenomenological psychological overview of learning and memory. Lately there have also been some fruitful, interdisciplinary efforts by scholars to integrate phenomenological philosophical insights (although in a highly critical manner) with cognitive-neuroscience (Gallagher and Zahavi, 2008). Now, if one would move away from the abstract notion or the metaphorical meaning of the term memory merely being something associated with modern day computers systems, cognitive science, or intellectual discourses in artificial intelligence and instead approach memory as something lived, then one would enter the experience of the horizon of the past. Then we are also truly in a different "order of reality", as Sartre (1956) would have claimed, and as human scientists we are entering phenomenological psychological aspects of such a phenomenon. If we want to move away from the narrow quest for the natural scientific facts and move in the direction of human meaning, it is also plausible that this path will lead us to discover something about our own motivation (in a phenomenological sense) and how we constitute a relation within our embodied-self-world-others (Giorgi, 1997).

I will not exhaust nor reiterate all the critique that has been prevalent among phenomenological human scientists and philosophers against the cognitive scientific and/or neurobiological models of memory here since it can be found more developed elsewhere (for a recent account, see for example, Gallagher & Zahavi, 2008). However, I find it essential to provide the reader with a critique against the general attitude towards studying the phenomenon of memory that is prevalent among contemporary natural scientists, as we are now almost a decade into the 21st century. Unfortunately (from a human scientific perspective), it seems as if mainstream psychological issues concerning human memory has found its permanent home in the natural scientific model. Eric Kandel, the 2000 winner of the Nobel Prize for his work on the biology of memory, captures today's research attitude as he writes:

> Imbued with new knowledge and confidence, biology turned its attention to its loftiest goal, understanding the biological nature of the human mind. This effort, long considered to be prescientific, is already in full swing. Indeed, when intellectual historians look back on the last two decades of the twentieth century, they are likely to comment on the surprising fact that the most valuable insights into the human mind to emerge during this period did not come from the disciplines traditionally concerned with mind – from philosophy, psychology, or psychoanalysis. Instead they came from a merger of these disciplines with the biology of the brain, a new synthesis energized recently by the dramatic achievements in molecular biology. The result has been a new science of mind, a science that uses the power of molecular biology to examine the great remaining mysteries of life. (Kandel, 1996, p. XII).

It does not come as a surprise that a biologist like Kandel would argue for his own scientific field to "examine the great remaining mysteries of life", nor is it surprising that a biologist would argue for a reductionistic model. What is surprising is the fact that we still are bound to experiments on a sea snail or a laboratory rat (that Kandel uses as his "research subjects") to "examine the great remaining mysteries of life". Note that Kandel, midway through the paragraph suggests the advances to be due to an interdisciplinary effort, although, in a way, undermining this effort by the recent "achievements in molecular biology".

From a phenomenological point of view that is interested in the lived, human meaning of a phenomenon, it is difficult to understand how we could ever enter the stream of consciousness of a rat or the world of a sea snail by comparing its biological structure and processes to a human being's. Many researchers in the field of memory tend to look at the phenomenon from a biological-behavioristic way, using animals as their "research subjects" (see for example, LeDoux, 1993; Davis et al., 1995; Cahill and McGaugh, 1998). The question is whether we learn anything from animal experiments about human memory as it is lived? According to Straus (1966, p.61), animal experiments:

> [...] can never test the re-call of the past as past. Animal experiments are necessarily confined to the study of recognition, for the most part of re-enacting, and this in the wake of vital needs renewed from day to day. Such doing or avoiding under the actual pressure of desire may require not more than a minimum of guidance; [...] it does not require a more or less exact replica of the training situation.

In other words, animal experiments on memory lack the necessary distinctions regarding the phenomenon under investigation. If we want to understand memory as it is lived, would it not be more appropriate to choose a method that began its investigation with human subjectivity? Although Kandel (2000) make some suggested inferences about human meanings in regard to the phenomenon of memory, he is also acting carefully, and at the end of his Nobel Prize lecture, he makes sure that all that we really know at this point from his research is the memory of a laboratory animal. This last point is essential because it gives us the essential distinction between what we are studying and what we strive to understand; and most important of all, implicitly, it is an encouragement for future interdisciplinary efforts. Could it actually be feasible in our day and time that the natural scientific method is still the owner of the exclusive rights to the "great remaining mysteries of life?"

Let us take a brief look at how brain-behavioral scientists study, for instance, the phenomenon of emotional memory. The biological theories of emotional memories are many. Most scientists, however, point to the amygdala as the anatomical structure that is involved in this phenomenon (LeDoux, 1993). Studies done on the impact of the amygdala in correlation with animal behavior have shown that this anatomical unit is a functional unit of most emotional related phenomena (LeDoux, 1993). The main claim of Davis et al. (1995), following research on rats, using a fear-potentiated startle paradigm is that, "A great deal of data now indicate that the amygdala and its efferent projections to the hypothalamus and brainstem form a central fear system" (p. 32). LeDoux & Muller (1997) claim that emotional memory can be understood from complex activity in the cells and synapses in the amygdala and its direct connections to other brain activity centers such as the thalamus and the cortex. Even older studies, for example, Kluver and Bucy (1937) and Weiskrantz (1956) provided empirical support for the amygdala's leading role of emotional processing in monkeys. Now, in what way have these brain-behavioral scientists clarified the complex issues surrounding the subjectivity of emotional memory? As can be seen in Davis et al. (1995) emotional memory is being represented by a fear-potentiated startle paradigm. Fear could be interpreted as an emotion and if one gets startled it can leave a memory of that fearful situation, and in a rational and operational sense then, these scientists are studying an emotional memory. And not to forget, a laboratory rat is supposedly experiencing this emotional memory. It is one thing to be interested in the biology of emotional memory; however, as soon as the term behavior is introduced and inferences are made to account for how human beings work, this is when we need to become critical. I can only agree with Giorgi (2004, p. 10), "[...] such studies should be viewed as being interdisciplinary and complementary to research that focuses on subjectivity, and not a substitute for them".

Phenomenologists have made a number of solid arguments against brain-behaviorists' types of scientific reasoning in the past and it seems as if they will have to continue to do so into the 21st century. As I mentioned earlier, Sartre's (1956, p. 280) words stand out as he pointed out, in his discussion on the body, that we cannot forget that we might be "[...] dealing with two essentially different orders of reality". In other words, we cannot be sure that a biological account can get us closer to an understanding of the lived meaning of human memory. As Giorgi (1989, p. 110) states, "To seek a physiological or chemical model is to try to understand memory externally and non-psychologically. An attempt to measure memory would be a quantification of it and would presuppose the lived experience". Straus (1966) reminded us of this that when psychology searched for the engram, a human being must still at the end read biology, no matter how sophisticated the nature of the inquiry. In other words, and as Straus (1966) points out, biology cannot read itself. And of course, it seems reasonable to clarify what is meant by a memory trace, before one starts to look for it (Strauss, 1966). To discover and describe the many human meanings present in a phenomenon like memory, we will instead have to go back to the source in which such meanings thrive; namely in the lived experience of a human being. In Straus' (1966, p. 99) words, "Human experience, the attitude of man toward the world and to himself, should not be assimilated to events within the organism [...] After many years of being accustomed to a scientific terminology, we have to relearn the mother tongue of human experience".

In general, the cognitive scientific view of memory is that it consists of mental images representing something from the past. In many ways, the cognitive model of memory has the same problem of approaching the phenomenon of memory as the biological; that is, both approaches are bound to the natural scientific paradigm and thus tend to force the lived phenomenon into the format of what Husserl (1998/1913) would have called a real object. Like most psychological phenomena, memory is a mixed object that has characteristics of an ir-real as well as a real object. To then force the phenomenon into a real object in order to stay with the natural scientific agenda is thus to put method before sense. What happens is that the lived aspects of the phenomenon become objectified and abstract (perhaps "dead" and misrepresented), and thus lose their original meanings for the sake of the cognitive scientist's motivation to stick to their own paradigm's sense of what it means to be objective. Giorgi (1989, p. 110) writes, "The cognitive approach is descriptive, but it is more faithful to the model, which is formal and abstract, and thus the description remains external to the lived experience". Hence, although the cognitive approach seems interested in human meaning, it sometimes fails methodically due to its attitude towards what it means to be scientific.

What happens then when the cognitive scientist is trying to fit the meaning of memory into the natural scientific formula? There are numerous problems, but let us take a look at the most foundational. Although this problem is quite obvious, it is worth noting here because it involves the notion of the choice of scientific, research method and hence it becomes relevant to our overall discussion. As most of us are familiar with, the natural scientific method was designed to make an inquiry into things (i.e., real objects); hence, natural scientists also tend to be very successful in its investigations of things. However, human subjectivity and consciousness is not necessarily motivated in the same way as a material thing that exists in space, time and is regulated by causality (Giorgi, 1997). Hence, what the cognitive scientist must do to make consciousness "thing-like" is to fit the whole subjectivity of remembering something into the format of a real object. What happens then is that memory becomes objectified and loses its human meaning. Memory is now abstract and "thing-like". The real problem here is that in making memory into a real object, it becomes very similar to another intentionality; namely that of picturing something. In doing so, the cognitive scientists have distorted not just our scientific understanding of memory, but also, in an implicit sense, our lived experience of remembering versus picturing something. Sokolowski (2000, p. 67), points this out:

> We might be tempted to think of memory in the following way: when we remember something, we call up a mental image of the thing and recognize this picture as presenting the same thing we once saw. In this view, remembering would be not all that much different from looking at a photograph of someone and recognizing who the person is and the setting in which the photograph was taken. The only difference would be that the photograph is in the "extramental" world, while memory is in the "intramental" world.
>
> This interpretation of remembering is very wrong. It confuses remembering with another kind of intentionality, picturing. It is not surprising that we tend to confuse these two types; it does seem that we have inner images in the mind's eye, and once we learn about the brain it seems inevitable that we are going to postulate some sort of projection of some sort of image on some sort of screen in the brain. But the incoherence of this interpretation becomes obvious when we consider the type of identity that occurs in remembering.

Sokolowski (2000, p. 67-68) continues:

> Suppose we are willing to say that we do not look at internal pictures when we remember; what else are we supposed to say? How can we express, from the transcendental viewpoint, what happens in remembering? If we do not look at inner pictures, why does it seem that we do, and how can we account for what seems to show up in our mind's eye or our mind's ear? Our reply to such questions can be put this way: what we store up as memories is not images of things we perceived at one time. Rather, we store up the earlier perceptions themselves. We store up the perceptions we once lived through. Then, when we actually remember, we do not call up images; rather, we call up those earlier perceptions. When these perceptions are called up and reenacted, they bring along their objects, their objective correlates. What happens in remembering is that we relive earlier perceptions, and we remember the objects as they were given at that time. We capture that earlier part of our intentional life. We bring it to life again. That is why memories can be so nostalgic. They are not just reminders, they are the activity of reliving.

Hence, forcing lived memory into the natural scientific realm confuses us not just scientifically, but also contributes to a distorted, everyday understanding of the phenomenon. In this way, the cognitive scientists have contributed to an abstract view of memory that has objectified or perhaps even de-personalized our understanding of this phenomenon and that has forced us into analyses built upon formal cognitive theoretical constructions in order to remain in harmony with the natural scientific paradigm. As Merleau-Ponty (1962/1945, p. 22) once pointed out, "To remember is not to bring into the focus of consciousness a self-subsistent picture of the past; it is to thrust deeply into the horizon of the past and take apart step by step the interlocked perspectives until the experiences which it epitomizes are as if relived in their temporal setting".

One aspect of showing why the psychology of memory also should be seen from a phenomenological point of view is that memorial events are more often than not connected by embodied re-awakenings (Giorgi, 1989). Embodiment is something that belongs to the living subject and to translate embodiment to the natural science paradigm, that is, to the biology of the body, is to distort the meanings present in the lived experience, and hence distort human subjectivity. After natural scientists have observed the biological structures and/or processes involved, they are forced to make interpretations based on these observations in order to present meanings that they can introduce back to the life world of human beings. Often the meanings must harmonize with the investigation, making the interpretations cognitive-scientific in character, and thus they tend to be abstract and distorted in relation to how they are actually lived. In other words, if we as psychological researchers want to remain within the sphere of natural science, we will have to make the phenomenon into a real object, and to follow up on our inquiry, we will have to construct meanings that are within the limits of our initial rationale and paradigm, resulting in cognitively-scientific based interpretations. The body as seen by natural scientists tends to become a body that is anybody's body, whereas the phenomenologist focuses on the lived body (See for example, Sartre, 1956). More specifically, as Merleau-Ponty argues, "[…] our physical body is not experienced by us as an object among other objects in space" (Moran, 2000, p. 423). This does not imply the dichotomy of individual versus the general, leaving the phenomenological to be the individual. Meanings can also be generalized and since phenomenology rests on the notion of inter-subjectivity (Zahavi, 2001; 2003), it is of utmost importance that the apparent dichotomy between my body and anybody's body instead is understood as the lived body versus the biology of the body. Thus, the lived body just like time-consciousness has a leading role in phenomenological theory. According to Moran (2000, pp. 424-425):

> […] my body occupies the "zero point", as Husserl had already described in Ideas II. […] The body, for Merleau-Ponty, has its own set of motivations […] The body discloses the world for us in a certain way. It is the transcendental condition for the possibility of experiencing objects at all, our means of communication with the world.

If one then is interested in psychological meaning, it is more rigorous to capture these meanings by returning to where these meanings are lived; that is, in our subjectivity. To distort or objectify the subjective just to remain natural scientific is to "make a mess" of veracity (cf., Sokolowski, 2008, p. 21).

Considering a Phenomenological Human Scientific Understanding of Memory

As we have seen in the above critique of the biological and cognitive scientific attitudes and approaches towards the phenomenon of memory, an essential aspect of human subjectivity and time-consciousness is the lived body. If we look at the lived body, it can make us self aware of our own sense of subjectivity. For example, in an emotional memory as we initiate a return to the perceptions in the original event in the past, we tend to re-live such emotions (Englander, 2007). That brings about not just the embodiment; however, for when we think about the memory, or perhaps dwell on it, or share it with somebody, we also (although not always explicitly) are present to a first-personal givenness of it. We are through our lived body connected to our lived time. In other words, it is as if the lived body reminds us of our own subjectivity through our lived time by connecting us to the past. Let us take a look at some examples provided by Giorgi (1989, p. 108) of how embodiment tends to show up in descriptions of memory.

> (Subject 4) As I recall this incident. I feel pain [...] I find that I really don't want to remember it, and yet it remains a vivid memory of a day in my life [...] Neither of us spoke, but as I sat there, I remembered as clearly today as then, and that I felt very close to him [her son].
>
> (Subject 5) It was sunset, and the warm breeze that had been drifting through my window all afternoon was becoming chilly. It sent a shiver through me [...] A similar cold breeze was coming in the house through the back screen door. The cold air sent a shiver through me, and as I got up to close the back door, I saw my *fiancé* coming up the back walk.
>
> (Subject 6) This event took place 31 years ago. A minimal amount of background seems necessary, and I feel a little anxious about getting to hard parts of the story; I start tightening up around my center [...] Bodily, when remembering about this, my head wants to sink down into my shoulders – I feel like closing up, disappearing [...] [Subject was required to leave a pet squirrel behind because of state laws and she abandoned it in a forest. Part of the description of the event at that time reads:] I can feel the cage wire hurting my fingers, and the difficulty of walking up that hill. I feel tight, like I am trying to keep from falling.

Giorgi (1989, p. 108) hence concludes:

> Because these are previously lived perceptual acts that are being reawakened, it is not surprising that there should be a bodily role. Often, the feelings that the awakened perceptual acts evoke reverberate back to the present and subjects re-experience in the present the feelings that are being evoked in memory. It is as though the body is the silent carrier of these meanings through feelings [...]

In other words, as a "communicator with the world", the lived body also earns the role of a communicator in the history of the subject, making it the possible "zero point" for some structures of the self to remain while we move through time, through life. Of course, this is not to claim that the body is the cause of everything, but rather the means for the possibility for a subject to have an experience (Moran, 2000).

When one remembers something it is experienced in the sense of the subject's own experience. Simply put, it is I, myself, who is doing the remembering and not somebody else, hence carrying that "warmth and intimacy" as James (1890/1950, p.650) once wrote. In a sense then, memory makes us connected in the present to our past and thus to our own primary sense of subjectivity through time. Even so, it is essential to stress that this sense of subjectivity is often pre-reflective. Zahavi (2005, p. 65) makes this point clear:

> When Husserl claimed that the experience is constituted in inner time-consciousness, he was not saying that the experience is brought to giveness by some other part of subjectivity, as if one part took the other as its object. Rather, to say that an experience is constituted in inner time-consciousness is to say that it is brought to awareness by its own means. It is called inner time-consciousness because it belongs intrinsically to the innermost structure of the experience itself. To put it differently, inner time-consciousness simply is the pre-reflective self awareness of the stream of consciousness (protention-primal/ presentation-retention) should consequently be appreciated as an analysis of the (micro) structure of first-personal givenness.

At this point, it starts to become clear that this first-personal giveness is a pre-reflective self-awareness and that it is directly linked by meaning to the lived body through emotional expressions.

Let us consider another example, an excerpt taken from an interview in a descriptive phenomenological psychological study (using Giorgi's method) on the phenomenon identified as *The Lived Persistent Meaning of an Early Emotional Memory* (for a more extensive account on this study, see Englander, 2007).

Perhaps this description is a bit longer than the previous one's quoted from Giorgi (1989) and can thus better serve as our primary example in explicating the embodied role and first-personal, pre-reflective giveness in emotional memory. The subject responds to the researcher's request for a description of a situation in which the subject remembered an early emotional event.

> This past week, as I guess I didn't express before one trigger that actually works within me that takes me back to my childhood happened on Tuesday, you know, after parking the car right off campus and walking around the back of the chapel, I was aware again as I mentioned of the flight pattern and an aircraft flying overhead and as I came around the corner what was happening was the reflection of the aircraft was in the pool outside the chapel and it was absolutely beautiful. And as I looked up what I see again beginning at the reflection and you've got overhead an aircraft in final approach to Seattle-Tacoma International Airport, and I tried to stop and figure out exactly what are the components that go into what I am feeling at that point in time. Because of studies of feelings and experience actually going back to the beginning of psychology, I tried to break it down into what I was behaving and what I was feeling, how I was affected, and see if I could do that. What I was feeling is very similar, surprisingly very similar to what I was feeling as a child. If you look at my behavior, it stops me. It's a break in my momentum of my walk. There's actually a physical response to it. And I think there is a physiological response as well as an affective response. Actually there is almost a warmth. If I allow which I did on that particular day to just rest with me, I physically slow down, I get a sense of almost warmth and almost a sense of longing, and a sense of reflection that is very comforting, very, very comforting. It gives me mentally and physical both ties it almost into a sense of peace. And that sense of peace allows me to transcend back to different portions of my life, and specifically because of our focus here to when I was a young child.

It becomes quite obvious that the subject is a psychology student and uses technical terms such as "trigger" and "physical response". In fact, at times, the subject comes through as providing a quasi-behavioral analysis while describing the experience. However, this will not be a methodological concern due to the fact that Giorgi's method accounts for all data because the goal of the method is even to describe the psychological meaning of a person's own interpretation of their experience.

Nevertheless, the embodied-self present in the experience can clearly seen from expressions like:

"If you look at my behavior, it stops me."
"It's a break in my momentum of my walk."
"Actually there is almost a warmth."
"I physically slow down [...]"

Now, let us return to a quote used earlier in which Giorgi (1989, p.108) writes, "It is as though the body is the silent carrier of these meanings through feelings [...]". One could perhaps argue that the lived body plays such a vital role since we had asked the subject to describe an emotional memory and one could also argue that the examples provided by Giorgi would also fit the description of an emotional memory although the subjects were asked the more general question to describe a situation in which he/she remembered something.

A particular aspect of Giorgi's (1985, 1997) qualitative method is that it includes in the situation the subject who experienced the phenomenon under investigation. In a sense then, the factual aspects of memory that natural scientific approaches to psychology is so interested in also lacks the life world context in which meanings are constituted, emotions are experienced, and feelings are felt, etc. Now, constructing a situation, that is, an experiment, in which measuring or testing is carried out in the experimental situation, is that which the natural scientific approach suggests. This means that its method is not "contextless". However, to control the situation in terms of trying to avoid the subjective involvement of the researcher and at times even the subjectivity of the participant points to the natural scientific agenda and also to the idea that a "thing" should exist in itself whether or not subjectivity is there or not. In other words, natural scientific psychology seeks the exclusion of subjectivity in order to assure factual objectivity, leading to a sense of objectivism. Ebbinghaus' classical experiment on memory using nonsense syllables could perhaps be seen as an example of this particular point. In the true natural sciences, such as the physical sciences, human subjectivity is not an issue, however, in a natural scientific psychology it cannot be avoided. Would it not then be more rigorous to take subjectivity into serious consideration as Giorgi (2004) does in regard to his methodology, instead of uncritically adopting the method and reasoning from the natural sciences? In order to discover human, psychological meaning, we also need to have a human being in a situation as it is lived, because human meaning is different from a natural scientific fact simply because meaning cannot exist in itself. Meaning depends on subjectivity. The critique of subjectivity depends on inter-subjectivity and not whether subjectivity is present in the first place (Giorgi, 2004). As Giorgi (2004, p.23) states, "In the human world, capturing the subjective as subjective is objective".

So far I have tried to point out the necessity of using a qualitative method, like that developed by Giorgi (1975, 1985, 1997), that critically incorporates the notion of subjectivity in order to capture the meaning of human memory. Evidently, I have been very critical towards natural scientific psychology in its attempt to establish psychology primarily as a natural science particularly because such an approach towards research does not address human subjectivity appropriately and critically in relation to the phenomena that are being studied.

Now, let us integrate the notion of reflective consciousness with the pre-reflective one, in order to address some methodological issues of the subjective realm of the human science researcher. By critically reflecting on the meaning of a phenomenon through using the phenomenological psychological reduction and imaginative variation, one might be accused of objectifying the phenomenon as it is lived by the research subject. Nevertheless, it is not my intention to go into this philosophical debate about reflection and objectification, since it can be found more developed elsewhere (see for example, Zahavi, 2005). It is useful, however, for the purpose of our discussion to cite a brief paragraph by Giorgi (2006) as he clarifies this issue by going back to Husserl. Giorgi (2006, p.105) states:

> [...] the very idea of a non-objectifying presence to consciousness is in Husserl. While often mistaken among social scientists, it is well known by Husserlian scholars that Husserl never said that intentionality is the essence of consciousness. It is an important characteristic of many acts, but it is not essential because there are aspects of consciousness that do not partake of it, e.g., hyletic data. More importantly in this context, however, is the fact that Husserl acknowledges that consciousness is reflexive as well as reflective. With reflexivity, consciousness is aware of itself independent of intentionality. This would provide a basis for a non-objectifying awareness of consciousness, but a proper understanding of certain types of reflection can perform the same function. Husserl mostly worked within the context of reflective phenomenology.

Giorgi (2006, p.103) also summarizes Zahavi's (2005) point that, "Husserl's reflective phenomenological method does indeed alter (not distort) the prereflective consciousness, but in a way that actually enhances it". This is exactly the point of describing the human scientific meaning in Giorgi's method, it explicates the meanings to be useful in the world of psychology, hence it provides us with eidetic knowledge and a generalizability of the results without distorting, that is, going beyond or reducing the pre-reflective giveness present in the raw data.

The human scientific researcher's ability to address the subjective realm might be difficult to comprehend for somebody not well acquainted with phenomenological theory. Let us consider a concrete example of a general structure of a memory-related phenomenon, i.e., a study of the lived persistent meaning of early emotional memories (Englander, 2007). The general structure is as follows:

> In the context of an early emotional situation in which a person's emotional equilibrium has been significantly challenged, a person incorporates the meaning of a present object as a personal value constituting a foundation of one's emotional life. The meaning of the object is perceived by the person as a constitutive of his or her emotional life and is fully accepted as part of the permanent perception of self that is frequently relived and never challenged. The early emotional situation is vividly remembered throughout life in similar or analogous emotional challenging situations in which the meaning of the object is present. The lived persistent meaning of an early emotional memory is revealed by the person's motivation to go to extraordinary efforts throughout life to maintain his or her emotional equilibrium using the meaning of the object as a thematic foundation for his or her emotional coping strategy. To maintain one's emotional equilibrium and to continue perceiving one's self as whole, the person structures daily activities as well as life-long goals in conjunction with the emotional coping strategy (based on the meaning of the object). The meaning of the object is directly used or avoided (as an emotional coping strategy) in real and potential situations in which a person's emotional equilibrium is, or could be, challenged. (Englander, 2007, p. 189)

By using critical reflection through the phenomenological psychological reduction and imaginative variations, the researcher attempts to describe the psychological meaning of the phenomenon, that is, the researcher makes the psychological in the raw data explicit that was implicitly given from the pre-reflective point of view of the research subjects. In a phenomenological sense then, the raw data is not distorted but offered a meaning from a psychological perspective as opposed to the lived perspective of the research subject. This is an essential point because it also implies another important aspect of subjectivity in relation to Giorgi's human scientific method; that is, it is no point in going back to the research subject to check to see if one's description of psychological meaning is valid, just because of the fact that the research subject is not a psychologist and is thus not acquainted with the psychological perspective. The critique has to come from the same inter-subjective level, namely that of fellow psychologists. This is not to say that a psychologist's opinions are valued more than that of their research subjects, which would clearly be an ethical dilemma instead of a methodological one.

Let us now take a closer look at the knowledge of memory that we can gain from such a structure and appreciate how it directly relates to our discussion on the necessity of addressing subjectivity in psychological research. From the above general psychological structure we can get a sense that people who have experienced this phenomenon constitute it as an essential part of their emotional self, as an essential part of their being, perhaps we could even go as far as saying that it belongs to the constitution of their identity. This is in harmony with what Giorgi has found in the work of J.N. Mohanty. Giorgi (2004, p. 16) states:

> The natural sciences, dealing with things, found it easy to accommodate the term "substance", along with its correlate, "accidents". Substance referred to what intrinsically belonged to a thing, made it what it was, and accidents were characteristics that were contingent. However, when it comes to understanding subjectivity, Mohanty (2000) has argued rather convincingly that identity is the better term, especially when it is a matter of speaking about what unifies subjectivity. Identity also refers to characteristics quite different from substance. Mohanty (2000, p. 84) notes that the identity of the subject is not pregiven and it has to be continually re-established and that it is never finished. One's ultimate identity is a higher order identity among various levels or specific types of identity that are established throughout the course of a life. The achievement of identity is irreal or invisible.

Giorgi (2004, p. 18) continues:

> Because of the relationship between the acts of the subject and the objects towards which the acts are directed, the subject has a stability that is beyond the changing contents of consciousness; it is something self-identical. The self-identity is related intimately to the inner experiences of lived time that end up constituting an enduring identical self.

Hence, in a phenomenological analysis like the one presented above on *the lived persistent meaning of an early emotional memory*, the essential issue of subjectivity is apparent. The basic notion of the self is part of the whole basic structure in which the lived body and time-consciousness interact on a pre-reflective level, making the subject in subjectivity possible (e.g., Zahavi, 2005). By making use of reflection in order to describe the psychological meaning, we can gain psychological insight into how we pre-reflective "define" ourselves through life.

If we turn to the whole notion of our personal identity that is of prime interest to, for example, a clinical psychologist or perhaps a personality psychologist, it seems difficult, from our discussion above, to avoid the lived emotional memory and the lived body in discussing this aspect of human psychology. If memory is just a collection of pictures or images like the cognitive scientist thinks, and the biological body is analogous to a thing, like a computer with software (schemas) a very extensive hard drive (nervous system), then where in this formula does human subjectivity fit in? Just like the psychological search for the engram, maybe the terms image, picture, software, and hard drive can at best be used as metaphors, appropriate for our present *Zeitgeist*.

The fact is that if we force the whole notion of the phenomenon of memory into the empirical format of a real object, we do miss out on its *ir*-real qualities that makes it into the mixed object that it is. What we neglect is the whole aspect of how it is connected to our subjective constitution of the self. As Sokolowski (2000, p. 70) concludes, "Just as the past object is brought to light again, so my past self as an agent of that experience is brought to life again. Through memory a distinction is introduced between the remembering self and the remembered self". Hence, we can conclude at this point that the "first-personal giveness", the pre-reflective consciousness allows us to be subjects. By remembering an emotional event, this primary sense of our subjectivity ("the zero point") is expressed through embodied reawakening that confronts us with our own development and self-awareness, and even at times, forces us to re-constitute a sense of our own personal identity.

Let us briefly return to the biological and/or cognitive scientific approaches and how, in general, such understandings differ from that of the phenomenological psychological. One could say that since the natural scientific approach does not start off from the subject and subjectivity, but instead from the "object", it is doomed to reach an abstract and a de-personalized account of the self. Take for example, testing a person's memory to reach a diagnosis. I am not saying that a diagnosis cannot help a person, mostly since a diagnosis among other things implies the meaning of getting possible help for something. Here, I am merely suggesting that in starting to understand lived memory and seeing the role of subjectivity of the self and the constitution of identity through time, we can also reach the active, meaning-constituting, human being in the quest to identify his or her own self-awareness. Is this insight something that we can "afford" to leave out in our attempt to help a person? The sense of self in phenomenology is thus something fundamental to the very notion of being human. Gallagher & Zahavi (2007) writes:

> To have a self-experience does not entail the apprehension of a special self-object; it does not entail the existence of a special experience of a self alongside other experiences but different from them. To be aware

> of oneself is not to capture a pure self that exists separately from the stream of experience, rather it is to be conscious of one's experience in its implicit first-person mode of givenness.

In other words, the cognitive-biological model is leaving out the basic sense of an experiencing self. "Translated", this theoretical stance becomes a third-person account that is derived from an already abstract third-person account and then later translated into psychological meaning accompanied by possible, therapeutic strategies. In this context of research, memory is external to the lived experience. In contrast, Giorgi's method can aid the researcher in describing the psychological meaning as derived from a first-person mode of giveness and, as we can see in the above line of reasoning, it can capture that psychological structure of lived memory, which brings us back to the lived body and which is a reminder of the pre-reflective sense of self in constituting our self-awareness and personal identity.

Discussion and Conclusion

The many aspects of subjectivity such as the pre-reflective self and the embodied re-awakenings so often present in the lived connection among memorial events cannot be accounted for by cognitive and biological scientists without losing their lived meanings. Their attempt to do so results in the loss of the lived meanings of memorial events. This is due mostly to the fact that a person's biology and cognitive schema are *dimensions* far too abstract in relation to the basic dimension of lived meanings. The natural scientific effort in psychology is too narrow in this regard. Thus, this strongly suggests that some answers to some question are better left to the human scientific psychologist. Giorgi's method can provide answers from within the human scientific realm of lived emotional memory and it can contribute to a re-direction of our psychological understanding of the phenomenon of memory. Note that it has never been my intention to claim that biologists or cognitive scientists are not conducting legitimate scientific research, nor has it been my attempt to degrade interdisciplinary efforts. In many ways, this account might also be interpreted as having had a focus primarily on the "individual" self. It is worth noting that phenomenological philosophy is inter-subjective (Zahavi, 2001). Simply put, without the other, there would be no individual and vice versa. The notion of the self is thus rooted in the whole sphere of an inter-subjective world. In other words, the value of subjectivity depends on inter-subjectivity. Nevertheless, it has been my purpose to highlight the possibility of a phenomenological approach to the psychology of memory using Giorgi's method and to show that in so doing we could interlock some of the possibilities for what it means to be an embodied-self who is experiencing oneself as a human being through lived time.

Now, how is this discussion of any value to the practicing psychologist? If we as clinicians want to therapeutically help a person to change, we cannot just think of changing that person's behavior or make them redefine their negative schemas to positive ones or to give them medication to alter their neural activity. We also have to be able to engage their sense of their own subjectivity, of that aspect that makes them human; that is, their primary sense of being a subject. For example, even though a person receives cognitive-behavioral therapy at the same time that he or she is put on an anti-depressant medication plan, this person can still remember him or herself as having been depressed and what that "depressed person" did in the past and thus, if our above analysis has something to it, the person now also has to deal with issues of identity and self-awareness through lived time. How does the cognitive-behaviorist deal with these issues? Do they simply encourage the client to do the cognitive exercises when they are experiencing the negative cues? Of course, cognitive exercises can be helpful; however, the effort seems short-lived if the embodied, pre-reflective self is not engaged more deeply. For example, even though an active effort to change one's negative thinking at the same time that one is on an anti-depressant medication plan directing one's life less self-destructively, the change still needs to be integrated into the self as a whole through lived time and the constitution of human meaning. In a phenomenological sense, cognitive strategies are as if my problem becomes "anybody's problem" and my body becomes "anybody's body". If say the least, with cognitive strategies, it seems that one becomes, in theory, an abstract subject who is manipulated in a way that is analogous to a machine that can be re-programmed.

It is also worth noting that the pre-reflective self can also be seen in more extreme cases of pathology. For example, even a person diagnosed with paranoid schizophrenia, hearing voices belonging to someone else, is by pre-reflectively recognizing this as happening to him/herself engaged in a "sense of ownership", i.e., I am hearing voices, "but the lack of self agency is missing", i.e., "someone else is putting them there" (Gallagher & Zahavi, 2008, p. 160). This sense of identifying one's pre-reflective ownership as a subject with the help of, for instance, the empathic engagement of a therapist seems crucial if one considers self awareness (and perhaps even self-worth) as an issue in the treatment process. Hence, I am not saying that recognition of the pre-reflective consciousness makes the client capable of solving his or her own problem. Rather, I am merely suggesting that we cannot avoid this basic sense of subjectivity if we want to recognize the subject who constitutes meaning in regard to his or her own self-awareness. Now, whether this will make for a more successful therapeutic outcome is another question belonging to another discussion.

It has been my attempt to show that Giorgi's human scientific research method can enhance our understanding of the phenomenon of memory partly because such a research strategy actively engages the concept of subjectivity. To reach out to this dimension of embodied subjectivity and lived time is to engage the self-initiated, pre-reflective psychological mobility of the person. Perhaps it is to engage our "zero point". As Zahavi (2005, p.67) writes, "Whereas we live through a number of different experiences, the dimension of first-personal givenness remains unchanging. It stands, to use a striking image from James, permanently, "like a rainbow on a waterfall" (James 1890, I/630), its own quality unchanged by the events that stream through it".

References

Brown, L. S. (1996). On the construction of truth and falsity: whose memory, whose history. In Pezdek, K. & Banks, W. P. (Eds.). *The recovered memory/false memory debate.* San Diego, CA: Academic Press.

Cahill, L. & McGaugh, J. L. (1998). Mechanisms of emotional arousal and lasting declarative memory. *Trends Neuroscience*, 21, 294-299.

Davis, M., Campeau, S., Kim, M., & Falls, W. A. (1995). Neural systems of emotion: the amygdala's role in fear and anxiety. In McGaugh, J. L., Weinberger, N.M., & Lynch, G. (Eds.). *Brain and memory: modulation and mediation of neuroplasticity.* New York: Oxford University Press, pp. 3-40.

Englander, M. (2007). Persistent psychological meaning of early emotional memories. *Journal of Phenomenological Psychology*, 38:2, 181-216.

Freud, S. (1899/1989). Screen memories. In Gay, P. (Ed.). *The Freud reader.* New York: Norton & Company, pp. 117-126.

Gallagher, Shaun and Dan Zahavi, "Phenomenological Approaches to Self-Consciousness", The Stanford Encyclopedia of Philosophy (Summer 2007 Edition), Edward N. Zalta (ed.), URL = <http://plato.stanford.edu/archives/sum2007/entries /self-consciousness-phenomenological/>.

Gallagher, S & Zahavi, D. (2008). *The phenomenological mind: an introduction to philosophy of mind and cognitive science.* London: Routledge.

Giorgi, A. (1975). An application of the phenomenological method in psychology. In A. Giorgi, C. Fischer & E. Murray (Eds.). *Duquesne Studies in Phenomenological Psychology II.* Pittsburgh, PA: Duquesne University Press, pp. 72-79.

Giorgi, A. (Ed.) (1985). *Phenomenology and psychological research.* Pittsburgh, PA: Duquesne University Press.

Giorgi, A. (1989). Learning and memory from the perspective of phenomenological psychology. In Valle, R. S. & Halling, S. (Eds.). *Existential-phenomenological perspectives in psychology.* New York, NY: Plenur, pp. 99-112.

Giorgi, A. (1997). The theory, practice, and evaluation of the phenomenological method as a qualitative research procedure. *Journal of Phenomenological Psychology*, 28, 235-260.

Giorgi, A. (2004). A way of overcome the methodological vicissitudes involved in researching subjectivity. *Journal of Phenomenological Psychology*, 35:1, 1-25.

Giorgi, A. (2006). Concerning the phenomenological methods of Husserl and Heidegger and their application in psychology. In Thiboutot, C. (Ed.). *Essais de psychologie phénoménologique-existentielle.* Montréal, Qué. CIRP, pp. 91-108.

Howe, M. L. (2000). *The fate of early memories: developmental science and the retention of childhood experiences.* Washington, D.C.: American Psychological Association.

Husserl (1991//1893-1917). *On the phenomenology of the consciousness of internal time* (Trans. Barnett). Dordrecht: Kluwer Academic Publishers.

Husserl, E. (1998/1913). *Ideas pertaining to a pure phenomenology and to a phenomenological philosophy, book one* (Trans. Kersten). Dordrecht: Kluwer Academic Publishers.

James, W. (1950/1890). *Principles of psychology vol. I.* New York: Dover Publications.

Kandel, E. R. (1996). In search of memory: emergence of a new science of mind. New York: W.W. Norton & Company.

Kandel, E. R. (2000). Nobel lecture – The Molecular Biology of Memory Storage: A Dialog between Genes and Synapses. Nobel Media - Nobelprize.org. URL = <http://nobelprize.org/nobel_prizes/medicine/laureates/2000/kandel-lecture.html >.

Kluver, H., Bucy, P.C. (1937). "Psychic blindness" and other symptoms following bilateral temporal lobectomy in rhesus monkeys. *American Journal of Physiology*, 119, 352-353.

LeDoux, J. E. (1993). Emotional networks in the brain. In Lewis, M. & Haviland, J. M. (Eds.). *Handbook of emotions.* New York: Guilford Press, pp. 109-118.

LeDoux, J. E. & Muller, J. (1997). Emotional memory and psychopathology. *Philosophical transactions of the Royal Society of London series B: Biological Sciences*, Nov 29, 352 (1362), 1719-26.

Merleau-Ponty, M. (1962/1945). *Phenomenology of perception* (Trans. Smith). London: Routledge.

Moran, D. (2000). *Introduction to phenomenology.* London: Routledge.

Sartre, J-P. (1956). *Being and nothingness: a phenomenological essay on ontology* (Trans. Barnes). New York: Citadel Press Kensington Publishing

Shapiro, F. (1995). *Eye movement desensitization and reprocessing: basic principles, protocols, and procedures.* New York: Guilford Press

Sokolowski, R. (2000). *Introduction to phenomenology.* New York, NY: Cambridge University Press.

Sokolowski, R. (2008). *The phenomenology of the human person.* New York, NY: Cambridge University Press.

Straus, E. W. (1966). *Phenomenological psychology.* New York: Basic Books.

Weiskrantz, L. (1956). Behavioral changes associated with ablation of the amygdaloid complex in monkeys. *Journal of Comparative Physiology*, 49, 381-391.

Zahavi, D. (2001). *Husserl and transcendental intersubjectivity: a response to the linguistic-pragmatic critique* (Trans. Behnke). Athens, OH: Ohio University Press.

Zahavi, D. (2003). *Husserl's phenomenology*. Stanford, CA: Stanford University Press.

Zahavi, D. (2005). *Subjectivity and selfhood*. Cambridge, MA: The MIT Press.

APPLICATION OF DESCRIPTIVE PHENOMENOLOGICAL RESEARCH METHOD TO THE FIELD OF CLINICAL RESEARCH

Barbro M. Giorgi, Ph.D.

Saybrook University
United States

Abstract

The literature on the psychotherapeutic practices reveals a high level of discord. On one hand there is a clamor for evidence-based research and on the other hand there are many serious criticisms about the nature of empirical research on the therapeutic practices. On one side there are the logical rules for conducting allegedly sound research and on the other hand there are the experiences of therapeutic practitioners which seem to be at odds with the accepted rules. It is suggested that this chasm can be bridged by phenomenological research strategies that are experientially congruent and based upon the discovery of lived meanings derived from the concrete descriptions of the participants, whether therapists or clients.

As I embarked on my studies in psychology, I was frustrated by my experience which could be simplistically summarized by "but it's not like that". All the theories I read in the textbooks held together beautifully as long as they remained on the page but the minute I tried to take them into "life" and tried to use them in order to understand myself or to understand others around me and our relationship to one another, the beautiful logic of the theory would collapse to one degree or another with me saying to myself "but it doesn't work that way".

This frustration continued all through graduate school and, I think culminated in the literature review for my dissertation. From the very beginning of my education I experienced a gap between what I was being taught about psychology, and life as I experienced it. When I started my literature review about the therapeutic process I then also came face to face with the gap between clinical practice "the way it really works", and the research results that are supposed to inform this clinical practice.

There was an overwhelming amount of research on the topic but almost every article I read complained about the general lack of relevance of research findings to clinical praxis. Some complaints concerned the lack of ecological validity. Research is being conducted under circumstances that are too different from the way therapy is being practiced, dealing with issues in ways that are too simplistic and approaching clients in reductionistic ways. Throughout the literature there was a sense of crisis. First, a sense that research is not sufficiently relevant to practitioners for them to even read the literature and secondly, a frustration over the lack of influence research was having on clinical training and the education of psychologists and, thirdly, a sense of urgency to show some clear and positive results in order to justify therapy, an urgency fueled by new economic and political pressures from managed care and third party payers. The literature was full of calls for new and different approaches to doing clinical research in order to overcome these issues. Some called for small variations, tweaking our methods a little and others were calling for a fundamental and radical paradigm shift.

The objections contained in the literature, and their sources, are summarized in Tables 1 and 2. Table 1 lists the types of objections being made about clinical research strategies, and Table 2 specifies the type of complaints being voiced concerning the lack of relevance of therapeutic research for therapeutic practice in general. I shall not dwell on these objections because most experienced clinicians are well aware of them, and besides, I want to concentrate on a key positive aspect that the phenomenological approach can bring to these issues. The key inference to be drawn from these two tables is that research into the therapeutic process is problematic, and because of this problematic status, this subfield of psychology should be open to novel strategies of research.

Table 1

The types of objections made about psychotherapeutic research over the last three decades by therapists/clinicians who conduct the research and their sources. Each source cited has at least one such objection, many have several, and a few contain them all.

Objections Concerning Strategies	SOURCES
Overemphasis on methodology in empiricist tradition Questioning of empiricist strategies and assumptions Disaffection with verification mode of research as only mode Therapeutic research should open up to other paradigms Major strategy shifts are required in therapeutic research Analogue therapeutic research is inadequate Therapeutic research has yielded noncumulative findings	Barlow, 1996; Bergin & Strupp, 1972; Budge, 1983; Elliott, 1983; Frank, 1979; Gelso & Fassinger, 1990; Goldfreid & Wolfe, 1996; Gottman & Markman, 1978; Greenberg, 1986; Horowitz, 1982; Hoshmond, 1989; Howard, Moras, Brill, Maritinovich, & Lutz, 1996; Meehl, 1978; Orlinsky & Howard, 1978; Persons, 1991; Rice & Greenberg, 1984; Rorer & Widiger, 1983; Sechrest, McKnight, & McKnight, 1996; Seligman, 1995; 1996; Sher & Truell, 1996; Singer, 1980; Wiggins & Pincus, 1992.

Table 2

The types of objections made about psychotherapeutic research over the last three decades by therapists/clinicians who conduct the research and their sources. Each source cited has at least one such objection, many have several, and a few contain them all.

Objections Concerning Clinical Relevance	Sources
Scientific rigor and clinical relevance are at odds	Anderson & Strupp, 1996; Elliott, 1983, 1995; Emmelkamp, 1981; Fishman, 1981; Gelso & Fassinger, 1990; Goldfried & Wolfe, 1996; Greenberg, 1986; Hayes & Nelson, 1981; Heller, 1990; Hollon, 1996; Howard, Orlinsky, & Lueger, 1995; Hugdahl & Öst, 1981; Levy, 1981; Magnusson & T^restad, 1993; Mahrer, 1997; Maletzky, 1981; McCullough, 1984; Mintz, Drake, & Crits-Cristoph, 1996; Norcross, 1997; Persons, 1991; Sechrest, McKnight, & McKnight, 1996; Seligman, 1996; Shapiro & Shapiro, 1983; Strupp, 1996; 1997; Tedeschi, Heister, & Gahagan, 1969.
Research conditions and practical clinical settings are at odds	
There are tensions in scientific-practitioner model	
Clinical research and clinical training are at odds	
There is mismatch between level of conceptualization of phenomena and level of typical measurement	
Decontextualized isolated variable studies are not ecologically related to clinical settings	

My own frustration increased as I reviewed more and more of the traditional literature. Not only were there no answers to my own clinical questions, but it became quite clear that we do not really know what happens to our clients in therapy or how come therapy works. I had to conclude that the state of affairs of clinical research is indeed problematic. Research results show, without a doubt, that therapy does work, *but*, there are no significant differences to be found either in terms of schools of thought or in terms of implemented tools or techniques. Much research has been conducted, but no theory or type of practice can be shown to be better than any other. And, while there is no discernible difference between different theories or techniques, there is, moreover, no difference between professionals, paraprofessionals or lay persons nor are there significant differences related to level of experience among professionals. In other words, research shows that therapy works but it makes no significant difference what theory or technique you use nor how much experience you have. This is a problem both from a research perspective as well as from the perspective of training and education.

As I proceeded in my review it also became increasingly difficult to arrive at some kind of understanding of what the various aspects of therapy are in traditional terms; i.e., what are the variables? The literature is full of arguments for various aspects of therapy for its success. The list is long and contains concepts such as "being heard", "safety", "correcting erroneous cognitions", "corrective emotional experiences", "cathartic experiences", "dealing with unfinished business", plus many other lists of critical factors. A more complete list of these factors is presented in Table 3.

Table 3

Summary of factors designated as helpful in psychotherapeutic research.

(Table derived on the basis of data from Mahrer and Nadler, 1986).

Criteria Used To Establish Good Moments	Helpful good moments
Outcome Criteria	- Voice quality was active, vivid and rich, energetic and expressive. - Client involvement and active engagement. - Willingness to communicate. - Commitment to change. - Trust in therapist. - Recognition of one's own responsibility, owning feelings and behaviors. - Clients who engage in warm accepting dialogue. - Support-seeking relationship with their therapist.

Normal Ways of Being and Behaving	- Mature behavior. - Reduction of defensive behavior. - Focusing on immediate experience. - Higher levels of cooperativeness; but also some disagreement and disapproval. - Emotional expression of feelings. - Depth of personal self-exploration. - Shift in self-concept.
Theories of Therapeutic Practice	- Free and realistic expression of basic impulses. - Heightened awareness of interpersonal consequences. - Heightened positive attitude toward self and others. - Search for felt meaning and inner understanding. - Heightened awareness of higher order personal relative to opening up of life options. - Open and direct expression of feeling and emotions. - Engagement in internal encounters with deeper personality processes. - Experiential sampling of concrete new ways of being and behaving. - Cooperative attitudes with therapist - Hard work on problems. - Achieving emotional insight. - Being in a state of emotional arousal and ready to apprehend new ways of seeing selves and others. - Accessing cognitions, feelings and impulses previously unavailable. - Sense of completion, i.e. feeling that something had shifted and that a problem ceased to exist.

Post-Session Evaluation	- Moments of heightened insight and understanding. - Moments of generalized good feelings such as trust, optimism, security, relaxation, warmth, acceptance and support. - Experiences of most intimate personal relationships, past or present. - Moments of personal insight, problem clarification and solution. - Moments of personal contact, reassurance and involvement with therapist. - Moments of lowered resistance in analytic relationship. - Decreased description of problems and increased insight into client's problems. - Expression of thoughts and feelings and discussion of their meanings.

Upon review, it can be seen that much of the literature emphasized a few particular aspects and suggested that this or that aspect was the most critical one. Some researchers indicated that the therapeutic relationship is the cornerstone of therapy while others would downplay the significance of the individual therapist and suggest that specific techniques account for success. Then, of course, there is the issue of *what is* successful therapy. Research can be broadly divided into process versus outcome research and this is linked to the issue of what constitutes successful therapy. A positive outcome such as a reduction of symptoms or symptom relief is one possibility, and so is increased functioning, increased insight and self awareness. More maturity and personal growth or a sense of deepened meaning of life and so on, are other possibilities. There is by no means any consensus as to what a positive result actually means or a consensus as to what should be examined. It seems that the philosophical and theoretical perspective of the researcher determines how and what is to be researched as opposed to a preexisting body of research findings or knowledge upon which to build further understanding. Some research emphasizes learning or modeling, intellectual insight, cognitive clarification and correction while others emphasize a human encounter in a "here and now" context or "in the moment" experience and still others take a spiritual approach and/or an embodied approach borrowing much from Eastern philosophy and its practices. Should the issue be symptoms, diagnoses and subsequent interventions, as in the medical model, or a more humanistic approach with a foundation in existential philosophy, or a biological, neurological perspective looking for genetic predispositions and biochemical solutions?

Yet another issue of how to approach clinical research is in terms of what time span to include. In the studies found in the literature the researchers have chosen a specific time period to examine such as a certain number of sessions, critical parts of single sessions, some of those decisions based on a numeric amount such as number of words as a cut-off point or number of minutes within a session, while others are based on content in the session such as emotional intensity, nature of the dialog between client and therapist and so on. Some studies take a somewhat longitudinal approach while others look at critical instances.

As a result of the literature review I felt more confused than ever and I was glad to have a phenomenological method as a research method at my disposal for a number of reasons and in a number of ways. [For details about the method, see Giorgi and Giorgi, 2003a; 2003b.] I will not be able to give full justice to the method here but I will highlight what I found to be some of the most important benefits of the very approach of the method in my study (von Knorring-Giorgi, 1998). First, let me describe briefly the data collection process and how this is relevant to the previous discussion. Phenomenology deals with concrete descriptions of experiences that participants themselves have lived through or experienced. This is critical because it saves the participants from having to know or understand why or how something works. In my study, I asked the participants to simply describe as concretely as possible their experience of a successful and lasting change that occurred within the therapeutic context for them. This did not require them to actually understand it but simply to describe it the way they had experienced it. This also meant, perhaps even more importantly, that I, as the researcher, did not have to know what to look for. I did not have to make decisions about whether it should be a certain number of sessions, whether to look at the therapeutic relationship alone or include the clients' lives outside of therapy or whether to include other significant people in the clients' lives. In a phenomenological study the researcher does not have to nor should he or she make such decisions. The research participants make those decisions and inform you about the various aspects that arc important to them and how they relate to the issue in meaningful ways. When a person goes about describing an experience or event to another, he or she will spontaneously give the listener all the necessary background information so that the experience can be understood in its context. Not only did this save me from having to design "the right kind of study" in terms of time frame and what and who to include, what questions to ask, but results also provided a much more integrated picture of the process than what I had found in the literature in general.

Interestingly enough, all participants started with childhood, not in great detail and not in terms of traumatic experiences but each participant found it necessary to describe their familial relations and how they had perceived themselves and the world entering into therapy in order for me to fully appreciate what the experience of change within therapy had meant to them. This was interesting in the sense that none of the current research on psychotherapy had incorporated this into their inquiries. And in the literature in general, when childhood experience is included in research it is often approached in terms of specific problems or trauma. In any case, in the clinical research I reviewed, childhood was almost completely excluded. This is, of course, quite natural. If the decision of what time frame to limit the study to is to be chosen by the researcher, it would seem to most researchers a daunting task to have to start at the very beginning and include everything in the participant's life that could be connected to a therapeutic change. Of course, there is certainly the awareness that humans are complex beings and that in every moment of our lives we also incorporate all of our past history and experience as well as all our future goals, hopes, fears and aspirations, but this cannot be easily accommodated in a research project and so it is usually set aside from the inquiry. Phenomenology, in contrast, can to some extent accommodate this aspect of humans. This is important from a phenomenological perspective because it espouses to be faithful to the phenomenon of inquiry such that if this is indeed "how human beings are" then they must be studied in such a manner. What makes this, at least to some degree, possible is that in a phenomenological study the researcher does not have to ask about everything in the participant's life that might be of importance, but rather the participant will make the decisions about where to start and what to include based on his or her own experience and include what is important to him or her and exclude what is not. This has the additional benefit of allowing for individual differences. In other words, what is important to one participant may not be to the next and most importantly, the researcher does not have to know this in advance. Another aspect that is critical here is the fact that the description is not about how the participants understood their own experiences but simply a description of "what happened" from their perspective. This means that the participant does not need to have a psychological insight into the processes involved. This is an important aspect of doing phenomenological research because it capitalizes on the human phenomenon of people generally being very good at "living life" or at "doing things" while much weaker at being able to "know" what we do or understand ourselves. Thus, in a description of a concrete lived experience so much more is revealed than would be possible if an explanation or an understanding of the experience was required. It is through the analyses of this concrete data that an understanding of the psychological meanings emerges.

Another concrete benefit of the phenomenological approach was that a particular important aspect of idiosyncrasy was not lost in the study. I will take a small but illustrative example from the findings in my study to demonstrate this point. In the literature the issue of safety in the therapeutic relationship was a common theme. Safety was also shown to be important in my doctoral research. The difference between how safety was discussed in the literature and what emerged from my study has to do with idiosyncrasy. The literature found safety to be an important aspect and then proceeded to outline what safety is for a client and how to achieve it in therapy. This study, however showed that this is not necessarily the best approach to the idea of safety in therapy. Safety was equally important to each of the participants, but what safety was and how it was achieved differed drastically from one person to the next. What makes this critical is that, in effect, what made one person safe would actually have threatened another. The implication of this is that we cannot, as therapists, attempt to understand in a generic manner, what makes a client safe and then proceed to provide the client with that generic sense of safety. Instead we must listen to each individual client and discern what exactly makes them feel safe and from there attempt to provide a tailor-made safety for each client.

This became especially evident in looking at two of the participants, both women, and recognizing that one of them needed to be nurtured and met with gentleness and warmth to feel safe, while the other woman felt safe because the therapist was confrontational and allowed her to also be confrontational. What is critical here is the *psychological meaning* of nurturing and of confrontation that each woman experienced. The woman who needed warmth and compassion was very capable and strong while feeling generally unloved and therefore felt neither cared for nor safe. The other woman instead was treated by significant others with warmth but was not allowed to stand up for herself and acknowledge her own desires and opinions, especially if these were in any way confrontational. The fact that confrontation was allowed in therapy and that she was not rejected or punished for being confrontational made her feel safe. Thus, we cannot answer the question of safety with a prescription such as warmth and understanding or with being confrontational and straightforward, but must look at the meaning that it holds for each client at the most private and idiosyncratic level. A phenomenological study seeks to uncover the specific meanings of concrete lived experiences and in this case the psychological meanings that essentially describe the therapeutic process. The risk of ending up with a "one size fits all" model that actually does not fit anybody all that well is therefore somewhat less of a risk in a phenomenological study than may be the case in general.

In more general terms the phenomenological method offers the possibility to address issues that are not easily addressed with traditional research methods; i.e., those phenomena that are both more subtle, more intangible and more complex. Phenomenology allows for research in areas where it may be impossible to know what the critical variables are in advance both in terms of the time period to examine and in terms of what aspects of the phenomenon to look at and what players or individuals or relationships to include, where it is (as it is in most human contexts) impossible to control for variables and isolate specific aspects from their lived context and still get ecologically valid results. Phenomenology is discovery-oriented rather than hypothesis-testing oriented and the researcher can therefore pose research questions where not many prior answers exist.

Perhaps the discovery aspect of phenomenological research should be emphasized more. The "hypothesis-testing" method is surely a tried and true method in science. It certainly works well where there is solid background knowledge and certain specifics have to be tested where true independence of variables exists. But a more open-ended, discovery oriented approach seems more adequate for phenomena that contain many individual differences and where genuine independence among the factors (variables) do not exist. In a "hypothesis-testing" method, one has to know, or presume to know, quite a bit before the role of a specific factor can be determined. The discovery approach does not assume specific a priori knowing. Rather, it more generally asks, "How is the phenomenon operating? What is going on that makes it work, when it does?" Such questions are far more important where interdependency among the so-called variables exist. The traditional experimental method assumes genuine independence of variables so that each variable can be modified without simultaneously affecting other variables. But that condition does not exist with experiential phenomena, where strong inter-dependency is the norm. As with all gestalts, if one modifies one factor, all of the others are spontaneously modified because of internal connections among them. Consequently, all experiential changes have to be understood holistically and, initially, idiosyncratically. In such an approach, the specific experiences of therapeutic change are directly discriminable because they are contextually understood. Generalizations have to be made relationally and contextually, not in terms of the effects of isolated variables.

An important part of the strength of this research approach as applied to clinical research is that results have ecological validity. What perhaps was most personally satisfying for me conducting this study was the response from other clinicians to the findings rather than meeting the skepticism so prevalent among clinicians *vis-à-vis* research my study has been greeted with enthusiasm from colleagues. I have also been pleased to find myself informed by the findings in my own clinical work and this is indeed the very reason for my passion for clinical research.

Finally, a concrete practical implication of my study was that the results indicated most of the same findings already in the literature, but more importantly, it also gave some indication of how the findings related to each other and the context in which therapeutic change occurs. The study was holistic, contextual and concrete, and yet generalizations were possible. To have conducted such a comprehensive study using traditional research methods would have been impossible given the scope of the study but because the participants gave a comprehensive picture of the event as it related to their entire life while also restricting themselves only to what was relevant, the phenomenological approach used in this study offered a more comprehensive picture than would, to some extent, otherwise have been possible.

References

Anderson, T. A. & Strupp, H. H. (1996). The ecology of psychotherapy research. *Journal of Counseling and Clinical Psychology, 64,* 776-782.

Barlow, D. H. (1996). Health care policy, psychotherapy research, and the future of psychotherapy. *American Psychologist, 51* 1050-1058.

Bergin, A. E.& Strupp, H. H. (1972). Changing frontiers in the science of psychotherapy. Chicago: Aldine-Atherton.

Budge, S. (1983). A critical look at the psychotherapeutic outcome research paradigm. *Psychotherapy: Theory, Research and Practice, 20,* 294-306.

Elliott, R (1983). "That in your hands": A comprehensive process analysis of a significant event in psychotherapy. *Psychiatry, 46,* 113-129.

Elliott, R. (1995). Therapy process research and clinical practice: Practical strategies. In M. Aneline & D. A. Shapiro, (Eds.). *Research foundations for psychotherapy practice.* Sussex, England: Wiley, pp. 49-72.

Emmelkamp, P. M. G. (1981). The current and future status of clinical research. *Behavioral Assessment, 3,* 249-253.

Fishman, S. T. (1981). Narrowing the generalization gap in clinical research. *Behavioral Assessment, 3,* 243-248.

Frank, J. (1979). The prestatus of outcome studies. *Journal of Consulting and Clinical Psychology, 47,* 310-317.

Gelso, C. J. & Fassinger, E. (1990). Counseling psychology: Theory and research on intervention. *Annual review of Psychology, 41,* 355-386.

Giorgi, A. & Giorgi, B. (2003a). Phenomenology. In J. A. Smith (Ed.) *Qualitative psychology: A practical guide to research methods* (pp. 25-50). London: Sage Publications Inc.

Giorgi, A. & Giorgi, B. (2003b). The descriptive phenomenological psychological method. In P. M. Camic, J. E. Rhodes & L. Yardley (Eds.). Qualitative research in psychology: Expanding perspectives in methodology and design (pp. 243-273). Washington, DC: American Psychological Association.

Goldfried, M. R. & Wolfe, B. E. (1996). Psychotherapy practice and research: Repairing a strained alliance. *American Psychologist, vol. 51,* p. 1007-1016.

Gottman, J. M. & Markman, H. J. (1978). Experimental design in psychotherapy research. In S. L. Garfield & A. E. Bergin, (Eds.). *Handbook of psychotherapy and behavior change: An empirical analysis.* New York: Wiley & Sons.

Greenberg, L. S. (1986). Research strategies. In L. S. Greenberg & W. M. Pinsof (Eds.). *The psychotherapy process: A research handbook.* New York: The Garfield Press, pp. 707-734.

Hayes, S. C., & Nelson, R. O. (1981). On the nature of the clinical-research gap: The problems with some solutions. *Behavioral Assessment, 3,* 235-242.

Heller, K. (1990). Social and community intervention. *Annual Review of Psychology, 41,* 141-168. Hollon, S. D. (1996). The efficacy and effectiveness of psychotherapy relative to medications. *American Psychologist, 51,* 1025-1030.

Goldfried, M. R. & Wolfe, B. E. (1996). Psychotherapy practice and research: Repairing a strained alliance. *American Psychologist, vol. 51,* p. 1007-1016.

Gottman, J. M. & Markman, H. J. (1978). Experimental design in psychotherapy research. In S. L. Garfield & A. E. Bergin, (Eds.). *Handbook of psychotherapy and behavior change: An empirical analysis.* New York: Wiley & Sons.

Greenberg, L. S. (1986). Change process research. *Journal of Counseling and Clinical Psychology, 54,* 4-9.

Hayes, S. C. & Nelson, R. O. (1981). Clinically relevant research: Requirements, problems, and solutions. *Behavioral Assessment, 3,* 209-215.

Heller, K. (1990). Social and community intervention. *Annual Review of Psychology, 41,* 141-168.

Hollon, S. D. (1996). The efficacy and effectiveness of psychotherapy relative to medications. *American Psychologist, 51,* 1025-1030.

Horowitz, M. (1982). Strategic dilemmas the socialization of psychotherapy researchers. *British Journal of Clinical Psychology, 21,* 119-127.

Hoshmond, L. T. (1989). Alternative research paradigms: A reviewed teaching proposal. *Counseling Psychologist, 17,* (1), 3-79.

Howard, K. I., Orlinsky, D. E., Lueger, R. J. (1995). The design of clinically relevant outcome research: Some considerations and an example. In M. Aneline & D. A. Shapiro, (Eds.). *Research foundations for psychotherapy practice.* Sussex, England: Wiley, pp. 3-47.

Howard, K., Moras, K., Brill, P., Martinovich, Z., & Lutz, W. (1996). Evaluation of psychotherapy: Efficacy, effectiveness, and patient progress. *American Psychologist, 51,* 1025-1030.

Hugdahl, H. & Öst, L. G. (1981). On the difference between statistical and clinical significance. *Behavioral Assessment, 3,* 289-295.

Levy, R. (1981). On the nature of the clinical-research gap: The problems with some solutions. *Behavioral Assessment, 3,* 235-242.

Magnusson, D. & Törestad, B. (1993). A holistic view of personality: A model revisited. *Annual Review of Psychology, 44,* 427-452.

Mahrer, A. R. (1997). What are the "breakthrough problems" in the field of psychotherapy? *Psychotherapy, 34,* 81-89.

Mahrer, A. & Nadler, W. P. (1986). Good moments in psychotherapy: A preliminary review, a list, some promising research avenues. *Journal of Consulting Psychology, 54,* 10-15.

Maletzky, B. M. (1981). Clinical relevance and clinical research. *Behavioral Assessment, 3,* 283-288.

McCullough, J. P. (1984). Single-case investigative research and its relevance for the non-operant clinician. *Psychotherapy, 21,* 382-390.

Meehl, P. (1978). Theoretical risks and tabular asterisks: Sir Karl, Sir Tonald and the slow progress of soft psychology. *Journal of Consulting and Clinical Psychology, 46,* 806-834.

Mintz, J., Drake, R. E., & Crits-Christoph, P. (1996). Efficacy and effectiveness of psychotherapy: Two paradigms, one science. *American Psychologist, 51,* 1084-1085.

Norcross, J. C. (1997). Emerging breakthroughs in psychotherapy integration. Three predictions and one fantasy. *Psychotherapy, 34,* 86-95.

Orlinsky, D. E. & Howard, K. I. (1978). The relation of process to outcome in psychotherapy, In S. L. Garfield & A. E. Bergin, (Eds.). *Handbook of psychotherapy and behavior change: An empirical analysis.* New York: Wiley & Sons, pp. 283-329.

Parsons, J. B. (1991). Psychotherapy outcome studies do not accurately represent current models of psychotherapy. *American Psychologist, 46,* 99-106.

Rice, L. & Greenberg, L. S. (1984). Patterns of change: Intensive analysis of psychotherapy process. N. Y.: Garfield Press.

Rorer, L. & Widiger, T. (1983). Personality structure and assessment. In M. Rosenzweig & Porter, L. (Eds.). *Annual review of psychology, 34,* 431-464.

Sechrest, L. McKnight, P., & McKnight, K. (1996). Calibration of measures for psychotherapy outcome studies. *American Psychologist, 51,* 1065-1071.

Seligman, M. E. P. (1995). The effectiveness of psychotherapy: The *Consumer Reports* study. *American Psychologist, 50,* 965-974.

Seligman, M. E. P. (1996). Science as an ally of practice. *American Psychologist, 51,* 1072-1079.

Shapiro, D. A. & Shapiro, D. (1983). Comparative therapy outcome research: Methodological implications of meta-analysis. *Journal of Counseling and Clinical Psychology, 51,* 42-53.

Sher, K. J. & Trull, T. J. (1996). Methodological issues in psychopathology research. *Annual Review of Psychology, 47,* 371-400.

Singer, J. (1980). The scientific of therapeutic practice: Question of value and ethics. *Psychotherapy: Theory, Research and Practice, 17,* 369-375.

Strupp, H. H. (1996). The tripartite model and *The Consumer Reports Study*. *American Psychologist, 51,* 1017-1024.

Strupp, H. H. (1997). Research, practice and managed care. *Psychotherapy, 34,* 91-94.

Tedeschi, J., Heister, D., & Gahagan, J. (1969). Trust and the prisoner's dilemma game. *Journal of Personality and Social Psychology, 79,* 43-50.

Von Knorring-Giorgi, B. (1998). A phenomenological analysis of the experience of pivotal moments in therapy as defined by clients. Unpublished Ph.D. Dissertation, Université du Québec à Montréal.

Wiggins, J. S. & Pincus, A. L. (1992). Personality: Structure and assessment. *Annual Review of Psychology, 43,* 473-504.

TRUTH AND THE RHYTHM OF PHENOMENOLOGICAL RESEARCH[28]

Steen Halling, Ph.D.

Seattle University
United States

Abstract

Researchers have a moral obligation to their discipline, to themselves, to their readers, and to the people whose lives they study. Their obligation is to present their methods, approach, and findings as honestly and as completely as they can. Moreover, they have an obligation to keep questioning and giving words to the unspoken and the lived, providing interpretations of what they have heard. The truths that researchers search for are elusive and can be spoken of in a multitude of ways. Truths in human life are elusive not because they are abstract or unreal but because they transcend us even as they touch us deeply. Phenomena such as friendship, grief, or love are realities at the core of human existence, realities that elude measurement, and it is to them that we bear witness as researchers within a human science orientation. The truths we articulate as researchers, however provisionally, are embodied truths; they are felt in our bones. In this chapter, I will elaborate on and support the above arguments by looking at specific instances of qualitative research along with examples from everyday life. I believe that however problematic it may be, the notion of truth is indispensable to our work, and that our understanding of this concept must be developed in the context of a dialogue with the actual work of researchers.

The old proverb, "Children and fools tell the truth", has been updated, in our postmodern age, to "only children and fools believe there is a truth to be told". No doubt we have good reasons to fear or consider deluded those who claim to have the truth and rationality on their side. And yet we cannot so quickly dispense with this notion either in research or in our everyday lives, anymore than rhythm can dispense with pauses or resting points. As Merleau-Ponty (1968) has said, "We would not know even what the false is, if there were not times when we had distinguished it from the true" (p. 5).

The claim that notions of truth or reality are not applicable or have to be significantly redefined within the context of the social sciences has been made by a number of writers in psychology who describe themselves as postmodernists. Since this is a diverse and vast ranging tradition, I will refer to a particular thinker within it, the social constructionist Kenneth Gergen, to illustrate how the notion of finding "truth" has been brought into question. In a 2001 article, Gergen argued for the positive influence of postmodernism within psychology, especially as a vehicle for furthering human liberation. From a social constructionist perspective, our behavior and experience are shaped by social and cultural factors, including language. In other words, our existence is socially and culturally constructed. This position (aside from the peculiar use of the word "constructed") may not seem either radical or problematic. After all, who would question that humans are historical and social beings? But social constructionists further assert that as culturally conditioned beings, social scientists are basically encapsulated within the confines of their own culture, including the subculture or frame of reference of their particular discipline (Gergen, 1989; Halling & Lawrence, 1999). This is in contrast to the modernist perspective which is characterized as believing that our access to universal or objective truth is entirely possible. Gergen (2001) essentially stated that all truths are "local truths". More specifically, he drew upon the philosopher Ludwig Wittgenstein's characterization of specific forms of human interactions as rule-bound language games to arrive at the following "redefinition" of truth: "to tell the truth, on this account, is not to furnish an accurate picture of what actually happened but to participate in a set of social conventions, a way of putting things sanctioned within a given form of life" (Gergen, 2001, p. 806). Later, Gergen adds, "the postmodernist proposes that arguments about what is really real are futile" (p. 806). This latter statement illustrates rather nicely what Barbara Held (2007) has pointed out in her critique of postmodernist thinkers in psychology, namely, that despite their insistence that they eschew making assertions about what is universally true, they do nonetheless make such pronouncements quite regularly.

It is not my intention to address these issues of reality and truth in the abstract. Rather, in following Merleau-Ponty's notion that in everyday life the false and the true are interdependent, I will explore the importance and meaning of truth in phenomenological research with specific reference to the activity and experience of researchers and students. I believe that doing this is critical given that experience has received little attention in the whole postmodernist discussion of research.

In my view, this neglect of experience is a telling feature of the postmodernist movement in psychology. On the one hand, there is a great deal of reference to acknowledging the subjectivity of researchers and research participants, to recognizing the value of qualitative research, and of the importance of listening to the voices of those who have been marginalized within a given society. On the other hand, if one looks more closely at the writings of social constructionists and other postmodernist thinkers in psychology, one finds little reference to actual human experience.

This neglect of concrete personal experience, surprisingly, is similarly evident in the relational psychoanalytic movement (also part of the postmodern landscape) even though this movement has a strong emphasis on the subjective and on developing concepts and understandings that are "experience near" (e.g., Stolorow & Atwood, 1979; Atwood & Stolorow, 1981; Stolorow, Atwood, & Orange, 2002). Mills (2005) explains this apparent contradiction:

> It may be argued that relational thinking dissolves the centrality of the self, extracts and dislocates the subject from subjectivity, decomposes personal identity, and ignores the unique phenomenology and epistemological process of lived experience by collapsing every psychic event into a relational ontology, thus usurping the concretely existing human being while developing the notion of contextualism into the abyss of abstraction. (p. 169)

As qualitative researchers we become involved with particular persons as we listen to or read their stories and develop an intimate knowledge of aspects of their lives. We have a responsibility to be as faithful as possible both to the research participants who entrust us with their stories and to the topic that we are investigating. It may not be self-evident what it means to be faithful to stories and to phenomena, but I trust that most of us would agree that our claims need to be rooted in data and that our interpretation or analysis has to be done with integrity.

Research as Lived Experience

Accordingly, let me turn to three examples related to phenomenologically oriented research to ground this discussion in actual practice. Although these examples differ in method and topic, they have in common that the researchers are themselves engaged with the experiences they are studying.

I begin with the work of Robert Coles, a child psychiatrist whose numerous writings exemplify par excellence the power of field research. In his book, *The Call of Stories* (1989), he quotes the memorable advice of a clinical supervisor during his early years of training:

> The people who come to see us bring us their stories. They hope they tell them well enough so that we understand the truth of their lives. They hope we know how to interpret their stories correctly. We have to remember that what we hear is *their* story [emphasis in original]. (p. 7)

This advice is as relevant to research as to clinical practice since research requires us to be faithful to the meanings of specific phenomena as well as to individual descriptions.

When Coles started his first research on "Children in Crisis", during the period of desegregation in the South of the United States in the 1960's, he himself was confronted by a crisis as he came to recognize that his assumptions about children, defense mechanisms, the relationship between the individual and society, and what it meant to be a researcher were inadequate to the task at hand. The limitations, and even the arbitrariness of his assumptions and concepts, became evident as he developed enough of a relationship with the participants in this historical drama – black and white, children and adults, rich and poor – to be entrusted with their life stories and their thoughts. As he put aside some of his own preconceived ideas, he was able to hear more of what they had to say (Coles, 1978). In this regard, we can affirm Gadamer's (1994) assertion that knowledge in the human sciences always has something of self-knowledge about it.

Early in his career as a researcher Coles spent considerable time with Ruby Bridges, a six-year-old girl. She was the first black student to attend a previously all white school in New Orleans during the time of court ordered desegregation. As Coles became aware that she was a religious child who prayed regularly, even praying for the mob that taunted her each morning as she came to school, concepts like denial and reaction formation came to his mind. When he asked Ruby why she prayed for these angry white people, she looked at him with surprise, and said "Don't you think they need prayin' for?" Slowly, Coles (1986) began to wonder if his psychoanalytic interpretations of her behavior were missing the mark, leading him to underestimate both her moral judgment and her emotional maturity. When he further asked her what she said in her prayers, she responded, "Forgive them God, because they don't know what they are doing" (Coles, 1992). Her answer left Coles speechless and I would say that this was a moment of truth in his research journey. It was a moment of discovery and of coming up against a reality that pushed back. Contrary to what Gergen (2001) has suggested, truth telling, as in Coles's work as a researcher, goes far beyond participating in a set of social conventions and expressing one's findings accordingly. That is, it is meaningful to speak of truths in qualitative research.

Over time, Coles came to understand more of how the lives of children and their families were inextricably interwoven with historical and cultural processes. He also recognized, before it became fashionable to speak of root metaphor or narrative structure, how language can either illuminate or conceal personal and political realities. In an early article, decrying the movement towards abstraction in psychiatry, Coles (1961) wrote:

> As the words grow longer and the concepts more intricate and tedious, human sorrows and temptations disappear, loves move away, envies and jealousies, revenge and terror dissolve. Gone are strong sensible words with good meaning and the flow of the real. (p. 110)

Each of his five volumes of *Children of Crisis* begins with a section on method. In reading them one is struck by how acutely aware Coles is of the enormous complexities and difficulties that researchers face when they seek to understand people with a cultural and ethnic background different than their own. "Until I began to spend time with Indian children, I had never really had to examine my dependency on words", writes Coles (1977, p. 45) as he tells of the development of a personal relationship with several Hopi families. To a significant extent, Robert Coles has undergone what the cultural anthropologist Richard Katz (1993) has described as the experience of vulnerability. This experience involves a radical questioning of one's world view and one's professional and personal common sense through becoming involved with people whose tradition varies dramatically from one's own. Such vulnerability, from Katz's perspective, allows for a deeper understanding of another culture and the recognition, at a personal and intellectual level, of the multiplicity of experienced worlds.

This notion of vulnerability emphasizes how the researcher is necessarily implicated in the subject-at-hand. Throughout his work, Coles reminds us of who he is, personally, professionally, and culturally, and of how the tradition of which he is a part both informs and limits his work as a researcher. In his study of how desegregation affected children in the South, Coles (1964) expressed his awareness of this perspectival dimension of knowledge. "Here I am trying to give prominence to the lives of these people, to their involvements with the *world* [emphasis in original] – but there has to be the qualification: as I have seen and known these lives and involvements" (p. 34).

As we read Coles's books, we come face-to-face with the many ways in which the lives of the people he writes about, such as migrant workers in the United States, are different from our own. At the same time, he keeps before us our common humanity by describing so concretely the children and adults that he meets and telling of their struggles, hopes, and self-understanding. It is through his engagement with their lives that the everyday realities of those of whom he writes become alive for us as we open up to what was previously beyond our own horizons.

The second example of research I want to turn to is a collaborative phenomenological study of the experience of despair in which I was involved several years ago. Our research group consisted of my late colleague Jan Rowe, myself, and four graduate students. We started out with the assumption that despair was a fundamental human experience rather than just a component of a particular psychiatric disturbance, namely depression, and as such could not be adequately understood merely as a symptom that might be eliminated by medication. We noted that despair was depicted in classics of literature, from the Bible to Shakespeare, as well as recognizing it as a recurrent theme in the lives of many people, including our own. Such a universal experience, it seemed to us, deserved to be studied as a phenomenon in its own right (Beck et al, 2003).

In studying this phenomenon, our group followed the dialogal phenomenological approach. This approach is one that Jan Rowe and I, along with several graduate students, developed, or perhaps more accurately said, came upon, when we began our study of forgiving another in the mid-1980's (Rowe et al, 1989). The basic characteristic of the dialogal approach is an open and ongoing conversation (Halling & Leifer, 1991; Halling, Rowe & Kunz, 1994; Halling, Leifer & Rowe, 2006). This conversation or dialogue takes place on two levels: among the researchers and between the researchers and the phenomenon. For a dialogal project to be successful, the phenomenon under study has to become present in the group through an ongoing focus on and attunement to descriptions of it. Although there are phases in the research, it is a process oriented more than a procedurally based method.

To help make the phenomenon come alive within the group, as well as to begin to identify our presuppositions, we started by writing our own descriptions of being in despair. This part of our research was very demanding as it required us to confront and to share those dark moments in our lives that we would just as soon not remember. Navigating this stage of our project was only possible because we listened carefully to each other and allowed ourselves to be in the darkness together.

Our next step was to do in-depth interviews with research participants. As we expected, it took some effort to find people willing to tell us about their times of hopelessness. Yet most of our participants found that telling their story, often for the first time, brought them a measure of relief or new clarity. This phase of "data collection" was followed by intensive discussions within our group of the stories we had written as well as the ones we had gathered through our interviews. Our goal was to articulate as clearly as possible the general structure or core of this important and disturbing experience.

This was the most challenging research project I have ever been involved in – the phenomenon of despair was indeed a partner in our project, and at times moving forward seemed impossible. Increasingly we wondered if we had been foolish in undertaking this study. Then we experienced a breakthrough, which we described as follows:

> We thus characterize our method by our openness to experiencing the phenomenon, talking about it with each other, listening to our participants talk about it, and observing where the topic itself was

> moving us as individuals and as a group of researchers. Indeed, it was when we had the strongest sense of being lost, of being groundless, that we came to realize that our process was revealing to us the very essence of hopelessness. As a group we became willing to live with ambiguity, because, in fact, that was what the phenomenon required. (Beck at al, 2003, p. 343)

This, then, is another example of a moment of truth, this time in relation to the researchers' engagement with a specific phenomenon. This phenomenon, however elusive and difficult to describe, presented itself in a powerful way and gave direction to the study. Our work was sufficiently rewarding, notwithstanding the difficulties along the way, that we decided as a group to do a second project, this time on psychotherapists' approach to dealing with despair as it arose in their work with clients (Beck et al, 2005).

My third example comes from the experience of teaching phenomenological research methods to undergraduates. It is an example that will be familiar to others who have taught phenomenology, whether in the classroom or in the context of a workshop. When I teach this class, I divide the students into groups of four or five based on particular topics that they want to explore. During our time together, the students spend a considerable amount of time becoming familiar with and using the descriptive phenomenological method developed by Amedeo Giorgi (e.g., Giorgi & Giorgi, 2003).

Working together in their groups, they apply the steps of this method to a description written by a young woman who had experienced religious disillusionment. This young woman, who was a research participant for a doctoral dissertation (Holtz, 1984), described being raised in a Catholic household and taking her faith very much to heart. When her *fiancée* applied to medical school, she continually and steadfastly prayed that he would be admitted. When he was denied admission, she was shocked and dismayed. Typically, the students who read this description are perplexed by her reaction and make various critical judgments about her. "Bracketing" judgments and preconceptions is an ideal that they might subscribe to in theory but, like the rest of us, they find it difficult to implement these principles in practice.

In a number of cases, students come to a kind of epiphany as they go through the process of breaking the description into meaning units, summarizing the psychological meaning of each unit, and so on. As they work with the story in this structured way, they start to realize that they have been evaluating this young woman's experience from their own point of reference instead of being open to her perspective and life context. Sooner or later a student says something like:

"Ah, now I get why she was upset that her boyfriend did not get into medical school when she had prayed so hard that he would be admitted. This showed her that the God she had so firmly believed in, a God who can be relied on to answer prayers of the faithful, did not exist". There is two-fold recognition, at least for some of the students – first, this is what is going on for this woman, and, second, in order to see her point of view, one must first recognize and move past one's own egocentric perspective. This example demonstrates that human beings are indeed capable of transcending their own perspective (Held, 2007, pp. 330-331), which is something that social constructionists have been reluctant to acknowledge. It is also a reminder, once again, of Gadamer's insight that knowledge and self-knowledge are interwoven.

Witness to Truth

I would like to suggest that phenomenological researchers are witnesses rather than just observers, as illustrated in the examples above. Even in the third example, where there is no direct contact between the students and the author of the description, there is an engagement with the world and the concerns of the other. We already have the concept of "participant observer", developed by the psychiatrist Harry Stack Sullivan (1953), among others. This concept that has been particularly helpful in reminding us of the way in which there is a mutual process of influence between psychiatrist and patient or researcher and research participant. However, the notion of witness takes us several steps further toward recognizing the profoundly historical nature of both research and truth. It also serves as a reminder that research "findings" may have a claim upon us as persons, professionals, and citizens.

In the Bible the word "witness", used either as a noun or a verb, appears almost two hundred times (Bromiley, 1979, p. 1086). In the New Testament in particular a witness was someone who had been present to a significant event (e.g., the death and resurrection of Jesus) and who could tell others about it. In the contemporary world, we are likely to think of the term witness more narrowly, associating it with someone who testifies in court. The role of a witness in this context is critical but also quite restricted because the one testifying is asked to speak only of what was he or she directly observed. At a minimum, a good witness is a person with basic perceptual competence, who paid close attention to specific events, and is subsequently able to recollect what he or she observed. Ideally the person was in an advantageous position to observe the pertinent events. A case may be decided primarily on the basis of physical evidence, but such a possibility does not bypass the centrality of the notion of witness. Physical evidence allows one to construct what a witness would have observed had one been present.

When we think more deeply and broadly about this issue, we recognize that it is the presence of a witness that makes an incident into a public event. Journalists and historians alike search for those who can authenticate or repudiate rumors and speculations. In turn, those who voluntarily come forward to tell what they have observed are often acutely aware that they have seen something of legal or historical importance. Witnesses may feel compelled to tell others what has happened so that it will not be forgotten; they are likely to bear the imprint of what they have observed. Thus, Robert Coles has testified before Congress about what he has witnessed about the lives of children and his advocacy for children grew out of his experience as a researcher.

In an essay on "Testimony and Existentialism", the French philosopher Gabriel Marcel (1946\1991) elaborated on the meaning of witness by contrasting the witness with the observer. While Marcel referred at some length to the witness in the courtroom, this was not his central concern. Rather, Marcel's aim in this essay was to present key aspects of his understanding of existentialism, contrasting it with Jean-Paul Sartre's philosophy. A number of the points he made are especially germane to the present discussion. First, he suggested that when we speak of observation, it is a matter of indifference who the observer is. Testimony, in contrast, is the witness of the whole person – it comes from the individual as such. Thus, for the witness there is the requirement that one make a commitment to testify before others, that one be personally willing to stand behind what one says.

In referring to the individual as such, Marcel (1946\1991) included personal identity, as that term is ordinarily understood as well as "the identity, in time and beyond time, of a being who is not exhausted by immediacy" (p. 92). Marcel took a position against a merely empiricist understanding of experience and of persons and pointed to the transcendent and open-ended quality of human existence. In Marcel's philosophy, wrote Gallagher (1982), "All truth, all assertion, arises out of a non-objectifiable ground and is sustained by the root which it maintains in this ground" (p. 120). This position is in sharp contrast to the social constructionist and postmodernist view that we are encapsulated by language and culture.

As Marcel (1946\1991) further developed these ideas, he wrote of testimony as "based on fidelity to a light, or, to use another language, to a grace received" (p. 98). He was careful to emphasize that there is nothing passive implied in the use of the word "receive". Surely, he suggested, there is a creative element in receptivity, an element of response and participation. Marcel strongly affirmed "our capacity to open ourselves to others" (p. 100).

Researchers, as I have shown in the examples above, are receptive to what they study. They may even be profoundly affected by the people they interview and the stories they hear. It is in this context that Katz (1993) wrote of vulnerability as part of the researcher's process and that Gadamer referred to self-knowledge. In the case of the students studying the process of phenomenological data analysis, their self-understanding changed insofar as they realized that understanding another required a breaking away from a hitherto unacknowledged egocentricity.

Truth and Transcendence

So far I have discussed how the notion of truth is relevant – and even critical – to the practice of phenomenological research. We have also seen how truth and transcendence show up in Marcel's discussion of the difference between the witness and the observer. In this section, I will discuss truth and transcendence as interdependent notions.

In his chapter on Edmund Husserl and "The Method of Eidetic Intuition for Psychology" (in this volume), Frederick Wertz affirms that phenomenological psychologists believe that it is possible, and vitally important, to arrive at understandings of the essence of particular phenomena. As he points out, this belief seems to fly in the face of what postmodernist thinkers within psychology have argued against for decades. These thinkers have contended that there is no possibility that humans can arrive at objective knowledge since all human knowing is shaped by language, culture, and, in the case of psychologists, implicit and explicit theoretical commitments.

Admittedly, the language of "essence" could all too easily be taken to mean that Edmund Husserl had in mind Platonic essence, a sort of ahistorical, metaphysical reality. One would not have to be a radical postmodernist to be dubious about the possibility of uncovering such otherworldly essences. But this, Wertz argues, is not what Husserl meant. Rather, "Psychology imaginatively varies examples of psychological life through potentially infinite variations in order to grasp the essential structural *possibilities of humans as actually they exist in the real world*" (2010, p. 275). Even so, the very idea that these essences can be grasped (however fallibly) directly through intuition, that they are not social constructions, intellectual or otherwise, is at odds with a postmodern sensibility. But it is not at odds with the experience of those who are engaged in research. A basic faith in the possibility of genuine discovery animated the activities of the researchers I have discussed above. Robert Coles came upon realities that he had not anticipated and my fellow researchers and I struggled with a phenomenon that had a life of its own, becoming caught up in its essential structure without explicitly realizing it.

This faith in the possibility of genuine discovery is also evident in the writings of Amedeo Giorgi whose psychology is indebted to Husserl's and Merleau-Ponty's work. Giorgi has consistently called for development of methods and options within psychology "so as to make greater fidelity to the researched phenomenon possible" (Wertz & Aanstoos, 1999, p. 291), and has persisted in advocating for the truths of phenomenology even in the face of lack of acknowledgment or response from within mainstream psychology (Giorgi, 2003). Fidelity requires, among other things, setting aside prior knowledge and assumptions as one attempts to arrive at an articulation of the "lived structure of the phenomenon in a particular type of situation" (Giorgi, 2008, p. 41). In one of his studies of learning, for example, Giorgi (1989, p. 101) arrives at two typical structures, reflecting two types of learning. One he describes as the "experience of adequate performance", (as in learning to drive a car) and the other is the "experience of learning by detecting inadequate assumptions", (as in learning that one should not take it for granted that one's employees are honest).

This study was open-ended in its approach in that learning was defined by the research participants; the researcher did not dictate either the type or location of the learning. Nor did the study attempt to confirm or test existing theories or research on learning in psychology. Rather, its goal was to address the experience of learning as lived in everyday life. The underlying assumption of phenomenological psychology is that it is indeed possible to arrive at an understanding that is, in a meaningful but qualified sense, true. As Wertz makes clear, this does not mean that this understanding is true for all times or places or that it is not subject to modification. Nonetheless it is a truth that is lived and that we can recognize as speaking to our own experiences of learning. To put it in non-technical terms, we are speaking of truth that emerges in one's openness to the phenomenon.

Openness takes us back to the second term in the heading for this section, that is, transcendence. In a 1992 article, Giorgi wrote of transcendence as a distinctly human characteristic. It means, he argued, that we are not just controlled by circumstances but can move beyond them. Similarly, in my own work, I have suggested "transcendence is akin to openness, a movement toward the new, and thus is a key feature of our humanity" (Halling, 2008, p. 178). However, precisely because transcendence is such an essential dimension of our existence we tend not to notice it except under special circumstances. Even when we have a "breakthrough" that brings us to a new perspective, we are more likely to be struck by what we open up to than the fact we are capable of opening up and moving forward. For example, in forgiving another person we come to experience the other as a fellow human being. We have moved beyond the preoccupation with (although not the memory of) the self as injured and the other as perpetrator. It is likely that we will more be focused on the new that we have discovered than the change in ourselves that makes seeing the new possible.

In terms of transcendence in the lives of researchers, we can think of Robert Coles, who, however deeply influenced by his psychoanalytic training and his assumptions about children, was nonetheless deeply touched by what the children with whom he spoke told him. This led him, as we saw, to revaluate his whole viewpoint on children's maturity and understanding. A new seeing and a new self-awareness came together. No one could accuse Coles of being among those who "fail to escape the cocoon of their own tradition" (Gergen, 2002, p. 464). Similarly, some of my students were also able move to a place where they recognized the narrowness of seeing the life of the other through their own viewpoint. Then they could see that this prevented them from being open to the world of the woman who had experienced religious disillusionment.

This leads us to a final question – how do truth and transcendence fit together? How do they presuppose each other? To attempt to answer this question, I will once again turn to an example, this time drawn from the writings of a philosopher. At the beginning of his book, *Radical Realism: Direct Knowing in Science and Philosophy* (1992), Edward Pols described an experience he had as an undergraduate. While sitting in his dormitory room, he had a sudden awareness of the furniture in his room as real and independent of him. As he wrote subsequently, he was at that moment…

> […] rationally aware of certain things that were in no sense products of my act of rational attention and I was also rationally aware (by virtue of the reflexivity inherent in that function) that those things were indeed independent of my rational attention. (p. X)

It is interesting indeed this philosopher takes his own experience seriously. Regrettably, Pols does not give a complete description of this epiphany as he remembers it but interweaves reference to this experience with, as he himself says, "the language of this present book" (p. X). His after-the-fact interpretation of his experience places him on the side of a modernist epistemology – we have direct access to realities that exist independently of us; hence the term radical realism. Yet his description affirms, one might say, both truth and transcendence. From a phenomenological perspective, an experience of an object as independent of oneself does not negate the notion of co-constitution, that is, the notion that what one perceives reflects the interdependence of the perceiver and the perceived, the subject and the object. Of course, this does not imply that the perceiver creates what is perceived. Here I turn to Martin Buber (1965) whose essay on "Distance and Relation" takes us beyond the modern/postmodern divide as he deals with this fundamental paradox of human existence.

Buber agued that being human involves a special way of being that can be described as a two-fold movement of setting at a distance and entering into relation. He further emphasized that these two movements, though separate, presuppose each other: "That the first movement is the presupposition of the other is plain from the fact that one can enter into relation only with being which has been set at a distance, more precisely, has become an independent opposite" (Buber, 1965, p. 60). Humans, in distinction to animals, have the capacity to imagine and experience the world as existing for itself, and as transcending their own existence. In this emphasis on distance and relation, it seems to me, Buber turned away from both a modernist and postmodernist perspective. His position is similar to Merleau-Ponty's (1945\1962), who seeks the middle ground between objectivism (the world exists independently of us and is the ultimate source of the real) and idealism (we construct the world through the activity of our minds).

Conclusion: Final Thoughts about Truth

Admittedly, phenomenologists do not often speak directly of truth. But it is fair to say that they implicitly take "truth" to be a meaningful notion, however difficult it is to define. As I have suggested in the title of this chapter, truth is akin to the pauses that are intrinsic to rhythm. In the studies of hopelessness as well as of desegregation and its effect on children, there were moments of recognition, times when the researchers stopped and took stock. These were moments when something was discovered, something that led the researchers to pause and reflect. In addition, as researchers we assume that there will be such moments of discovery, whether they emerge gradually or appear suddenly, as epiphanies. But it is not just that we assume that we will discover something new; rather, we actively work to make this possible. Our methods of gathering and of analyzing data are guided by the notions of truth and discovery. We want to be faithful to the stories we are told, as Robert Coles' supervisor suggested. This desire is based upon a moral obligation to our research participants as well as a commitment to our integrity as researchers.

Let me conclude with some final comments about truth. The well-known American psychologist Jerome Bruner argued in 1986 that the notion of truth should be dissociated from narrative and stories. He suggested that there are two distinct although also complementary modes of thinking or ways of knowing. There is storytelling (narrative thinking) and argumentation (propositional thinking). The second mode of knowing, which he also referred to as paradigmatic or logico-scientific, "deals in general with causes and in their establishment, and makes use of procedures to assure verifiable reference and to test for empirical truth" (Bruner, 1986, p. 13). As Hermans, Kempen, and van Loon (1992) summarized Bruner, "Arguments are intended to convince someone of their truth; stories are intended to convince someone of their lifelikeness" (p. 26). This distinction may have some validity if one is contrasting physics with fiction. Yet it is quite literally a distinction that will not hold up in court, any more than it is viable in the human sciences. The witness is asked to tell the truth, not just a plausible story, and researchers strive for fidelity, not just coherence, in writing their reports. As Polkinghorne (1988) pointed out in his book on *Narrative Knowing and the Human Sciences,* "without the notion that the story is about something outside the discourse itself, it would lose its force as a selection from possible events and its power to intrigue us" (p. 92). Moreover, the concern for truth is part of everyday human life. As my colleague Brayton Polka (1990) has argued, truth and existence are mutually implicated:

> Truth, we must constantly realize, is not an object, on analogy with the objects or things of nature, but the subject of our lives, the self which we share with others as they share it with us. Interpretation, we must constantly realize, is not a method among other methods, but it is the method of our lives, the method by which we engage others' selves as they engage us (p. 332).

Polka squarely places truth within a social and historical context; this is not a turn to relativism any more than it is a return to objectivism. As Wachterhauser (1994) has said in his discussion of Gadamer's hermeneutics, "truth is always part of our experience in such a way that we always presuppose truth" (p. 4). Robert Coles also used the word truth. He sought to be faithful in his analyses and descriptions to the stories and the lives of the people that he had studied and had come to know. A guiding assumption of philosophers of dialogue such as Buber (1965), Gadamer (1986\1989), and Jaspers (1932\1970), and of dialogal phenomenology as we have practiced it at Seattle University, is that truth emerges in the context of human conversation (Halling & Goldfarb, 1991). Once more, truth references the experience of coming to an understanding of something that one is in relationship to and trying to do justice to that understanding. Within the context of dialogue, it refers to a deeply felt, communal experience of, "yes, this is how it is." This understanding of truth as historical is in contrast to positivistic notions of truth as independent of us. But it is also in contrast to much of postmodern thought which in rejecting truth in human affairs embraces a position that is simply the mirror opposite of the positivism that it has rejected (Sass & Woolfolk, 1988).

The truths that researchers search for are elusive and can be spoken of in a multitude of ways. Truths in human life are elusive not because they are abstract or unreal but because they transcend us even as they touch us deeply. Phenomena such as friendship, despair, grief, or love are realities at the core of human existence, realities that elude measurement, and it is to them that we bear witness as researchers within a human science orientation. The truths we articulate as researchers, however provisionally, are embodied truths; they are felt in our bones.

References

Atwood, G. E. & Stolorow, R. D. (1981). Experience and conduct. *Contemporary Psychoanalysis, 17*, 197-208.

Beck, B., Halling, S., McNabb, M., Miller, D., Rowe, J. O., & Schulz, J. (2003). Facing up to hopelessness: A dialogal phenomenological study. *Journal of Religion and Health, 42, 339*-354.

Beck, B., Halling, S., McNabb, M., Miller, D., Rowe, J. O., & Schulz, J. (2005). On navigating despair: Reports from psychotherapists. *Journal of Religion and Health, 44*,187-205.

Bromiley, G. W. (Ed.). (1979). *The international standard Bible encyclopedia, Vol. IV*. Grand Rapids, MI: Eerdmans.

Bruner, J. (1986). *Actual minds, possible worlds*. Cambridge, MA: Harvard University Press.

Buber, M. (1965). Distance and relation. In M. Friedman (Ed.). *The knowledge of man: Philosophy of the interhuman* (pp. 59-88). New York: Harper and Row.

Coles, R. (1961). A young psychiatrist looks at his profession. *Atlantic Monthly*, July, 108-111.

Coles, R. (1964). *Children of Crisis. Vol. I: A study of courage and fear*. Boston: Little, Brown.

Coles, R. (1977). *Children of Crisis. Vol. IV: Eskimos, Chicanos, Indians*. Boston: Little, Brown.

Coles, R. (1978). *Children of Crisis. Vol. V: Privileged Ones*. Boston: Little, Brown.

Coles, R. (1986). *The moral life of children*. Boston: Houghton Mifflin.

Coles, R. (1989). *The call of stories: Teaching the moral imagination*. Boston: Houghton Mifflin.

Coles, R. (1992). How our sense of social class shapes our sense of social justice. Presentation given as part of the Seattle Arts and Letters Lecture Series, Seattle, WA. April.

Gadamer, H. G. (1989). *Truth and method*. (2nd rev. edition). (J. Weinsheimer & D. Marshall, Trans.). New York: Crossroads (Original published 1986).

Gadamer, H. G. (1994). Truth in the human sciences. In B. R. Wachterhauser (Ed). *Hermeneutics and truth* (pp. 25-32). Evanston, Ill: Northwestern University Press.

Gallagher, K. T. (1982). Marcel, Jaspers, and the modes of truth. *Philosophy Today*, (Summer), 118-125.

Gergen, K. J. (1989). The possibility of psychological knowledge: A hermeneutic inquiry. In M. J. Packer & R. B. Addison (Eds.). *Entering the circle: Hermeneutic investigations in* psychology (pp. 239-259). Albany: SUNY Press.

Gergen, K. J. (2001). Psychological science in a postmodern context. *American Psychologist, 56,* 803-813.

Gergen, K. J. (2002). Psychological science: To conserve or to create? *American Psychologist, 57,*463-464.

Giorgi, A. (1989). Learning and perception from the perspective of phenomenological Psychology. In R. S. Valle & S. Halling (Ed.). *Existential-phenomenological perspectives in psychology* (pp. 99-112). New York: Plenum.

Giorgi, A. (1992). Whither humanistic psychology? *The Humanistic Psychologist, 20,* 422-438.

Giorgi, A. (2003). Lessons for the future from the margins of psychology. *Journal of Phenomenological Psychology, 33,*179-201.

Giorgi, A. (2006). Concerning variations in the application of the phenomenological method. *The Humanistic Psychologist, 34,*305-319.

Giorgi, A. (2008). Concerning a serious misunderstanding of the essence of the phenomenological method in psychology. *Journal of Phenomenological Psychology, 39,* 33-58.

Giorgi, A. & Giorgi, B. (2003). The descriptive phenomenological method. In P. M. Camic & L. Yardley (Eds.). *Qualitative research in psychology* (pp. 243-272). Washington, DC: American Psychological Association.

Halling, S. (2008). *Intimacy, transcendence, and psychology. Closeness and openness in everyday life.* New York: Palgrave Macmillan.

Halling, S. & Goldfarb, M. (1991). Grounding truth in the body: Therapy and research renewed. *The Humanistic Psychologist, 19,* 313-330.

Halling, S., Kunz, G. D., & Rowe, J. O. (1994). The contributions of dialogal psychology to phenomenological research. *Journal of Humanistic Psychology, 34,* 109-131.

Halling, S. & Lawrence, C. (1999). Social constructionism: Homogenizing the world, negating embodied experience. *Journal of Theoretical and Philosophical Psychology, 19,* 78-89

Halling, S. & Leifer, M. (1991). The theory and practice of dialogal research. *Journal of Phenomenological Psychology, 22,* 1-15.

Halling, S., Leifer, M., & Rowe, J. O. (2006). The emergence of the dialogal approach: Forgiving Another. In C. T. Fischer (Ed.). *Qualitative research methods for psychologists: Introduction through empirical studies* (pp.173-212). New York: Academic Press.

Held, B. S. (2007). *Psychology's interpretive turn: The search for truth and agency in theoretical and philosophical psychology.* Washington, DC: American Psychological Association.

Hermans, H. J. M., Kempen, H. J. G., & van Loon, R. J. P. (1992). The dialogical self: Beyond individualism and rationalism. *American Psychologist, 47,* 23-33.

Holtz, V. (1984). Being disillusioned as exemplified by adults in religion, marriage or career: An empirical phenomenological investigation. *Dissertation Abstracts International,* 45, 11B. (UMI No. 8500881)

Jaspers, K. (1970). *Philosophy, Vol. II.* (E. B. Ashton, Trans.). Chicago: University of Chicago Press. (Original work published 1932)

Katz, R. (1993). Respect and vulnerability in research. Appendix A. in *The straight path: A story of healing and transformation* (pp. 352-367), Reading, MA: Addison Wesley.

Marcel, G. (1991). Testimony and existentialism. In *The philosophy of existentialism* (pp. 91-103). (M. Harari, Trans.). New York: Citadel Press. (Original work published 1946)

Merleau-Ponty, M. (1982). *Phenomenology of perception.* (C. Smith, Trans). New York: The Humanities Press (Original published 1945).

Merleau-Ponty, M. (1968). *The visible and the invisible.* (A. Lingis, Trans). Evanston, IL: Northwestern University Press (Original work published 1964)

Mills, J. (2005). A critique of relational psychoanalysis. *Psychoanalytic Psychology, 22,* 155-188.

Polka, B. (1990). *Truth and interpretation: An essay in thinking.* New York: St. Martin's.

Polkinghorne, D. E. (1988). *Narrative knowing and the human sciences.* Albany, NY: SUNY Press.

Pols. E. (1992). *Radical realism: Direct knowing in science and philosophy.* Ithaca, NY: Cornell University Press.

Rowe, J. O., Halling, S., Davies, E., Leifer, M., Powers, D., & van Bronkhorst, J. (1989). The psychology of forgiving another: A dialogal research approach. In R. S. Valle & S. Halling (Eds.). *Existential-phenomenological perspectives in psychology* (pp. 233-244). New York: Plenum.

Sass, L. A. & Woolfolk, R. L. (1988). Psychoanalysis and the hermeneutic turn: A critique of narrative truth and historical truth. *Journal of the American Psychoanalytic Association, 36,* 29-454.

Stolorow, R. D. & Atwood, G. E. (1979). Faces in a cloud: Subjectivity in personality theory. New York: Aronson.

Stolorow, R. D., Atwood, G. E. & Orange, D. M. (2004). *Worlds of experience: Interweaving philosophical and clinical dimensions in psychoanalysis.* New York: Basic Books.

Sullivan, H. S. (1953). *The Interpersonal theory of psychiatry.* New York: Norton.

Wertz, F. J. & Aanstoos, C. (1999). Amedeo Giorgi and the project of a human science. In D. Moss (Ed.). *Humanistic and transpersonal psychology: A historical and biographical sourcebook* (pp. 287-300). Westport, CT: Greenwood Press.

Wertz, F. J. (2010). The method of eidetic analysis for psychology. In T. F. Cloonan & C. Thiboutot. (Eds.). *The redirection of psychology: Essays in honor of Amedeo P. Giorgi.* Montreal, CAN: Éditions du Cirp, Les Collectifs du Cirp, Volume 1.

Note

1 I am grateful to Mical Sikkema for commenting on an earlier version of this chapter. Her suggestions helped me to become clearer about what I wanted to say.

PLAYING WITH POLARITIES OF EXISTENCE: TOWARD UNDERSTANDING A PIVOTAL PASSAGE IN THE LIFE AND WORK OF ROLLO MAY

Mufid James Hannush, Ph.D.

Rosemont College
United States

Abstract

In this chapter the author applies an existential-dialectical-phenomenological (EDP) method toward understanding two so-called case histories, which in reality are self-analyses, in the works of Rollo May. In these two self-analytic case histories, May describes a pivotal passage in his life which richly anticipates the major themes of his prolific and productive contributions to existential-humanistic psychology.

In a 1987 interview with the author (Hannush, 1999a), Rollo May responded to a question regarding a clinical vignette that appeared in one of his writings by affirming, on the one hand, that the patient, Philip, in this case history was May himself in disguise and, on the other hand, by adding that the case history was a composite that contained, *at least*, some autobiographical elements. Here is what May had to say:

> Yes, I am Philip, incidentally. Philip is, as he is presented that book [*Freedom and Destiny*], a composite of different characters and that part of it is certainly me. It's amazing how much they are alike, isn't it. I never realized that. Once I write something I forget it and I may write it over again. (Hannush, 1999a, p. 133)

After publishing my interview with Rollo May and confirming my hunch that there was a striking resemblance between the case history of "Philip" and the life history of May himself, I came upon Robert H. Abzug's discovery that Rollo May had also disguised himself behind the case history of "Charles D", that appeared in a much earlier publication, entitled *The Springs of Creative Living: A Study of Human Nature and God* (May, 1940). According to Abzug (1999),

> May's case history of Charles D. is literally one of self-analysis. From beginning to end, with only minor details changed, Charles D.'s history is Rollo May's history. Many of the quotations from Charles D. come

> almost verbatim from May's own diaries and letters, and the specific events reported, with names and places changed, come directly from his own experience. (p. 66)

Now Abzug had interviewed May, and, as indicated in the above quotation, seemingly had access to May's "diaries and letters". In fact, Abzug was intending to write a biography of May which has not materialized as of today. Abzug does not say, as does May in my own interview with him regarding the case of Philip, that May himself owned up to the fact that he was Charles himself. The inference, however, seems incontrovertibly and unambiguously clear.

In this chapter, I will apply an existential-dialectical-phenomenological (*EDP)* method to these two so-called case histories or self-analyses in an effort to understand a pivotal passage in Rollo May's life (Hannush, 1999a; see also Bilmes, 1978; De Carvalho, 1999; and Schneider, 1999) which richly anticipates the major themes of his prolific and productive contributions to existential-humanistic psychology (See Hannush, 2002, Chapter Five; 2001; 1999b).

Method

The existential-dialectical-phenomenological (*EDP*) method outlined here is a variation on a method that I first developed under the guidance and mentorship of my dissertation director, Amedeo Giorgi, in 1981. The method was originally tailored to the rigorous study of linkage between the lives and works of John B. Watson and B. F. Skinner (Hannush, 1983). It was later applied toward understanding the autobiographical work of the American novelist Richard Wright (Hannush, 1985). Recently, in another version, it was applied once more to understanding cultural tilts (Hannush, 2007). The theoretical underpinning of the *EDP* method is described in my article, "An Existential-Dialectical-Phenomenological Approach to Understanding *Cultural Tilts*: Implications for Multicultural Research and Practice" (Hannush, 2007). In the present study, four *methodological steps* are adapted to the nature of the present project. But before describing these steps, a brief definition of the term "dialectics" is in order.

Leslie Baxter and Barbara Montgomery distinguish between "dialectics-as-ontology" and "dialectics-as-epistemology". "Dialectics-as-ontology refers to a view of reality as the dynamic interplay of opposing forces [or polarities], whereas dialectics-as-epistemology refers to a method of reasoning by which one searches for understanding through the clash of opposing arguments [or forces]" (Baxter and Montgomery, 1996, pp. 18-19). This kind of methodical understanding aims at elucidating the essential complementarity between seemingly oppositional and conflictual polarities, such as separateness versus connectedness. In this dialectical sense, seeming functional opposites define, require, and lend meaning to each other. Without connectedness, there can be no separateness. The initial tension-producing imbalance provides an opportunity for the achievement of balance-producing complementarity between what first appeared as mutually exclusive opposite forces (For a more in-depth discussion of dialectics, see Hannush, 2007).

Four Methodological Steps

1. After familiarizing himself thoroughly with the life and work of the subject, Rollo May, and the two so-called case histories or self-analyses in particular, the researcher captures the heart of the life narrative as described by the subject, while remaining faithful to the subject's language.
2. The researcher distills the subject's narrative into concise language.
3. The researcher embarks upon the transitional step of moving back-and-forth between the language of the subject, as distilled in Step 2, and a description of the subject's life narrative through the language of dialectics. Here the researcher is attempting to be selectively attuned to and focused on those dialectically thematic tensions in the life narrative that the subject is struggling with and attempting to resolve. For example, the researcher tries to answer the question, "Are there polar needs or desires that the subject is attempting to resolve which at first appear as opposites and mutually exclusive, but, at a deeper level, prove to be complementary?"
4. The researcher moves toward capturing essential life themes from a dialectical perspective. The researcher retells the life story of the subject in dialectical terms.

Rollo May: A Brief Biography

Rollo May, the first son of six children, was born in Ada, Ohio on April 21, 1909. May described his parents as austere disciplinarians and anti-intellectuals. He was "raised in the Protestant culture of the small-town Midwest by a devout mother and a father who was a YMCA field secretary" (Abzug, 1999, p. 60). When May's oldest sister had a psychotic episode, his father attributed it to too much education. After receiving his Bachelor of Arts degree, with a major in English, from Oberlin College in 1930, he spent three years teaching at Anatolia College in Thessaloniki, Greece. In Europe, he traveled, painted, and studied psychology at Alfred Adler's seminars in Vienna. After returning to the United States, he pursued a divinity degree at Union Theological Seminary. There he studied with Reinhold Niebuhr and with Paul Tillich, who became a mentor and a life-long friend. "Under Tillich's tutelage in particular, he had plunged into Nietzsche, Kierkegaard, Berdyaev, and other Christian radicals or critics of the faith" (Abzug, 1999, p. 60). May's deeply religious orientation, in relation to which his interest in philosophy and psychology were subordinated, is revealed in a diary entry written in 1936: "But religion especially is in crying need of its leader. I am fitted to be that leader. I feel called to it [...] The world calls – I must give" (Abzug, 1999, p. 60).

> Between 1940 and 1947, May confronted death at the hands of tuberculosis and, almost simultaneously, gave up an established career in the Christian ministry for the riskier trade of psychological counseling. These two events together constituted an extraordinary turning point in May's life, one that drove him in search of a more authentic confrontation with life. (Abzug, 1999, p. 59)

After taking time off from Union Theological Seminary to work as a student counselor at Michigan State University, he returned to earn his degree in 1938. After his graduation, he married and accepted a position as a minister in a New Jersey church. In 1942, having become deeply dispirited, he resigned his ministry position and started his doctoral work in psychology at Columbia University. After recovering from his contracted disease of tuberculosis, May opened his counseling practice in 1945. He earned his doctorate degree from Columbia in 1949.

Overworking and overextending himself, May attributes the fact of his succumbing to the disease of tuberculosis to "'trying to be something I wasn't'" (Abzug, 1999, p. 61). Additionally, May provides the explanation of having found "spiritual reality" in his counseling work and not in his work as a pastor in a suburban church as a reason for his career shift and change of calling.

In my interview with Rollo May (Hannush, 1999a), May states that upon seeing Arthur Miller's *Death of a Salesman* he was shaken to the core of his being. In response to my invitation to reflect on this, he says this: "You see, the salesman, Willie Loman, was like my father. [...] I thought that at the time I saw this drama that the drama was written about my father" (p. 130). Like his father, a Loman-like tragic figure, May had believed in the Horatio Alger myth – that if you worked hard, then you will achieve success. At a critical junction in his life's journey, a *pivotal passage* that will be central in this study, May had become conscious of the contradictions and opposites within himself and, with uncanny acuity, he glimpsed the presence of these contradictions and opposites in the American culture.

> I knew American characteristics – such as generosity, friendliness, courage to risk an experiment, energy – of which I was proud despite the fact that they go hand-in-hand with their opposites such

> as violence and money-mindedness [...] Loyalty to my country made all the stronger my hatred of national violence and spiritual vacuity. (Hannush, 1999a, p. 130)

In the interview, May describes his parents as having been strict and sexually repressed mid-westerners. May had this to say about his father's attribution of May's older sister psychotic breakdown to "too much education": "I sensed how inhumane and destructive this remark was" (p. 130). May appropriated what he calls mid-western character strengths of courage, generosity, hard work, perseverance, and experimental risk-taking, but at the same time describes himself as having been "to some extent maimed by the disease of anti-intellectualism" which he hated (p. 131). He grew up surrounded by "a kind of religious evangelism" of which he was a part and at the same time, he grew to hate. But even though he grew not to like it, it had given him "a kind of strength". Similarly, he describes his father in ambivalent terms. Although insensitive and anti-intellectual, he was a psychologically strong man. May has this to say about his father's insensitivity: "[My older sister] was a very pathetic person and she suffered a great deal, and he [my father] never had much sympathy for her" (p. 131). May says further of his father: "[From] my father I got the idea that life is serious, that one ought to do the best one can, one ought to serve other people the best one can – all these are aspects of being. I would not have used the word "being" then, but I later realized that it fitted my background" (p. 134). The word "being" itself he appropriated from Paul Tillich. May here links his personal and vocational passionate preoccupation with the quest for understanding our sense of being – the main concern of his life.

May describes his mother, who was orphaned as a child, as a "strong woman [...] [who] had a very bad temper" (Hannush, 1999a, p. 132). "[My parents] used to fight a lot. She was also very courageous. She raised six children and I have to admire her for this kind of courage. Nevertheless, I never got along very well with her" (p. 132).

Reflecting on the year in which he experienced a "nervous breakdown" while teaching English to Greek students in the spring of his second year at Anatolia College, May says, "As the year went on I found that my habits and principles, coming from a typical small town, mid-western childhood, such as hard work, fidelity, honesty and so on, stood me less and less [...]. [The] rules, principles, values by which I used to work and live simply did not suffice anymore" (Hannush, 1999a, p. 132). He came to the self-discovery that he had to let go of his moralistic and rigid principles and learn to be appreciatively attuned to the beauty of and kinship to life in the here-and-now.

Application of Method

METHODOLOGICAL STEP ONE

After familiarizing himself thoroughly with the life and work of the subject, Rollo May, and the two so-called case histories or self-analyses in particular, the researcher captures the heart of the life narrative as described by the subject, while remaining faithful to the subject's language.

Rollo May as "Charles D." (May, 1940)

The case of Charles D. is described in the second and third chapters of May's book, *The Springs of Creative Living.* In Chapter Two, which is entitled "But What Kind of Meaning?", "Charles" first appears under the sub-heading, "Authoritarianism – Thou Shalt and Shalt Not". Charles, we are told, is in his early thirties. He sought counseling because he was ambivalent about his marriage decision. He belonged to a mid-western family. His parents are described as intelligent, hard-working. But most of all, they were continually concerned about "moral details" and with "strong character". Additionally, they displayed "a great aversion" toward sexuality. More than that, their marriage is described as not having been a happy one. He recalls several quarrels that occurred during his boyhood.

As a college student, Charles was deeply religious. He focused his energies on developing his "character". But even though he had "rich religious experience" in his junior and senior years, "his outstanding memory of his college life was one of loneliness and isolation". Although he was generally liked, he did not establish close friendships. And even though he had several girlfriends, he was not able to "move into sound love". His non-coital sexual play and masturbatory activity were followed by deep feelings of guilt.

May also describes the Charles of this period as being "highly moral in the authoritarian sense". He set up rules – regarding time management, study habits, physical exercise, health, and so on, and resolutions and focused his energies on meeting them. A diary entry contained a maxim to follow in order to develop his character: "keeping my body at its best, giving attention only to what is right, controlling my will". Interestingly, when he tried to combat his loneliness by making rules to be more friendly, he ended up making himself "more self-conscious". Similarly, his resolutions to cease masturbating only intensified his "temptation to masturbate".

After graduating from college, Charles taught at an American college in Egypt. He fell in love with an American girl, who lost interest in him, which he attributed to his inability to express his affection for her. During the first two years there, he continued to focus his energies on building his character, "making and remaking resolutions about his life and work". His ultimate resolution was to become Christ-like. His deepest desire was to appropriate the Christian attitudes of patience, sympathy, strength of purpose, moral strength, and devotion to the call of teaching. Again, even though he was generally liked by his colleagues, "his loneliness increased". In spite of his vacillation between the joy of solitude and the heavy burden of isolation, he "clung tenaciously to his religion". His belief in God was "most important" for him in this period of his life. He felt that he was God's "special representative. He wanted to have an impact on the "character development" of his students. Still, in this endeavor he felt self-conscious. He came to the realization that the students were discretely laughing at the teachers, including Charles. They perceived them as idealistic hypocrites who were unable to practice true Christian love. He came to the realization that "our emphasis on character development was defeating itself" and that it was a "self-centered" endeavor. Instead of connecting him to others, it was closing him off from others. It dawned upon him that something was wrong and that his "life had not been real, solid, genuine".

It was at this time that Charles experienced a "nervous breakdown". The *"breakdown occurred simultaneously with the realization that the meaning by which he had been living was destroyed"* (May, 1940, p. 47). To find a cure, he had to find a "new meaning", a new life scheme. In the previous year, sensing the impending failure of his life style, he had "thrown himself into his work with increasing vigor" in a desperate effort to shore up his previous pattern. "The human being fights hardest for his psychological pattern just before it collapses" (May, 1940, p. 47). May describes this life style as an "*authoritarian* kind of life". An authoritarian person, says May, attempts to live by rules and principles external to himself. The authoritarian individual, continues May, "finds his true meaning in life in subjecting himself and his desires to this [external] structure [or authority] by dint of a strong will" (May, 1940, p. 48).

The case history of Charles continues under the next subheading, entitled "Romanticism – The Full and Free Life". After a one month rest and a "partial treatment by a psychotherapist", Charles comes to the realization that his moralism had been used by him as means of shoring up his prestige and pampering himself. He had consequently become focused upon himself. What he needed was to "forget" himself, to let himself go, by letting his rigid rules go. He needed to set himself free by pursuing the "spontaneous life". This he came to call his "romantic period". He joined a group of roving musicians. His inhibitions subsided, as his "senses came to life". He fell in love with an attractive and talented American girl, who similarly was reacting "against a too rigorous background". He was no longer hesitant and timid, for he approached this relationship with "courage and freedom". Upon returning to his teaching he separated from her "successfully". His orientation toward work changed. He did not take it too seriously. He was no longer overly conscientious. He made more close friends and "fell in love with five different women", who had a difficult time separating from him. But now, with his new orientation, this "was not his worry". He now worshiped "experience" and Walt Whitman's writings became his "bible".

Still, Charles wanted to "contribute to his fellow-man". He came to the conclusion that he could help others, who had been failed by religion, overcome their "restrictive dogmas" and their fears by understanding themselves through psychoanalysis and thus cultivate the courage to "let themselves go in love". But at the same time he also started to doubt the applicability of his new vision of understanding and love to resolving larger issues, such as the emotionally-laden irrational conflict between the nations of Europe.

Charles returned to America to teach and to assume the mental and financial responsibility that fell upon him after his parents were divorced. He began to realize that "the Whitmanesque view" did not account for the tragic elements of human experience, of the "dance of life". Consequently, his doubts regarding his new meaning or purpose in life intensified. Although he was "still falling in and out of love, even with college girls whom he taught" (May, 1940, p. 54), he had more difficulty surviving these affairs. In a diary entry, he writes, "Life is too much for me". After succumbing to an illness and taking two months to recover, he changed his job and "moved along a plateau for two years" until he had to face "the marriage decision" which necessitated his seeking counseling.

May now reflects on the dialectical tension between authoritarianism – with its emphasis on determinism and rigid external structure and romanticism – with its emphasis on freedom and self-expression from the inside out: "It is significant that Charles D., in his earlier partial psychotherapeutic treatment, absorbed the romantic self-expressive emphasis without the corresponding structure to serve as a balance" (May, 1940, p. 55). May retrospectively ruminates that structure provides the necessary complementary pole to "a creative dialectic of human personality". Just like Jean Jacque Rousseau, Charles (May) finds a contradiction in himself and in human life, "which gives a tragic depth to human existence":

> Rousseau was rebelling against sterile rationalism of the eighteenth century French drawing room, and Charles D. was reacting against Pharisaic authoritarianism. In the very reaction, however, one uses the structure one attacks as a pivot-point. [...] Some "play of opposites" is necessary to give a dynamic balance to personality. (May, 1940, p. 58)

The next subheading is entitled "A Dialectic of Personality", of which the previous sentence in the quotation is an example. Here Charles's dialectical dilemma is described in the following terms: "Charles D. [...] became *more* rigid in his authoritarianism as he felt it collapsing under him, and he pushed ahead to more experience when his romantic way of life was tottering" (May, 1940, pp. 58-59). Charles paid a mental health price for not being able to find a balance and hold a flux between determinism and freedom. Charles "fell into ill-health when he assumed himself to be either entirely determined (as in the authoritarian stage) or entirely free (as in the romantic period)" (May, 1940, p. 60). He lacked the creativity and courage to "avail himself of his freedom and the humility to place himself in accord with the structure of life" (p. 60).

May continues to delve into Charles's case history in Chapter Three of his book, *The Springs of Creative Living*. In the subheading entitled "Charles D.'s Crisis", May describes in further detail Charles's decisional dilemma: To marry or not marry Helen R. It is a classic approach-avoidance, emotion-laden conflict. The emotions run the gamut from passionate enthusiasm, to jealousy, to fear and flight. Helen is described by Charles as being attractive, well-educated, and comes from a good familial background. But, she is also described as not "sufficiently high type" and did not have a "strong" enough of a personality. To avoid following the divorce pattern set by his parents, Charles was resolved to "keep his ideals high". Yet at other moments he ruminated, "Perhaps he could help her develop after marriage to be the "strong" kind of personality he could love" (May, 1940, p. 64). As May sees it, Charles not only intellectualized, but also spiritualized his problem by elevating it to the "altruistic sphere". By hiding behind a façade of "unselfishness", Charles is hiding his selfishness. His superiority is masquerading as unselfishness. May reflects on Charles's indecision in the following manner:

> As had been his habit in previous emotional disturbances, he filled his diary with introspective searchings of his mind and heart, trying to decide intellectually whether or not this was the girl he should marry. This endeavoring to settle emotional problems via the intellectual route is a common error in our modern culture, and one of the central contributions of modern depth-psychology is in pointing out that the major problems of life are emotional rather than intellectual and need to be "clarified" rather than settled by logic. (May, 1940, p. 62)

In the section entitled "Weakness and Strength", May describes Charles's ambivalence as a "*weakness-strength dilemma*". Because Charles is insecure (weak) himself, he cannot tolerate Helen's weakness. He wants Helen to embody the strength he lacks. Charles's idealism and sense of specialness and superiority compensated, according to May, for Charles's weakness. His idealistic striving toward perfection was stimulated by Helen's imperfection. Again, May reflects on Charles's problematic situation:

> Being soundly in love means a direct movement of the total personality, in which one person reaches out toward another on all levels without bothering much about the perfections and imperfections involved. One can define love as that attraction which appeals to one's strength rather than to one's weakness, that attraction which is not a compensation for one's own inferiority and not a means of finding neurotic dependence. (May, 1940, p. 68)

May, once again, links Charles's personal dilemma to our common cultural dilemma: "The weakness-strength dilemma is fairly common in our culture" (May, 1940, p. 66). May then asks, "What was the real flaw in Charles D.'s personality which had kept him from making a successful marriage decision?" (May, 1940, p. 70). His answer is that "he could not achieve a [balance in the] polarity between his *freedom* and *determination*" (p. 70). Charles could not accept that to a certain degree he was determined. He could only gain his relative freedom when he simultaneously accepts his determination.

"He could not relax and accept the facts of creation" (May, 1940, p. 71). Charles could not accept that he was partly determined by his body, by people in his environment, and by his destiny, which included the facts of life and death. Thus he could not fully enjoy pleasures such as eating or sexual love. He could not make use of his determination or necessity as way to cultivate his character. He could not use these determining forces in a creative fashion. Consequently, he could not use his freedom to mold his own character development. Instead of accepting these determining forces and thus gaining relative freedom, he enslaved himself by insisting on perfection – "he must choose perfectly and the girl must be perfect" (May, 1940, p. 71). He assumed a God-like position of superiority by judging Helen "minutely" and by assuming responsibility on her behalf. "He acted as though he were the arbiter of her destiny" (p. 71). After discovering all this in therapy and thus achieving "clarification", Charles was able to accept his own imperfections and "could make his marriage decision healthily and courageously" (May, 1940, p. 72). His marriage decision came several weeks after his therapy ended: He "proposed to Helen and she accepted" (p. 69). A year after Charles's marriage, he said to his therapist: "It turned out to be an excellent marriage [...]. [It was] certainly worth the neurotic agonies I went through at the time of my consultations" (pp. 69-71).

In the last section of Chapter Three, entitled, "Making One's Own Decisions", May states that to be free does not mean giving expression to one's impulses and desires without selectively keeping them in check.

> This was Charles D.'s mistake: he acted as though freedom consisted of promiscuous flowing out of oneself in dominating others. The failure of this concept of freedom is shown in his inability to make decisions. He was not autonomous; he was in reality enslaved by his need to dominate. There is no such thing as "pure" freedom – we can only use our freedom to decide *for* and *with* other people and things. (May, 1940, pp. 73-74)

Rollo May as "Philip" (May, 1981)

On January 14, 1987 I interviewed Rollo May at his home in Tiburon, California. In that interview (Hannush, 1999a) the following question-and-answer transpired:

M. J. Hannush:

Dr. May, in a chapter entitled, "One Man's Passage" in your book *Freedom and Destiny* [May, 1981], you present a detailed description of a case history of a man named "Philip". Toward the end of Philip's story you make mention of the following: "For some reason not clear to me at the time but obvious later, Philip then told me about his three years at Robert College in Istanbul where, on his graduation from college, he had gone to teach. The second year there he had felt pain-fully lonely due chiefly to the isolation in a foreign land where the English-speaking group was small and boring, and teaching English to Turkish boys was not that absorbing. Philip had followed his usual defense. He threw himself into his work with even greater zeal, but the harder he worked the more isolated he felt. Finally he collapsed and had to go to bed for a couple of weeks. This he called his nervous breakdown. He then changed his life style, he told me. He began to draw, he wandered around drawing poppies in the fields and old mosques in Istanbul, he gave up his habit of rigidly planning his life and began to take flow of energy as it came, but all without aim or sense of direction, isolated, feeling often like nonentity since all of his old ways of proving his worth no longer worked". Dr. May, this is almost identical to your own early life story…

R. May:

"Yes, I am Philip incidentally. Philip is, as he is presented in that book, a composite of different characters and that part of it is certainly me. It is amazing how much they are alike, isn't it. I never realized that once I write something I forget it and I may write it over again." (p. 133)

After graduating from Oberlin College in 1930, with a Bachelor of Arts' degree in English, May spent three years as a missionary teacher at Anatolia

College, in Thessaloniki, Greece. In his case history of "Philip", May simply substituted "Turkey" for "Greece".

In this case history, which is entitled, "One Man's Passage", May divides the life narrative into seven sections, the titles of which are intriguing:

1. *The Fear of Abandonment.*
2. *The Acknowledgment of Destiny.*
3. *The Confronting of Mother.*
4. *Little Philip.*
5. *Anger as a Path to Freedom.*
6. *The Green-Blue Lad.*
7. *Loneliness and Rebirth* (May, 1981, p. V).

Philip is described as being in his middle fifties when he enters therapy. He is gripped by jealousy because his partner and lover of several years, Nicole, expressed a desire to feel free to seek simultaneous relations with other men. She had threatened to act upon this unless Philip married her, which he was reluctant to do because of his two failed previous marriages. Philip is an architect; Nicole is a writer. They both have children from their previous marriages. As May, the therapist, listens to Philip the client he comes to construe an image of Philip as "a man of powerful idealism, reaching upward toward the sky which promised freedom, but at the same time unintegrated with and hopelessly bound to the mud [of the earth]" (p. 25). The reader is told that although the relationship between Philip and Nicole started off on a very harmonious accord – where there was tenderness, warmth, sexual enjoyment, and intellectual stimulation, there had also been an episode of betrayal, whereby Nicole had connected with a former intimate college friend with whom Nicole had fallen in love while on a trip to put her children in school. "Philip's world collapsed" (p. 26). But after a period of six weeks "Nicole got over her infatuation [...] [and] was back in love with Philip" (p. 26). Because of his "need for security" (p. 26) Philip did not question Nicole's promise of future fidelity. He offered her further financial support to keep her contented in his relationship with him.

But it was a second episode of infidelity that triggered Philip's seeking of therapy. Between episodes, Philip had his doubts about Nicole's allegiance to him and her motives for staying with him. But in an entry in a diary he says, "But I am very lonely" (p. 27). Upon his discovery of the second betrayal, Philip tries to be more accepting and accommodating of Nicole's actions. He asks himself, "Are we living in a new age, [...] when promises and rules and roles are all thrown overboard?" (p. 28). Although May the therapist does not say this directly to Philip, he feels that these so-called "*principles* [or beliefs] seemed to me to be rationalizations with a masochistic feature" (p. 28).

After a short hopefulness-restoring hiatus, yet a third incident transpired. May asks, "Why didn't Philip break off this relationship?" (p. 29). The feeling of love is not a sufficient answer, May writes. He describes Nicole as needing her "space" and "freedom" (p. 29). What, May asks further, accounts for Philip's inaction, paralysis, or passivity? Jealousy, he states, has been Philip's "Achilles heel all his life" (p. 29). And this includes his earlier two marriages, even though he was the one who initiated the divorces. May conjectures that, although Philip has been unaware of it, the roots of his jealousy started in the very early years of his life. Because of the time limitation imposed on the length of therapy – six weeks, May mentions that he had to use certain therapeutic techniques that he did not typically use. Although May does not name these techniques, the reader can surmise some of them from May's description of his therapeutic mediations. "One of my tasks in therapy with Philip was to get across to him that this struggle he was engaged in was bound to be self-defeating [...]. I pointed out to Philip how hanging on to this way of life [searching for women that will undo his childhood losses] was also hanging on to his mother" (pp. 33-35). In other words, May found himself using a didactic-interpretive therapeutic technique because of the short-term nature of the therapy. It is also possible that the use of the empty chair therapeutic techniques may not have been something May typically used in a naturally unfolding joint therapeutic journey. "At my suggestion, Philip had a conversation with his dead mother in my office. In the fantasy, his mother was sitting in the opposite chair" (p. 37). Or, in the same vein, asking Philip to bring a childhood photograph of himself and instructing him: "Philip, this little boy is in that period which you walled off, encapsulated. Please call him back to mind now. Have him sit in this other chair. Talk to him, and let him talk to you" (p. 39). And yet again, May instructs Philip to "*Imagine Maude* [his sister] *sitting in the chair now. She's been dead for two moths. Tell her what you really felt*" (p. 43). And lastly, May instructs Philip in the last therapy session: "*Please close your eyes and imaging yourself back at that time in your life* [his three years at Robert College in Istanbul] [...]. *Be that young man who had that "breakdown"* [...] *What is he doing?*" (p. 49).

1. *The Fear of Abandonment* (pp. 30-32):

May describes Philip's mother as having been a borderline schizophrenic. She was emotionally unstable and given to hysterical blowups. In her treatment of Philip she oscillated between tender, loving care and cruelty. Philip had an older sister who was without doubt a schizophrenic. She later spent time in a mental hospital and had subsequently died just before Philip started therapy.

Philip thus grew up in a home with two unpredictable women. He came to see his early mission in life as involving vigilance toward his mother and sister and rescuing them when the need arose. "Philip would understandably not be free, but rather would require that he be continuously on guard or on duty" (p. 30). May remarks that Philip was to reenact the vigilance he acquired early in life in his relationship with Nicole. He adds the following comment: "Freedom in such a situation would be like Michelangelo's half-finished statues of slaves: *freedom within the bonds of slavery*" (p. 31).

Just like his mother, Nicole alternated between being lovingly tender and brutally cruel. Her brutal honesty about her infidelities made her harshness doubly difficult to bear for supposedly she was acting upon the "principle" of truthfulness. Her unpredictability simply repeated an "old pattern" established early in Philip's life. In fact, May conjectures that it probably was critical to Nicole's attractiveness in Philip's eyes. Having learned that his survival as a child was contingent upon assuming responsibility for his mother and his sister, he now found himself having difficulty breaking himself free from the burden of excessive responsibility toward women.

> Another reason he could not break free was his sense of responsibility for the woman; his survival as a child had depended on how he responded to his mother and sister. Both of his previous marriages had been with women who "needed" him. He had a strong sense of duty to take care of women; the more crazily they behaved, the stronger was his need to take responsibility for them. These things were in some way twisted into the cords that bound him to Nicole and enslaved him. (p. 31)

Philip has been visited upon by "destiny" in the form of Nicole (p. 31). But instead of seeing it as a "roadblock", May views it as "an opportunity – indeed, a requirement – to work through the remaining problem with his mother and sister" (p. 32). It is only by seizing this opportunity that Philip will be enabled to achieve "personal freedom" (p. 32). A neurotic problem, which is a part of a larger complex whole, can be "fateful" in that it surfaces at a time in one's life and demands attention and resolution. From this perspective, it is a blessing in disguise. In his last therapy hour, Philip links his transformation in therapy to his transformative experience that followed his so-called "nervous breakdown" in Turkey [in reality, Greece]. "Philip subconsciously associated that [best] summer with his present moment [in the last therapy session]" (pp. 50-51). May interprets this as an expression of a therapeutic movement "from despair to joy".

As a child, Philip had felt the pain of loneliness. Additionally, he had experienced guilt at being healthy while his sister suffered from schizophrenia. This repressed guilt surfaced at times through the symptom of physical pain,

pain in the neck. A (physical) symptom does not arise by sheer "accident", but rather is a revelation of one's "inner destiny" (p. 32).

2. *The Acknowledging of Destiny* (pp. 32-37):

May begins this section by asking Philip to bring a photograph of himself dating back to the first two years of his life. Upon inspecting the anxious vigilance in the child-Philip's eyes, May infers that Philip "must have imbibed with his mother's milk the fateful "truth" that one cannot basically trust the world" (p. 33). A "schizoid mother" and a sister with a disturbed mind made up Philip's world in his first two years of his life. Philip had to adapt to this difficult destiny. Philip survived by developing an interpersonal pattern of placating and pleasing others and an ability to detach himself when in danger and keeping his real thoughts secret. Paradoxically, it was this acquired "talent" that included "hypersensitivity" to the intentions and desires of others – an almost "psychic quality", that contributed to the making of a successful architect and a likable person, especially in the eyes of women-lovers. "But one cannot make such compromises without penalty. The penalty came from the fact that whenever a relationship got below a certain depth, Philip became panicky" (p. 33). May likens the process of acquiring this compensatory relational style to the imprinting of a duck to a rabbit who repeatedly nipped [the duck] to drive it away to no avail. He then interjects, "I [Rollo May] felt like crying out to the duck [Philip], *For God's sake, go away and find your own mother! Don't continue just being bitten and hurt*" (p. 34). Even in his fifties, May reflects, Philip still looks "in the face of every woman he meets with the silent question: Are you the one who will make up for my loss?" (p. 34)

One of May's goals in therapy was to help Philip realize the futility of this self-defeating search for a "good mother" to compensate for the "bad mother" of his early years. His primary challenge as a therapist was to assist Philip in confronting and reconciling himself to his fate or destiny. He points out to Philip that to hang on to his mother is to hang on to a relational pattern. The missing mother cannot be restored. By blindly and repeatedly attempting to transform the bad mother into a good mother, Philip is hitting his head against a stone wall. He is at the same time cutting himself off from new and alternative possibilities. Simply stated, Philip was losing his freedom.

May points out that not only was Philip damaged by his fate, but a gift was also bestowed upon him by his early destiny. May asks rhetorically, "Would Philip have developed these talents which led to his high status in the world of architecture if he had not experienced such a disturbed family life?" (pp. 35-36). Agreeing with Alfred Adler, May adds that creativity can emerge as a compensation for early trauma. Freedom and creative possibilities, May muses, may be born out or in spite of the burden, loneliness, and pain of early childhood and adolescence.

Creativity may be the result of the disproportionate disparity between early disappointment and high aspiration. May concludes this section by saying that he wanted to assist Philip in accepting his destiny not "*in order* to achieve creativity [...] but simply because it *is*" (p. 37).

3. *The Confronting of Mother* (pp. 37-39):

May then encourages Philip to engage in an imaginary conversation with his dead mother and then to assume the role of his mother in the conversation. From this fantasy exercise, Philip gets in touch with his fear of his mother, of having to prevaricate in order to survive. Additionally, Philip asserts this stage of filial fright has come to an end. Through role reversal he learns that his mother, who had been orphaned, was a courageous woman who passed on her courage to her favorite son, that she did her best in taking care of a large family, and that, although she did not verbalize it, she took special pride in his achievements. The exercise ends upon Philip's expression of gratitude toward his mother.

4. *Little Philip* (pp. 39-41):

Next, May encourages Philip to talk to "Little Philip" (as he appears in his photograph as a little boy) and allow the latter to talk back to him. Little Philip tells of "how frightening it was to exist day by day in that atmosphere in the house with two hysterical zombies. It was constant inconstancy, unpredictability, insecurity, and especially loneliness" (p. 39). Little Philip had to be constantly vigilant "for the times they'd get upset". May encourages the adult Philip to view Little Philip as a guide, a friend, a comforting companion, and a protector; to perceive this part of himself as having not succumbed, but succeeded in the face of his problems. The adult Philip is thereafter grateful for this momentous reunion with his abandoned early self. His feelings of loneliness, emptiness, anxiety, and jealousy begin to subside. The adult Philip exhorts, "I'm not abandoned any more!" (p. 41). Accompanying this discovery is "the awareness of new possibilities". This is the beginning of "accepting [radical] acceptance" and the movement toward freedom. "Although this does not alter the original lack of basic trust, it does *surmount* it in the literal meaning of that term" (p. 41).

5. *Anger as a Path to Freedom* (pp. 41-44):

Next, May addresses Philip's repression of anger. He helps Philip learn the difference between unhealthy or pathological and healthy or integrative anger. Whereas unhealthy anger "curtails one's freedom", healthy anger "makes freedom possible". May then focuses on an incident in the relational life between Philip and his girlfriend, Nicole. In this incident, Nicole is cruel toward Philip, but Philip is not feelingly responsive to her cruelty. Here is May's response to this incident:

> *The reason you don't feel it is you can't admit your own cruelty – cruelty to* yourself *most of all. Today you are surprisingly like the little boy begging Maude* [Philip's sister] *and Mother, "Slap me, beat me, anything you wish, so long as you let me keep on living here!" Yes, I know that back in that home you had to be deceitful to survive, you had to cover up what you really felt and thought. You surrendered your freedom. You always tried to foresee what the other person's reaction would be before you spoke. You hid behind such laudable words as "responsibility", "dutiful", "noble son", and so on. But you must have hated those roles with Maude and your mother.* Philip: *Christ, yes!* (May, 1981, p. 43)

Thereafter, May makes two additional links. He connects Philip's repression of anger to his fear of losing control, as did his sister and his mother, thus becoming over-controlled. May also links Philip's denial of his own feelings to his desire to take care of his sister and his mother. *"You always prefer to be hurt rather than to take care of yourself even if it hurts someone else"* (p. 44). These linkages, May tells Philip, carry over into his relationship with Nicole.

6. *The Green-Blue Lad* (pp. 45-48):

At this juncture in therapy, the green-blue lad, who seemed not to have a precise age, appeared in Philip's fantasies. He personified Philip's anger. This lad was energetic, honest, open, and spontaneous. He stimulated Philip's sense of humor, for the lad was almost always on the verge of laughter. This inspired Philip to begin taking life more lightly, something he had not done throughout his life. He now was able to laugh at those times when he felt troubled and defeated. This orientation brought with it a sense of strength and self-efficacy. It opened up new possibilities. At the same time, Philip was getting in touch with his healthy feeling of integrative anger. Simultaneously, his feelings of abandonment and jealousy disappeared. When, "in therapy, he got angry at his mother in his fantasy, this led him, to his great surprise, to reveal how he secretly was appreciative of his mother's care for him and her gifts to him" (p. 46). Philip was now able to anchor his anger in the objective conditions which precipitated the anger – his mother's own difficult childhood and her having to take care of a large family without assistance, for examples.

Having confronted his destiny, Philip recovered his anger as a source of strength. "Passivity will not do" (p. 47). Philip is freed from perceiving himself as too "precious". Philip's newly found anger was freeing. Through its constructive expression, he gained important insights and was empowered to confront his destiny. "As Beethoven cried, "I will seize fate by the throat!" And out came the fifth symphony" (p. 48).

7. *Loneliness and Rebirth* (pp. 48-51):

This section focuses on Philip's last hour in therapy. In this final session, May asks Philip about his loneliness. Through a free associative response, Philip connects loneliness to honesty and the absence of mothering. May responds,

> *Isn't that the loneliness we all experience at times, the kind that is inseparable from the human condition? If you dare to be honestly yourself, you will be lonely. At each moment in our self-consciousness we are alone. No one else can genuinely come into our sanctum sanctorum. We die alone. No one escapes. This is destiny in the deepest sense. When we recognize this, then we can overcome the loneliness to some extent. We recognize that it is a human loneliness. It means we are all in the same boat, and we can then choose to, or not to, let others into our life. Lo and behold, we then have used the aloneness to be less lonely.* (p. 49)

Suddenly Philip, for "some reason not clear at the time but obvious later", interjects the following story:

> *Philip then told me about his three years at Robert College in Istanbul, where, on his graduation from college, he had gone to teach. The second year there he had felt painfully lonely, due chiefly to the isolation in a foreign land where the English-speaking group was small and boring. And teaching English to Turkish boys was not that absorbing. Philip had followed his usual defense: he threw himself into his work with ever greater zeal. But the harder he worked, the more isolated he felt. Finally he collapsed and had to go to bed for a couple of weeks. This he called his "nervous break- down". He had then changed his life style, he told me. He began to draw. He wandered around, drawing poppies in the fields and old mosques in Istanbul. He gave up his habit of rigidly planning his life and began to take the flow of energy as it came. But all without aim or sense of direction, isolated, feeling often like a nonentity since all his old ways of proving his worth no longer worked.* (p. 49)

After being encouraged by May, by way of a fantasy exercise, to tenderly embrace himself as a young man, and having responded feelingly to this invitation, Philip continues his story.

> *By accident [that summer, while on vacation] I met a group of fifteen or sixteen artists traveling and doing art as a group, and I got a job with them as a sort of fancy handy man. I traveled and made sketches with them all through the villages along the Caspian Sea. This was the birth of my becoming an architect.* (p. 50)

Philip goes on to describe that period "the best summer" he ever had, the summer where he fell in love and lost his virginity "with the greatest of joy." May reflects that having surrendered "his rigid and compulsive" expectations of life, Philip was able to open himself to "unexpected possibilities" including being surprised by joy. May links the movement "from despair to joy" in this story to a similar movement in this last hour of therapy. May then concludes with his thoughts on the phenomenon of despair. Despair, he says, which can be viewed as an opportunity, can result in insight that in turn can lead to change. He "hoped that Philip would experience his despair constructively" for it can lead to the discovery of one's hidden talents. Despair can eradicate our fear and open us up to new possibilities and a new freedom.

METHODOLOGICAL STEP TWO

The researcher distills the subject's narrative into concise language.

May (M1) as Charles (S1)

S1 (May as Charles) is ambivalent about marrying: he wants and does not want to marry. S1 reflects upon his college and post-college years. He views himself as deeply religious. He focuses his energies on developing his character. S1 is ambivalent about sexuality: he wants to experience the pleasure of auto/heterosexuality, but he wants to avoid the consequential guilt. S1 focuses his energies on setting up rules and resolutions such as keeping his body in shape, giving attention only to what is right, controlling his will, and becoming more friendly – the latter to combat his loneliness. S1 discovers that the more and harder he tries to live up to his resolutions, the more he fails.

Again, upon graduating from college and becoming a missionary teacher, S1 focuses his energies on building his character. He wants to acquire Christ-like virtues. His aim is to cultivate the virtues of patience, sympathy, strength of purpose, moral strength, and devotion to the call of teaching. His belief in God is very important to him for he holds to the conviction that he is God's "special representative" [May's words]. In time of turmoil, he tenaciously clings to his religion. Yet again, S1 discovers that the more and harder he tried to develop his character, the more he failed. He comes to the realization that his emphasis on character development is defeating itself. Instead of feeling connected to others and feeling less lonely, he feels closed off from others. He comes to the conclusion that something is wrong: that he did not feel selfless, real, solid, and genuine.

Upon the realization that the meaning by which he has been living is collapsing, S1 suffers a nervous breakdown. He had thought that with hard work he could shore up his previous psychosocial pattern that he now labels as an authoritarian way of life where he tried to live by rules and principles external to himself. He now realizes that he had tried to find meaning in life by subjecting himself and his desires to an external structure of authority through the exertion of sheer will. He had believed that his life was mostly determined by forces outside himself. This old belief pattern provided him with a short-cut security at the cost of repressing his desire for and affirmation of life, which included his erotic and other instinctual desires. For the sake of short-cut security he was attempting to squeeze all of life and living into a few rules and principles, for he was afraid of life itself. In the end, his soul became sick. He could not free himself from his ingrown prejudices and he could not transcend his self-centeredness which was lurking behind the façade of his seeming unselfishness.

S1 now viewed his moralism as a means of shoring up his prestige and as a way of pampering himself. He focused upon himself. He realizes that what he needed was to forget himself, to let himself go by letting his rigid rules go. He needed to set himself free by pursuing a spontaneous life. He calls this his romantic period. He approached his romantic relationships with courage and freedom. His orientation toward work changed. He ceased to take life too seriously. He worshiped experience. Walt Whitman's writings became his bible.

Still S1 wanted to contribute to his fellow-man. He wanted to help others, whose religious beliefs had failed them, to acquire the courage to let themselves go in love. But he also started to doubt the applicability of his new vision to the resolution of larger issues such as conflict between nations. He came to the realization that his Whitmanesque view did not account for the tragic elements of human experience. Consequently, his doubts regarding his new meaning or purpose in life intensified.

M1 (May as psychotherapist) interjects and reflects on the dialectic between past authoritarian lifestyle and present romanticist life-style. He assesses that as a result of his earlier partial psychotherapeutic treatment, S1 absorbed, reactively, the romantic self-expressive orientation to living without the corresponding structure to serve as a balance. M1 ruminates that structure provides the necessary complementary pole. Consequently, he was not able to acquire the leeway necessary for the play of opposites in order to achieve relative balance in his orientation to life. Just as he became more rigid in his authoritarian orientation as he felt it collapsing, he pushed ahead in his romantic way of life as it was collapsing. He lacked the creative courage to avail himself of either the structure of determinism or the freedom of spontaneous possibilities.

According to M1, when S1 was faced with a major life-decision – whether or not to marry and lacking this dynamic balance between freedom and determinism, he became frozen in a posture of ambivalence which he labeled as S1's "weakness-strength dilemma". While in the grip of his ambivalent stance toward Helen, he experienced a range of emotions that ran the gamut from passionate enthusiasm, to jealousy, to fear and flight. Because S1 was insecure (weak), himself, he could not tolerate his girl-friend's weakness. He wanted Helen to embody the strength he lacked. He used his sense of idealism, specialness, and superiority to compensate for his own inferiority. His sense of idealistic striving toward perfection and his domineering attitude toward Helen was stimulated by Helen's imperfection and seeming dependence. S1, as M1 sees it, could not accept and make creative use of the determining forces in his life – including the imperfections it bestowed upon him and consequently could not feel free. He thus enslaved himself by insisting on perfection. He wanted to look for the perfect woman or a woman he can make perfect. Additionally, M1 introspects, S1 engaged in two more self-deceptive and self-protective maneuvers in his approach to Helen and the question of marriage: 1. He hid behind the façade of selflessness or unselfishness to conceal his self-centeredness or selfishness; 2. He endeavored to settle his deeply emotional problems intellectually, which M1 says is a common error in Western culture. All this explains why S1 was ambivalent about this potentially life-transforming decision.

May (M2) as Philip (S2)

S2 (May as Philip) is in his fifties upon entering therapy. He is described by M2 (May as psychotherapist) as an idealistic man, whose idealism promises unlimited freedom, yet it is an idealism that is unintegrated with reality. S2's presenting problem is that he is gripped with feelings of jealousy and betrayal by his girlfriend, Nicole. Additionally, S2 is paralyzed by a sense of inaction and passivity in his relationship to Nicole. Because of his need for security, M2 adds, S2 bends backwards to accept and accommodate Nicole's intermittent infidelity. M2 traces the roots of S2's jealousy, which has been his Achilles' heel all his life, to the early years of his life.

M2 provides his reader with a summary of S2's early life and upbringing. He describes S2's early life project as that of being vigilant in relation to, standing by, and rescuing his mentally disordered mother and his sister. M2 reflects that part of S2's early destiny was not to be free, for he was always on guard or on duty. As a child, S2 learned that his survival was contingent upon assuming responsibility for his mother and sister. M2 adds that S2 was to reenact the vigilance he acquired early in life in his relationship with Nicole. Nicole's unpredictability, he tells us, repeated an old pattern established early in S2's life. Similarly, S2 had reenacted the same life drama in his two previous marriages with women who "needed" him and for whom he assumed responsibility. M2 interjects that therapeutic movement occurred when S2 was able to transform his early, fateful, and destined roadblock to freedom, which surfaced in the present in the form of painful loneliness and painful psychosomatic symptoms, into an opportunity for achieving personal freedom.

M2 tells us that as a consequence of his early upbringing, S2 was unable to develop a basic trust in his world. In order to survive, S2 had to develop an interpersonal pattern of placating and pleasing others and an ability to remain detached from others when in danger and keeping his real thoughts secret. Paradoxically, M2 reflects, S2's hypersensitivity to the desires and intentions of others became a "talent" that contributed to his choice of vocation and his becoming a likable person, especially in the eyes of women-lovers. The mental health cost came from the fact that whenever a relationship got beyond a certain depth, S2 experienced panic. M2 tells us that even in his fifties, S2 searched for a compensation for his early loss of secure attachment in the faces of mother-like women.

M2 set a therapeutic goal the aim of which was to help S2 realize the futility of the self-defeating search for the good mother to replace the bad mother of his early years. M2 wanted to help S2 confront and reconcile himself to his fate or destiny. M2 points out to S2 that to cling to the fantasy of finding a good mother is simultaneously a blind and repetitive clinging to a maladaptive relational pattern acquired early on in life for the purpose of survival. By hanging on to such a pattern, S2, in the eyes of M2, was cutting himself off from new and alternative possibilities and thus undermining his own freedom.

M2 points out to S2 that his early wounding fate was at the same time the source of his talent which has led to a successful vocation. In spite of the emotional cost, it was the source of his creativity. M2 assisted S2 in accepting his fate not because it contributed to his creativity, but because it simply *is* his destiny.

Through M2's therapeutic mediations and encouragements, S2 became in touch with the other side of his deep ambivalence toward his mother. S2 is enabled to resurrect not only his filial fright, but also his filial gratitude. He was now grateful for the courage his mother demonstrated and bequeathed upon him as a psychosocial inheritance; for doing her best as a mother under difficult circumstances; and for bestowing upon him the status of a special son of whom she was very proud.

Through M2's further therapeutic interventions, S2 is enabled to uncover and get in touch with his very early self, a self that was abandoned early on in his life, an untainted self that became a guide, friend, protector, and a comforting companion. With the discovery of this part of himself, S2 becomes more radically accepting of his freedom and destiny, of his strengths and limitations, of opportunities and immovable barriers. He is more aware of new possibilities, feels less enslaved, and more enabled to surmount, but not alter, his original lack of basic trust.

M2, thereafter, addresses S2's repressed anger and helps him learn the difference between unhealthy or pathological anger and healthy or integrative anger. Whereas disintegrative anger curtails one's freedom, he tells S2, integrative anger opens up one's freedom. M2 then links S2's repressed anger and the consequent surrendering of his freedom to his original fear of and responsibility for his mother. In assuming the early roles of a responsible rescuer and a dutiful and noble son, S2 had simultaneously repressed his rage and surrendered his freedom. Additionally, M2 links S2's repression of anger to his fear of losing control, as his mother and sister had lost control, thus becoming over-controlled. Lastly, he links S2's denial of his own feelings to his desire to take care of his mother and his sister instead of taking care of himself. This taking-care relational orientation is carried over into his relationship with Nicole.

Once more M2 succeeds in enabling S2 in getting in touch with his integrative anger, his healthily angry self, a self which is energetic, honest, open, and spontaneous. This healthily angry self stimulates S2's natural propensity toward humor, laughter, and openness to new possibilities. This healthily angry self became a source of strength and self-efficacy. S2 began to take life more lightly, something he had not done throughout his life. In addition, his feelings of jealousy and abandonment began to significantly subside. And, once again, he became evermore appreciative of his mother's care for him and her gifts to him. He was now able to see the objective conditions that contributed to his mother's difficulties and thus modulated his original repressed anger. M2 comments at this juncture that having confronted his early destiny, S2 was able to recover his healthily integrative anger as a source of strength. He was no longer frozen in a passive posture. Passivity, as a life orientation, no longer sufficed. S2, in M2's judgment, found freedom in confronting his destiny. By giving constructive expression to his healthily integrative anger, S2 not only gained important insights, but more importantly he felt freed and empowered.

In the last hour of therapy, M2 asks S2 about his loneliness. In response to S2's free associative link of his loneliness to honesty and the absence of mothering, M2 points to the inseparability of loneliness from the human condition. To dare to be honestly oneself is to feel lonely. To be self-conscious is to be alone. No one can enter fully into our subjective world. No one can die for us. This, M2 tells S2, is our existential destiny. And if we recognize our human loneliness, which no one escapes, we can overcome it to some extent.

It is at this juncture that S2 narrates to M2 the story of his post-college years. He tells M2 about his three years at Robert College in Istanbul, Turkey. He had gone there to teach upon graduation from college. In the second year there he felt painfully lonely. He felt isolated in a foreign land. He felt alienated from the small English-speaking group that surrounded him. Moreover, teaching English to Turkish boys was not challenging enough. S2 fell back upon his familiar defensive strategy: he tried to work harder. But the harder he worked the more isolated he felt. Finally, he suffered a nervous breakdown.

Finding that his old ways of proving his worth were not longer working for him, S2 changed his style of life. He abandoned his old habit of rigidly planning for the future. Instead, he tried to live spontaneously. He did this, however, without a sense of direction. He still felt as a nonentity without a sense of direction. By sheer coincidence, that summer, he joined a group of traveling artists who employed him as a handy man. He began to draw, which prophesized the direction of his future vocation as an architect. It proved to be a most wonderful summer filled with joy and pleasurable sexual adventure.

Reflecting on this story, M2 states that having surrendered his rigid and obsessive expectations of life, S2 was able to open himself to unexpected possibilities and joyful surprises. M2 then links the movement from despair to joy in this story to a similar movement that had occurred in S2's therapeutic journey in general and in the last hour of therapy in particular. Despair, he tells S2, can be viewed as an opportunity which can yield insights that in turn can lead to therapeutic change, the discovery of hidden talents, the eradication of fear, and the openness to new possibilities and freedoms.

METHODOLOGOCAL STEP THREE

The researcher embarks upon the transitional step of moving back-and-forth between the language of the subject, as distilled in Step 2, and a description of the subject's life narrative through the language of dialectics. Here the researcher is attempting to be selectively attuned to and focused on those dialectically thematic tensions in the life narrative that the subject is struggling with and attempting to resolve. For example, the researcher tries to answer the question, "Are there polar needs or desires that the subject is attempting to resolve which at first appear as opposites and mutually exclusive, but, at a deeper level, prove to be complementary?"

May (M1) as Charles (S1)

M1 observes that S1, who is in his early thirties, is experiencing a deep ambivalence (a "yes" is opposed to a "no") and an intense decisional anxiety regarding the question: "to marry or not to marry?" Upon reflecting on his college and post-college years, M1 sees more clearly that, as a younger S1, he experienced ambivalence regarding his sexuality. Looking back, he now perceives that there was a tension or split between his struggle to assert his morally resolute will (mind) and his untamable sexuality (body). Additionally, M1 sees that S1 was torn between being right versus being wrong and between being sociable and being lonely.

Again, gazing back, M1 now realizes that S1 experienced an intense tension between developing his character - by cultivating the virtues of patience, sympathy, strength of purpose, moral strength, and devotion to the call of his vocation, and thus attaining existential success, on the one hand, and failing in spite of trying hard to cultivate his character, on the other hand. In his aim to achieve true selfhood he ended up by feeling false: selfish as opposed to selfless; unreal as opposed to real; fragile as opposed to solid; fake as opposed to genuine; and ordinary as opposed to special.

M1 concludes that the reason he, as S1, finally suffered a mental collapse, a nervous breakdown, or a soul sickness, was because he was torn between two basic desires. On the one hand, he wanted to live up to or have control over, what he later discovered were, his rigid, authoritarian, externally-imposed rules, roles, responsibilities and principles (basic beliefs) by the sheer exertion of his will. On the other hand, he wanted to live freely. He felt caught between being self-conscious and self-forgetful; between being cautious and surrendering to his impulses; between taking life too seriously and taking life lightly; between living life the deliberate way and living life the spontaneous way. At that juncture in his life, after the emotional breakdown, S1 had, temporarily, swung from the authoritarian style of life to the romantic life-style for he knew not how to bridge these two basic and seemingly conflictual and contradictory desires.

The lingering sense of guilt over the tension experienced between his seemingly self-centered new orientation to life and his not-yet silenced desire to contribute to his fellow-man creates deep doubt in S1's new meaning or purpose in life.

M1 ruminates on the reason why S1's new orientation failed him. M1 concludes that S1 was unable to play with the polarities of his existence. S1 was unable to find a balance between his new self-expressive orientation and its corresponding complementary structure. S1 followed the same strategy for rescuing his new way of relating to the world that he used in his attempt to revive his old way of operating in the world. He pushed ahead in his romantic way of life as it was collapsing. He was unable to avail himself of a leeway that would allow him to straddle both worlds of structure and spontaneity for he lacked the courage and creativity to envision possibilities on both ends of the spectrum.

It is no wonder then, according to M1, that when S1 was faced with a major life-decision concerning marriage, he became frozen in a posture of ambivalence that M1 labeled as the "weakness-strength" dilemma. Under "strength", he subsumed S1's quest for idealistic perfection which promised to bestow upon him a sense of security, specialness, and superiority. Under "weakness", he subsumed his inferiority-and- insecurity-triggering imperfection that would render him ordinary. It was this dynamic and unresolved tension that contributed to his frozen posture and inclined him to abhor Helen's unpalatable imperfection and dependence. S1 entrapped himself in his own imperfection, which he projected upon and persecuted in Helen, by insisting on his quest for perfection. In his quest for perfection, S1 was unable to accept and make creative use of his limitations, including his imperfections. Additionally, M1 introspects, S1 hid his self-centeredness or selfishness behind the façade of selflessness or unselfishness as he endeavored to settle his deeply emotional problems intellectually. All this, according to M1, explains why S1 became frozen in his ambivalence posture and was thus rendered unfree.

May (M2) as Philip (S2)

S2 enters therapy in his middle fifties. According to M2, one reason why S2 is gripped with feelings of jealousy and betrayal by his girlfriend is that he is caught in the inaction/passive pole in the existential tension with the opposite, action/active pole. Moreover, from M2's perspective, S2 is also caught in the idealism pole in the existential tension between idealism and reality. Additionally, he is trapped in the struggle-toward- freedom pole in the existential tension between this striving toward freedom and the acceptance of one's limitation. In other words, because of S2's inability to come to terms with these polarities of existence, he is frozen in an inactive and passive stance. M2 further traces this indecision-producing imbalance to S2's original insecure relationship with significant others, especially his mother and older sister.

According to M2, S2's early destiny, which constituted an intrinsic part of his early life's limitations, was not to be free. This early destiny bestowed upon and burdened S2 with the original project of taking care of his unpredictable and disordered mother and older sister. Instead of being the recipient of care, S2 vigilantly assumed the prematurely responsible role of the protective and rescuing care-giver and care-taker. S2 was to repeat and reenact this dramatic relational pattern with his two former wives and his present girlfriend, Nicole.

Because of this early destiny, M2 reflects, S2 was unable to find a balance between trusting and cautiously mistrusting his world, between becoming securely attached and healthily detached from significant others in his world, between moving pleasingly toward others and moving discerningly away from others, and between moving pleasingly toward others and taking an assertive stance toward others. Still, paradoxically, in spite and because of the original loss (of basic security and at-homeness in the world), S2 acquired a gain: the acquisition of the talent of intuiting and being attuned to the intentions and desires of others which rewarded him with acceptance, admiration, especially from women, a talent that contributed to his choice of and subsequent success in his future vocation. To help S2 in his therapeutic movement toward change, M2 guides S2 in achieving the dual task of accepting his fate and destiny, on the one hand, and initiating and embarking upon an alternative path to the old repetitive pattern established early in life, on the other hand.

M2 points out to S2 that he is to accept his early wounding fate not because it contributed to his creativity and success in his vocation, but because it simply *is* his destiny.

To further his acceptance of his mother, M2 helps S2 integrate his emotion-laden internalized images of her by assisting S2 in getting in touch not only with aspects of the bad mother, but also aspects of the good mother – her courage, her haunting painful past, and the special status she had bestowed upon him, for which S2 is now grateful.

To further his acceptance of himself, M2 assists S2 in integrating his earliest untainted self with the later, but still early tainted self. This allowed S2 to derive guidance, protection, comfort, and companionship from this earliest, pure part of himself. It permitted this pure, life-loving self to radiate light into the darker corners of the self. With this acceptance, and the acceptance of acceptance, S2 is enabled to become aware of new possibilities and to surmount, but not alter, the original loss.

M2 turns S2's attention toward his anger – his original repressed rage and the resulting surrender of his sense of freedom in the face of his fear of his mother's and his sister's unpredictability and of his early burdensome responsibility toward taking care of his mother and his sister. M2 enables S2 to differentiate integrative from disintegrative anger, connecting the former to a sense of mastery and freedom and the latter to surrendering one's feeling of freedom and one's sense of control. Furthermore, M2 links S2's preoccupation with being overly-controlled to his original fear of the unpredictability of his mother and his older sister.

M2 then assists S2 in balancing his over-controlled self with his spontaneous self – a self that is in touch with his integrative anger, a self that is energetic, honest, and open, a self that has a natural propensity toward humor, laughter, and openness to new possibilities, a self that is resilient and efficacious. Through the gradual achievement of this kind of balance, S2 is empowered to take life more lightly, become significantly less tormented by feelings of abandonment and jealousy, become more appreciative of his mother's care for and gift of courage to him, and become more of an active modulator of, rather than a passive responder to, life's happenings. In confronting his destiny, S2 is enabled to find his freedom. In facing his passivity, he finds the strength to become an initiator and active participant in the stream of life.

In the last hour of therapy, M2 helps S2 confront his loneliness. M2 points to the distinction between psychological and existential loneliness, the former of which is linked to the early absence of good-enough mothering and the latter of which is part of the human condition. To be self-conscious and honestly oneself is to be alone and lonely. That is our human destiny. Recognizing and accepting this enables us to overcome our existential loneliness to some extent.

[It is at this juncture that S2 relates (in point of fact M2, under the guise of S2, repeats, though in a very abbreviated fashion) the story of his pivotal experiences subsequent to graduation from college. The story is very similar to the one related by M1 as S1. These experiences take place in Turkey, instead of Egypt. While away from teaching, instead of joining a group of roving musicians, S2 joins a group of traveling artists. It was at this time that S2 envisions his future vocation as an architect. As in S1's story, as related by M1, S2's narrative moves from despair to joy.]

In reflecting on S2's narrative in the last hour of therapy, M2 concludes that having surrendered his compulsive, driven, rigid, future-oriented planning style, S2 is able to open himself to joyful surprises and unexpected possibilities. Even despair, M2 tells S2, can be viewed as an opportunity which can yield insights that in turn can lead to therapeutic change - the discovery of hidden talents, the eradication of fear, and the openness to new possibilities and freedoms.

METHODOLOGICAL STEP FOUR

The researcher moves toward capturing essential life themes from a dialectical perspective. The researcher retells the life story of the subject in dialectical terms.

May as Charles (May, 1940)

At approximately the age of thirty-one, May is attempting to understand the person he was in a pivotal period of his life when he was in his early twenties. From the beginning, May constructs a dialogical relationship between himself as analyst, therapist and subject (the "I") and himself as analysand, client, and object (the "me"). At the age of thirty-one, he is attempting to understand his present ambivalence toward marriage. He attributes it to a deeper and earlier, unresolved ambivalence. By pursuing its roots, he uncovers long-standing dialectical dilemmas: He could not reconcile the demands of his moral mind and the call of his conscience and religious-spiritual vocation with the demands of his sexuality and the requirements of socialization. He comes to the understanding that his frantically effortful attempt, as a younger self, to become a "good" person simply backfired and led to a so-called nervous breakdown. The younger May could not resolve the dialectical tension between being unselfish and selfless and being selfish and self-centered; between being genuine and true to oneself and being false and pretentious; between being special, as God's representative, and being ordinary; between being spontaneous and free and being self-conscious and excessively cautious; between an externally-driven authoritarian way of living and internally-driven expressive-and-romantic way of life.

After the emotional breakdown, the younger May decides to pursue the expressive-romantic life style and leave behind the authoritarian style of life that had failed him. However, in spite of his best efforts, he experiences residual guilt-producing tension between his self-serving romanticism and his deep desire to serve his fellow human beings. The older May ruminates that one reason why this new romantic orientation toward living failed his younger self is because he had been unable to play with the polarities of existence. He was unable to avail himself of elbow room that would allow him to make creative use of both ends of the continuum and thus meeting simultaneously his needs for spontaneity, self-expression, and romanticism, on the one hand, and his needs for structure, order, and limits, on the other hand.

The older May provides another explanation as to why his new self-expressive life-style failed him in his early twenties. He labels it as the "weakness-strength" dilemma. Under seeming strength, he subsumes his early quest for idealistic perfection which promised the payoff of a sense of security, specialness, and superiority. Under seeming weakness, he subsumes his "inferiority and insecurity triggering" imperfection which would render him ordinary. The universal tension with which May is struggling here is: specialness [when stripped from a sense of superiority] *versus* ordinariness [when stripped from a sense of inferiority].

Above and beyond these explanations, the thirty-something May concludes that an additional reason as to why the younger version of himself was unable to come to terms with the tension-producing polarities of his existence was that he endeavored to settle his deeply emotional problems intellectually. In other words, he had failed to achieve a balance between his intellectual and his emotional side. He had sided with the intellect. He had used his intellect as a means of rationalizing his skewed approach to understanding his relational existence. All these reasons, the older May now realizes, contributed to his frozen posture in facing the question of marriage.

May as Philip (May, 1981)

[The publication dates of these two case histories or self-analyses, do not necessarily reflect the actual dates of publications – 1940 and 1981 respectively. In the first self-analytic work May (Charles) is thirty-one years of age; in the second (Philip), he is in his middle fifties. There is a gap of forty-one years between the dates of publication. But there is approximately only a twenty-four year gap between the claimed ages of Charles and Philip.]

Although May is now supposedly in his middle fifties when he engages in his second self-analysis, he revisits the same pivotal period of his life and once again confronts repeated residual themes with which he struggled as a young man in his early thirties. His presenting problem is, once again, a decisional dilemma: to continue or discontinue his relationship with the emotionally important woman in his life.

The middle-aged May ties his confusion-producing indecision to his stuckness between wanting to be free and accepting his limiting destiny; between trying to live up to his ideals and needing to remain anchored in reality; and between finding himself frustratingly frozen in a passive posture and desiring to assume an active stance by taking initiatives that will resolve his dilemmas. May traces his indecision-producing imbalance to his early insecure relationship to his mother and older sister.

May subsumes his early destiny – his early upbringing which shackles him with the fate of unfreedom, under "limitations". Our psychosocial maturation requires of us to find a balance between being properly taken care of and acquiring the capacity to take care of others. Because as a child May was not taken care of properly, he was stuck in the premature position of assuming the role of a care-taker – first, taking care of his troubled mother and older sister and, later, taking care of the other important women in his life.

Because of this early destiny, May was not only unable to find a balance between being taken care of and caring for others, he also did not learn to be (securely) attached and also to be healthily separated from the important others in his life. Correlatively, he did not learn to negotiate the terrain of open-heartedly and trustingly moving toward others and cautiously assessing or judiciously moving away from others.

May also recognizes that from primary losses can emerge secondary gains and liabilities can be transformed into strengths. To rise above his original dialectical dilemmas – to be taken care of or take care of; to trust or not to trust; to be attached or separated, the young May adopted the interpersonal strategy of pleasing others. He developed the talent of intuiting and being attuned to the intentions and desires of others, a talent which contributed to his acceptance, popularity – especially with women, and his choice of his future vocation, which opened the floodgates to his creativity and success.

May is in search of a new balance between acceptance and change for he had paid a heavy mental health cost for his secondary gains. In order to change and find an alternative path to the old repetitive patterns he had established early in life, May had to accept his early wounding fate simply because it *was* his destiny. He had to accept his mother as she was: bad and good. He needed to acknowledge her basic lack of presence and provision at the same time that he needed to affirm her strength and resilience, her courage with which he identified and which he internalized and the special son status she had bestowed upon him.

To facilitate further his radical acceptance, May turned the focus toward self-acceptance. Just as he had come to accept the good mother and the bad mother, he came to accept the good (spontaneous) self and the bad (skewed) self. Sensing that he had habitually tilted toward over-valuing his intellect and under-valuing his emotion, May shined a truth-disclosing beam of light on his deeply buried feeling of anger. By focusing on and comprehending his anger, May learned the distinction between empowering and disempowering anger. He learned that his disempowering anger was related to his fear and helplessness in the face of inadequate and unpredictable mothering. This un-repressed rage was now linked to his emotional and behavioral over-control and the skewing of the needed balance between freedom and spontaneity, on the one hand, and the need for modulated control and healthy surrender, on the other hand.

May was now able to use his empowering anger to make contact with his forgotten spontaneous self, a free and joyful self that had been there from the very beginning. From this true self May now derived comfort, companionship, energy, guidance, and protection. This authentic self, he discovered, was efficacious, honest, open, and resilient. It was a self that had a natural propensity toward humor, laughter, and openness to new possibilities that life had to offer. It was a self that was capable of taking life more lightly. It was a self that was an initiator, a participant, and a responder in the stream of life. It was a self that was more at home in the world.

May then applies his newly acquired sense of radical acceptance to his incessant and intermittent experience of loneliness. He comes to the recognition that there is a difference between intrapersonal and interpersonal loneliness. He traces the roots of his intrapersonal loneliness to the early absence of good-enough mothering. He attributes the origin of existential loneliness to our human condition. It is a byproduct of our self-consciousness and our search for authentic selfhood. This enables May to overcome his excruciating loneliness to some extent.

Thereafter, May reflects on his past way of being in relationship to how he lived time - his compulsive, driven and future oriented planning mode of living. By surrendering his desire to control the future, May is now able to become more present in the here-and-now and thus is open to the future's surprises, joyful or otherwise. May concludes his self-analysis by juxtaposing his hope for and despair about the future. Even despair, he comes to realize, can be viewed as an opportunity which can yield insights that in turn can lead to change, a change that includes the discovery of hidden talents, the modulation of fear, and an openness to new possibilities and freedoms.

Discussion and Conclusion

What our *EDP* method yields is a portrait of Rollo May as a young man evolving into a middle-aged man struggling mightily, creatively, and courageously to perfect himself as a human being. We see him, simultaneously, as a serious and playful, childlike and adult-like, playing with polarities of existence in his pursuit of the endpoint of self-perfectibility, integration, and wholeness, while realizing that we can never be totally mature.

May's rigorous reflections on his existential identity hover over his movement toward wholeness. We witness how May's maturing identity is a byproduct of an acute perception and awareness of his own unconsciously accumulated skewed modes of being in the world with others. This delicate mental and emotional operation is entered into and embarked upon with humility and compassion. In spite of repeated slippages, May tries to minimize the projection of the negative elements of his identity onto emotionally important others. He is seemingly able to integrate his affect with his reason so as to un-skew himself and thus achieve a precarious balance in other domains of his relational life.

In the pivotal period of his life, May is jolted out of his unconscious habitual behaviors and biases. He discovers the hard way – by suffering a nervous breakdown, that the self he had constructed through hard work and adherence to rigid structure was nothing more than an egocentric identity. He further discovers that a mature identity cannot be gained through the loss of the identity of emotionally important others. Neither can it be attained by attempting to control others or by being overly controlling of oneself.

Through deep and intimate self-reflection, May does not shy away from confronting his own dark demons – including his dark dread of the void which discloses itself in the form of loneliness. Against this backdrop, he becomes aware of his radiant core. Through contacting this luminous core and through his efficacious use of anger, May overcomes his perplexing and paralyzing passivity. He becomes active, alive, and, more or less, integrated. He feels freer and true to himself. He is life-affirming and more intrapersonally and interpersonally open. Above all, he opens himself up, again and again, to the untapped opposites within himself.

May plays repeatedly with the Spontaneity versus Superego polarity. The superego he is burdened with is the weighty conscience of his early childhood, adolescence, and young adulthood. Through this kind of repeated play, May restores his aliveness, his ability to be surprised by joy, by his love of life. Through play – playing with sensations, images, ideas, emotions, memories, in/action and relational tendencies, losses, life-narratives, and more, May is able to work through the stages of early adulthood and middle adulthood. Through play with opposites, May is exploring new identity elements and creating a new life narrative, which solidify his sense of self. Through such play, his early roles are comprehended, his past reinterpreted, and alternate future possibilities are anticipated. Through this kind of play, May is enabled to free himself of earlier restrictions that he imposed upon himself in the domains of intimacy and work. He is able to move more easily and freely within an acknowledged and affirmed set of limits that included his early destiny. Play gave him the leeway or elbow room to transform the seemingly mutually exclusive opposite elements in his identity into complementary polarities. Thus, modulated spontaneity can now go hand-in-hand with a lighter superego, a mature conscience. This gentler, kinder, and wiser superego becomes one's best friend rather than one's antagonistic inner executioner. This mature conscience is a life-affirming energizer.

Throughout his two self-analyses, May plays with the polarities of his existential identity, polarities such as freedom versus destiny, connectedness versus separation, and taking care of others versus being the recipient of care. Through this kind of serious play, which blurs the line of demarcation between work and play, he is able, relatively speaking, to bridge these polarities. By bridging these polarities he gives himself the clearance, elbow room, or leeway necessary for change. He is able to let go of old ways of thinking, emoting and doings things.

Through these playfully serious self–analyses, which themselves are a byproduct of a balanced achievement of the polarity, Playfulness versus Seriousness, May becomes acceptingly aware of his strengths and limitations. These polarities were at one time experienced as irreconcilable opposites: Strengths versus Limitations. He is able to ingeniously see the coherent continuous thread between the polarities that were central in the making of his own identity, in particular, and the polarities that typified American, western, and existential/universal identities, in general. He is able to view his own familial and cultural inheritance, retain valuable elements – such as his mother's courage and his father's desire to contribute to one's fellow man, and discard harmful elements, such as weighted conscience and the American valuation of appearance and pretense and devaluation of emotion. At the same time, he comes to the realization that every human identity, regardless of the family and culture in which it is embedded, is condemned to a struggle that aimed at finding a balance between universal polarities of existence, such Freedom versus Destiny or Connectedness versus Separation.

Still, the task of creating or constructing an individual-familial-cultural-existential identity is a daunting, difficult, and never fully completed life-project. The visual metaphor that captures the precariousness of this life endeavor is that of the tight-rope walker. It is hard because it requires of May to understand his own unconscious self as he repeatedly reviewed his past, especially the pivotal period of his life, where he suffered a nervous collapse. However, he was helped and strengthened in his quest for a mature identity by learning from and identifying with mentors and friends such as Paul Tillich (May, 1973). Tillich became an existential exemplar for May.

May is able to free the better side of himself to do battle with his demons and doubts, realizing at the same time that this dark side was shared by all. He succeeded in creating helpful images and sign posts in his writings for all of us. May pushed himself to think in terms of a familial, cultural, historical relative view and at the same time take himself into a higher, universal view. He is able to see into himself and his situation simultaneously. Through his insightfulness and the use of his emotions, he is moved, like an archeologist, to excavate his own constructed identity in a decisive and disciplined manner, intuitively trusting what he feels is beautiful or ugly, good or bad, truthful or distorting. It is through such rigorous digging that he uncovers the unconscious underpinnings of his desire to control himself and his emotionally important others. It is through such painful excavation that he finds a relative balance to the dialectical dilemma of Control versus Surrender.

Through agonizing soul search, May comes to understand that we all have a lower self; that there is an irrational, lower, and self-serving essence in all of us. It is this emotion-laden insight that, at least in part, enables him to become accepting of himself and emotionally important others and affirming of his wider identity with its contradictions and paradoxes. Acceptance for May has a pervasive spread effect. He comes to radical acceptance. With the acceptance of acceptance comes the paradoxical capacity for change. Thus he achieves the relative resolution of the dialectical dilemma of Acceptance versus Change.

What contributes to the making of May such an incisively insightful self-analyst is that he is able to listen for negatives in his own thoughts, emotions, speech, and behavior, negatives that are repugnant. Such awareness then prepares him to change these negatives into positives. Ultimately, he wants to conduct himself in a manner that transcends what he labels as his egocentrism. By contributing to his own self-perfectibility, May is able to hold himself together, to attain a precariously balanced self. He is then able to transmit to others – his readers, existential principles of worthy living.

Through reflection, May leaves behind regrets and resentments and achieves acceptance and perspective that are a byproduct of knowing where he stood in existential space. This kind of knowing is not only passionate, but also aesthetic and ethical. It is a type of intimate reflection that provides him with a deep sense of resilience. It gives him the strength to confront the dialectical dilemma of Passivity versus Activity. It enables him to move from the regressive push of passive innocence to the growth-and-change-producing pull of active responsibility or responsible action, guided by his love, beauty, goodness, and truth – his love of life, thus overcoming the dichotomy of Yes versus No to Life. Like Beethoven in one of his latest compositions, May would affirm this resounding ending, uttered against the backdrop of attunement to still Presence: Affirming Life; Accepting Life's Limits; and Changing through Acceptance.

The existential-dialectical-phenomenological (*EDP*) method has made it possible to analyze May's two so-called case histories, which in reality are self-analyses, in a way that has enriched our understanding of the slippage of life into work and back into life again. The *EDP* method has served as a fitting instrument of illumination that has enlightened our grasp of the dialectical relationship between the life and work of Rollo May. Beyond that, the *EDP* method has proved to be not only an effective research instrument, but also a therapeutic tool that can assist us, as it did intuitively for May, in playing with the polarities of our own lives in our quest for authentic existence. It promises to potentially transform our ambivalence in the face of our intolerably conflictual contradictions into tolerable ambiguities and thrust us forward, as it did for May, into the realm of creativity.

References

Abzug, R. H. (1999). The Deconversion of Rollo May. *Review of Existential Psychology and Psychiatry*, XXIV, Nos. 1, 2, & 3, 59-70.

Baxter, L. A. & Montgomery, B. M. (1996). *Relating: dialogues and dialectics*. New York: Guilford.

Bilmes, M. (1978). Rollo May. In *Existential-phenomenological alternatives for psychology* (R. S. Valle and M. King, Eds.). New York: Oxford University Press.

De Cavalho, R. J. (1999). Rollo May (1909-1994): A Biographical Sketch. *Review of Existential Psychology and Psychiatry*, XXIV, Nos. 1, 2, & 3, 51-58.

Hannush, M. J. (2007). An Existential-Dialectical-Phenomenological Approach to Understanding *Cultural Tilts*: Implications for Multicultural Research and Practice. *Journal of Phenomenological Psychology*, 38, 7-23.

Hannush, M. J. (2002). *Becoming good parents: An existential journey*. Albany, NY: State University of New York Press.

Hannush, M. J. (2001). Empowerment in Parenting. *Review of Existential Psychology and Psychiatry*, XXVI, Nos. 2 & 3, 181-199.

Hannush, M. J. (1999a). An Interview with Rollo May. *Review of Existential Psychology and Psychiatry*, XXIV, Nos. 1, 2, & 3, 129-141.

Hannush, M. J. (1999b). The Development of the Self in the Light of the Existential-Humanistic Psychology of Rollo May. *Review of Existential Psychology and Psychiatry*, XXIV, Nos. 1, 2, & 3, 73-103.

Hannush, M. J. (1985). The methodology of phenomenological psychobiography: The case of Richard Wright's Black Boy revisited. *Journal of Phenomenological Psychology*, 16, 39–68.

Hannush, M. J. (1983). The mirage of value-neutrality in the behaviorisms of J. B. Watson and B. F. Skinner: The nature of the relationship between personal and professional value areas. *Journal of Phenomenological Psychology*, 14, 43–90.

May, R. (1981). *Freedom and destiny*. New York: Dell Publishing.

May, R. (1973). *Paulus*. New York: Harper and Row.

May, R. (1940). *The springs of creative living: A study of human nature*. New York and Nashville: Abingdon – Cokesbury Press.

Schneider, K. J. (1999). Rollo May: Liberator and Realist. In Donald Moss (Ed.). *Humanistic and transpersonal psychology: A historical and biographical sourcebook*. Westport, Connecticut: Greenwood Press.

TOWARDS A PSYCHOLOGY OF HOMO HABITANS: A REFLECTION ON COSMOS AND UNIVERSE

Bernd Jager, Ph.D.

University of Quebec in Montreal
Canada

Abstract

Traditionally, psychology has sought to emulate the natural sciences by understanding and describing the human world and the human person as mere aspects of an all-encompassing natural and material universe. Where astronomers would observe stars and biologists frogs and bees, psychologists would scientifically study a particular biological species called Homo sapiens. *In the last instance, these astronomical, biological, geological and psychological studies all were meant to contribute to the study and mastery of a natural and material universe. It remains always possible, however, to conceive of psychology in a very different way as a discipline that takes as its ultimate object, not a natural and material universe, but the unique being of homo habitans, together with the non-dissociable human and divine cosmos where alone that being can fully manifest itself. Within that perspective we would come to understand natural science and the study of the material universe as one particular way of inhabiting a human and divine cosmos. In following this train of thought we would come to think of the natural sciences as chiefly associated with the workaday world, understood as the domain where homo habitans pushes back the limits imposed on it by a natural and material universe. By contrast, it is only within the domain of festive encounters that our eyes are opened to the true range and variety of the cosmic world and its inhabitants. Where the workaday world brings us natural science and technology, it is the world of festive encounters that gives birth to poetry, film, music, dance and thought. A psychology that allies itself with the natural sciences will pursue the goal of mastery of a material universe and thereby empower the workaday world. But only a psychology that draws its inspiration from festive encounters and that allies itself with the arts and the humanities will be able to fully explore a human and divine cosmos and thereby evoke the festive appearance of homo habitans.*

> The sages tell us, Callicles, that heaven and earth and gods and men are held together by community (*koinônia*), by friendship (*philiā*), by orderliness (*kosmiotēs*), temperance, and justice; that is why they call the whole of this world by the name of order (*kosmos*).
>
> – Plato, *Gorgias.*

All psychological questions ask implicitly about the genesis of a human world and our response to that fundamental question will frame our understanding of ourselves and our world. A natural scientific psychology understands the human world as a mere fragment contained within what it supposes to be a more original and more encompassing material universe. It similarly understands questions about our humanity and the human world as part of a larger natural scientific inquiry whose ultimate object is a scientific and technological understanding of a material universe. Within this perspective, the ultimate aim of such disciplines as psychology, sociology or anthropology is to restrict that inquiry to those aspects of human reality that can be linked directly to the functioning of a natural scientific universe.

All natural and human sciences are thus accorded their respective object of study. Botany chooses plant life as its object and zoology that of animal life. Sociology takes human societies as its object while psychology is accorded the franchise on individual and group behavior. But these objects all are thought of as forming part of the one ultimate object, understood as the physical universe studied and formally described by physics and astronomy.

These studies all presume that the cosmos, or the human and divine world in which we are born, live and die, forms but a small and inconspicuous part of the infinitely larger, and ultimately more important universe studied by the natural sciences. It follows that within this scientistic worldview our own common, everyday experience of the human and divine cosmos can lay claim to real knowledge only insofar as it is possible to directly link that experience to natural scientific revelations. This naturalistic belief system excludes from the start any systematic inquiry into a uniquely *human* world that as such is irreducible to, and ontologically distinct from the universal and material world revealed by biology, physics and astronomy.

It is important to realize that this scientistic understanding of human reality made its entry into modern life not as the result of a profound insight or conviction, but rather in imitation of a research strategy that had been highly successful in the natural sciences. Human scientists thought to repeat the triumphs of physics and astronomy by learning to regard human beings as material objects and the human world as a minor province in the kingdom of a material universe. Human scientists aspired to look at all things human the way astronomers taught us to look at stars and chemists recommended us to look at salt or water.

There is no reason to discredit this naturalistic approach to understanding our world and all that it contains, nor is there any reason to assume that it should be restricted to the natural sciences. This way of regarding and understanding is as old as mankind and can be credited with easing the burdens of labor and helping us achieve greater control over our natural environment. Nor can we maintain that it cannot lead to important discoveries in the human sciences or that it cannot improve our understanding of a human world. A scientific and materialistic investigative strategy becomes harmful to the human sciences, and to our collective intellectual and cultural life, only when it de-legitimates and atrophies other ways of regarding and thinking about the human world.

We have proposed that all psychological questions grow out of a particular understanding or pre-understanding of the genesis of a human world. The pre-understanding that guides the present inquiry maintains that our humanity is born with the building and inhabitation of a first human abode. Being human represents a certain distinctive way of inhabiting the earth. Humanity is bonded to the earth in a distinctive way that differs profoundly from the ways birds are attached to their nests or bees to their hives. Human beings move from one place to another in ways that are radically distinct, not only from stars moving in the sky or clouds drifting across the landscape; but also from animals moving away from or towards their shelter.

The distinguishing trait of human habitation is that it establishes and honors thresholds that are distinguished from natural or artificial barriers. The latter can be mastered by brute force or intelligent planning; the former can be crossed only by mutual agreement between a host and a guest. The threshold therefore represents a symbolic relationship that as such has distanced itself from a world of instinct, appetite and brute force. The threshold separates the human world from the animal world and opens a horizon of neighborly dwelling. As such it opens a world of dialogue, of prayer and sacrifice as well as of love and friendship. The threshold draws human beings away from the purely instrumental world of physics and the natural and instinctual worlds of plants and animals and opens to us a specifically human or cosmic world that is held together by myriad forms of conversation. It remains always possible to refuse to honor a threshold and to treat is as mere challenge to our strength or wit. The threshold opens a world of good and evil, of obeying the law of the threshold and of refusing to honor it. With dwelling arrives trespass and transgression; human vice finds no echo in the natural world.

A threshold embodies the typical and unique ways human beings are linked, both to the earth and the heavens, and to their earthly and heavenly neighbors. It represents a limit that all at once separates and binds human beings to what surrounds, undergirds and overarches their existence. Approached this way the threshold constitutes the ultimate foundation of a human world reflected in all building projects from the most primitive cave or hut to the most magnificent palace or city. We might even consider these buildings themselves as mere variations on the theme of the threshold, whose essential function is to hold separate and distinct worlds together.

This same threshold that separates us from and binds us to the earth and the heaven also governs our relationships to others. This is reflected in our most *basic* cosmogonic myths. We may think of Adam and Eve as making their entrance into a specifically human world at the moment they consented to take care of the Garden, thereby expressing their resolve to be good neighbors to each other and to their divine creator. They thereby bound themselves to the earth while yet refusing to fuse with it and to become wholly part of it. Nor did they as yet aspire to the position of their divine creator, whose Spirit "moved above the face of the waters" (Gen.1.1.). They understood that to become human means to bind oneself in a specifically human way to what surrounds, overarches and support our life. This specifically *human* bond forms the core of what is meant by the expression "to dwell on earth".

The birth of our humanity is therefore inadequately represented by the image of a first, ape-like creature assuming the upright position, or by the biological mutation that created an opposable thumb. Nor is it fully captured by a biological capacity to perform work or to fashion tools. A human being is not first and foremost a *homo erectus*, a *homo ergaster* or a *homo faber*, but he is first and foremost a *homo habitans*, a "being that became human by virtue of dwelling on earth".

It would be incomprehensible to suppose that the place where *homo habitans* took the first steps, spoke the first words and entered for the first time into specifically neighborly relationship, could have been a natural and material universe. Such a universe is governed exclusively by the laws of nature and as such cannot make place for a threshold and hence for a human body, a home, a temple or a city. Mankind's native habitat should be thought of as a *cosmos*, understood here as a unique and hospitable site that is made coherent, not merely by natural law, but by the law of the threshold that governs all human and divine interactions.

If we understand the cosmos as the home of divinity and the birthplace of humanity, we come to understand the natural universe as a partial and imperfect reflection of that larger cosmos. Within that context we come to think of natural science as itself a particular, ascetic form of dwelling that gives us an abstract and partial vision of the cosmos in the form of a natural universe. This universe highlights certain, otherwise invisible aspects of the cosmos, while it necessarily obscures others. It is one of the peculiarities of a natural scientific perspective that the objective observer, who adopts it and becomes absorbed in it, loses sight of the larger "cosmic" world that gives context and meaning to his explorations. Natural science therefore presents the natural universe as *sui generis* and as the absolute and ultimate source and foundation of all that is.

It appears that the universe of science can be made to appear in all its clarity only at the moment when the observer has drawn a veil over his own life and distanced himself completely from the inhabited world in which he lives and works. That universe appears then as wholly independent of the lived world. Yet the complete autonomy and absolute self-sufficiency of the physical universe is belied by the fact that it can be made to appear only to observers who inhabit a more encompassing human and divine cosmos. Every observation of the natural universe and every measurement and interpretation of a scientific fact presupposes an inhabited cosmos and silently evokes the miracle of its creation. If we understand natural science as the emergence of a natural, material and autonomous universe against the obscured background of a human and divine cosmos, we may understand phenomenology as the reappearance of that cosmos against the darkened horizon of an isolated, modern natural universe.

What does it mean to dwell?

We think of a cosmos as an inhabited world that is shaped and ordered by customary limits and divided by hospitable thresholds in such a way that human and divine encounters become possible. The fundamental order of the cosmos is therefore a *moral* order, guided by custom and ritual and governed by a threshold that both separates and symbolically unites human and divine neighbors.

As we have maintained above, all inhabitable structures, from homes to temples to cities, have the hospitable thresholds as their ultimate foundation and they reflect thereby a specifically cosmic rather than a merely universal order. This cosmic order separates and joins the sexes, the generations, and heaven and earth in such a way that they remain distinct and yet form a meaningful whole. We may therefore think of man and woman, of heaven and earth and of past, *and* present and future generations as *all* related to each other in the manner of neighbors.

To be a *neigh-bor* means "to dwell" (*buan*) "nearby" (*neah*) (E. Klein, op. cit., see under "neighbor") the other in such a way that one has to cross a threshold and perform the proper ritual to come into the presence of one's "near-dweller". As we have seen, the cosmos, understood as a *neighborly* world, is reflected or replicated in all inhabitable structures. A house, a temple or a city is not only marked by a threshold; it also shows an absolute and material limit that is made manifest in the foundations, the roof and the walls.

We may think of the walls that separate one house or one town from the next as representing a painful, original division that cannot ever be completely healed or overcome. Yet this division must be accepted as a condition for building a human life and dwelling in a human way. We are reminded here of the birth of an infant, understood as a first and painful separation from an all-providing mother. We think here also of the Genesis myth of Eve's creation out of a rib taken forcibly from Adam's chest and of the story of Adam and Eve being dismissed from Paradise. We find this theme of a fateful, original separation also elaborated in the Aristophanic myth as it is told in Plato's *Banquet.* This myth represents the birth of mankind as the result of a punishment meted out to an earlier non-human race of arrogant giants who refused to maintain neighborly relations with the gods. To curb their arrogance Zeus cut each of them in half, thereby hoping to make them more responsive to both the gods and to each other. This operation was at first unsuccessful because the separated halves found no way to interact with each other and thereby to create a human world. As a result they turned melancholy and succumbed to loneliness and despair.

The gods then reshaped the halves so they could face, talk and make love to each other. It then became possible for these new creatures to dwell together and to relate to each other in the manner of neighbors. It is in this way, so tells us the myth, that human beings were born.

Myths about the genesis of humanity are at the same time cosmogonic myths that tell about the creation of a divine and human cosmos. In the light of the Biblical and Platonic myths we come to understand the building of walls and the construction of houses, domains and cities as acts of material affirmation of an original, divine act of separation that broke a perfect world apart and thereby opened the prospect of a divided, yet neighborly cosmos. If the walls express consent to separation, we may think of thresholds as clearing the way to human and divine encounters, to love and friendship and to the coming into being of a human community.

It appears thus that the very structure of an inhabitable domain repeats, at the time of the construction of its walls and thresholds, a cosmogonic narrative that tells of the coming into being of a human world marked by neighborly relations. Every threshold that guards an inhabited domain repeats the myth of a primordial and perfect unity that preceded the building of walls and the creation of individual human beings. The walls speak of the disturbance of that unity, while the threshold speaks of a subsequent miracle of love and desire that reunites separate human beings and permits them to build together a human world.

We should note here that a cosmic or inhabitable space always refers to a space and a time that is inherently dual or plural, insofar as inhabitable worlds or domains necessarily point to *neighboring* ones. Within a house or a city we are never totally enclosed since the walls are interrupted by windows and doorways. An inhabitable domain therefore inevitably evokes actual or potential worlds that make it part of a larger context and accord it a meaning. To inhabit a home means to inhabit at the same time a neighborhood, a city and a world. We cannot truly inhabit a cosmos without maintaining viable relations with neighbors and neighboring worlds.

An ancient Greek proverb boldly proclaims that it is not possible to be human in isolation from other human beings. "*Eis aner oudeis aner*" can be translated as "one man, detached from his relationships to others is no longer fully human". If we extend the logic of that proverb we reach the conclusion that a house that offers no pathways to other houses, and that therefore lacks neighbors, is not a place fit for human habitation. That same logic also reminds us that if the earth were to become completely detached from the heavens, it would no longer be able to shelter human beings in a human way.

The essential dynamic of a cosmos concerns ongoing relationships between what we might call cosmic or *neighboring* pairs. The first of such a cosmic pair would be the earth, understood as the dwelling place of mere mortals, and the heavens, understood as the dwelling place of divine and immortal beings. The relationship between heaven and earth would thereafter be recreated in the bond between mortal and immortal beings or in that of host and guest, man and woman or native and stranger.

When the living sever their ties to the dead or when mortals no longer recognize what is divine, or when neighbors cease to have any interest in each other, the human world necessarily returns to an archaic and uninhabitable state. That archaic state can be symbolized by a house without windows, or with doors that remain shut to familiars and strangers. To confine one's life to such a place would effectively mean to lose one's humanity.

Cosmic order refers to the order of *co*-habitation. This order makes it possible for divine and mortal beings, for the living and the dead, for strangers and the native-born, for men and women and for members of succeeding generations to find common ground amidst profound differences. Such a cosmic order opens to us a world in which we live our individual and separate lives while yet being joined together by hospitable thresholds.

The antithesis of a cosmic order comes about with the destruction of thresholds and with the rise of barbarous societies that cannot bridge differences or interact in a fruitful manner with their neighbors. Such destruction turns the human world into a hostile enclave of competing material bodies that interact solely on the basis of brute force and the laws of nature. Cosmic order stands thus in the sharpest of contrasts to the uninhabitable order of a natural universe that is ruled entirely by a logic of material forces.

The cosmos reveals itself most clearly in a festive reunion of those who share a life together. The modern workaday world isolates us from the times, places and practices that reveal the cosmos and draws us ever closer the abstract universal world revealed by the natural sciences. Moreover, the sphere of work inherently stands apart from the festive world of revealing encounters. To enter it we to leave the circle of family and friends to face a world that does not specifically welcome us and where we survive and triumph by dint of our courage and wits and in the sweat of our brow. While we enter this indifferent world in the hope of mastering and improving it, we keep aloof and are careful to not to reveal our vulnerabilities. The world of work has become for us a world of stealth, method and strategy where we match our wits and our strength against an indifferent, soulless nature.

Descartes (1913), the father of the modern techno-scientific age, had as his Latin motto "*Larvatus prodeo*" (p. 213) meaning: "masked I advance". In assuming this stance he readied himself to enter hostile territory where disguise would be his best defense. Such an approach is fully adequate to the project of scientific discovery, but not to that of exploring a human and divine cosmos. Modern scientists have adopted this masked strategy to explore the natural universe and it is possible that in doing so they not merely followed in the footsteps of Descartes, but repeat an age-old pattern of stealth and subterfuge associated with hunting and warfare. Our modern scientists thereby show kinship with the first Neolithic hunters who left their comfortable settlements to enter the purely natural worlds of primeval forests and savannahs in pursuit of their prey.

Scientific observations become clouded in the presence of an all too evident display of human interest and desire. The practice of science, like that of hunting, demands stealth and anonymity and leaves no place for personal disclosure or individual manifestations. To rightly observe a natural universe the observer must for the moment lay aside his personal life, his age, his language, his sex and his dearest held beliefs. Only masked and skillful hunters know how to advance on their prey, and only anonymous scientists know how to wrest the secrets from a resisting natural and material universe.

We have established that thresholds are symbolic limits which embody the law governing human and divine relations. In contemplating a house, a temple or a city we note that portals and thresholds are places of vivid and personal interactions, while the walls evoke a silent world of fateful separations and separate destinies. Together they create a space of dwelling that fosters community while simultaneously bestowing on each person a separate life. The threshold not only separates and binds human beings; it also marries a private, intimate and personal realm to an outside, public and workaday world. The interior space of a home is like a harbor from which ships sail forth in all directions and to which they return to bring their gathered treasures.

The threshold that divides and then joins an "inside" to an "outside" sets in motion a dynamic of leave-taking and home-coming that inaugurates the temporal rhythm of work and play and of an active and contemplative life. This dynamic shows us that a home cannot exist apart from the path that leads from its doorsteps to the doorsteps of another house or another realm. This pathway interconnects not only neighbor to neighbor, but it also creates a link between a familiar world and the worlds unknown that surround it. We reinforce and elaborate such a path when we leave the intimate supportive circle of family and friends to enter the workaday world, or to undertake voyages to foreign shores.

It appears therefore that an inhabited space, no matter whether it forms part of a house, a city or a cosmos links together separate and distinct worlds that thereby are transformed into a symbolic or cosmic whole. We speak here of a "symbolic" whole because its parts are all at once held apart and kept together by virtue of an interconnecting threshold. The word "symbol" originally referred to a "pledge" or "token" that usually took the form of a coin or a piece of pottery that was broken in pieces so that each of the contracting parties would be in possession of part of the original whole. Only an inhabited world that is divided and reunited by thresholds can produce and use symbols and create symbolic wholes.

From whatever angle we approach the house or the city, it reveals itself invariably as a cosmos, understood as a place where the original, absolute separation symbolized by walls, becomes humanized through the addition of windows and portals that grant it access to neighboring realms. A house and a city become inhabitable by virtue of having joined together an inside and an outside, a heaven and an earth and a self and another. Building a house, a city or a temple is therefore never solely a question of labor and technical skills. Neither should we understand an inhabitable structure solely as a technical instrument that protects us from the naked elements. The building of houses, temples and cities should first and foremost be understood as a poetic achievement that repeats the genesis of a human world. As Mircea Eliade (1965) has so forcefully reminded us, a house is not, in the phrase of Le Corbusier, *une machine à vivre* but, on the contrary, "it forms a whole that imitates the exemplary creation of the gods, the cosmogony" (p. 55).

To enter a cosmos means to enter a world that cannot ever be fully encompassed by a single stance or point of view but requires exchanges with others. To disclose the cosmos we cannot remain stationary but must journey and accept a rhythm of coming and going, of entering and leaving, of living and dying. It is this temporal order that gives the hospitable cosmos its astonishing richness. This richness cannot be captured by violence and it is obscured by dreams of total possession and complete understanding. Persons and *things* make their true appearance only after we have renounced dreams of conquest and become reconciled to the fact that cosmic realities are destined to forever escape our categories and elude our grasp. A human and divine cosmos cannot be encompassed or controlled; it can only embrace us and be embraced in turn.

About the Meaning of a Modern Universe and an Ancient Cosmos

A close examination of the term "universe" reveals that it makes reference to unity (*unus*), and to a motion of spinning or turning (*versus*, past participle L. *vertere*: "to turn"). Perhaps the original image was that of a unified world spinning around a central axis. It is thought that the Roman rhetorician Marcus Fabius Quintillianus introduced the adjective *universalis* as a way to Latinize the Greek *katholikos*.

The Greek concept makes no reference to turning or spinning, nor does it to any other mechanical action capable of unifying a world. It speaks instead of seeing a particular thing or action in the light of a greater, preordained whole. If we translate *katholikos* syllable by syllable we come to understand it as a way of way of seeing or understanding something "according to" or "in the light of" or "in view of" (*kata)* "a whole" (*holos*). The Greek *holos* is etymologically related to the Latin *salvus*, for "saved", "preserved" and "safe" (Klein, 1971; see under "universal" and "catholic"). We are invited here to think of the whole that remains unchanged as we shift our focus and turn our attention from one thing or situation to another. The whole here referred to maintains its character and identity even when parts are added to it or subtracted from it. When we see a particular thing in the light of a larger and more stable whole (*holos*), we see it against the background of something that remains unchanged and that therefore is seen as something "preserved" or "saved". It is clear that neither the Greek *katholikos,* nor its Latin translation *universalis* can be thought to refer to anything resembling a modern, natural scientific universe.

The concept of a modern natural universe was described by Husserl's student, Alexandre Koyré (1973, p. 11) as: "an open, indefinite and even infinite universe that is unified and governed everywhere by the same universal laws and in which all constituent parts belong to the same ontological level". We already noted that the modern natural universe, understood as a completely self-sufficient, continuous and undivided world, leaves neither place nor time for a hospitable threshold. Such a universe encompasses a space and a time that *has ceased to refer beyond itself to another world.* It has become a space and time that can be observed and measured, but that can no longer be *inhabited.*

We may contemplate a universe, theorize at a distance about how it functions, probe it with our instruments and manipulate its substance in our scientific and technological laboratories. But all these probes and investigations cannot transform it into a place of dwelling. We can live a human life only within a time and space divided by thresholds. Within that space and time every door and portal is guarded by the god Janus who sits astride its lintel and looks in two directions at once. We can only live in a world that manifestly points to other worlds.

We think here of a child looking up from the intimate space of his bedroom to the starry heavens above. These stars evoke mythic narratives and poetic reflections that create a bridge between a comfortable personal world and a wondrous and distant *other* world. That same child may later discover the stars that guide sailors on their journeys, or that announce the seasons and determine the rhythms of public life. It is only much later, when the child has learned to take distance from the intimate space of home and hearth and mustered the courage to move beyond the paths and trails of public space and time, that he will be able to discover the mute and passive stars of astronomy and take delight in exploring the strange coherence of a material universe. But the stars of astronomy and the material logic of a natural universe can manifest itself only to someone who will return home after having explored the uninhabitable wilderness of a natural universe. To delight in the stars of astronomy is a privilege that is accorded only to those who continue to have access to the stars of myth and poetry.

If we are to understand *homo habitans* and are resolved to describe a lived human world in which it becomes possible to practice astronomy we are compelled to look beyond the natural universe and beyond the techno-scientific concepts and principles that were developed to explore and manipulate it. This cannot mean that we should ignore the natural universe or remove it from our intellectual horizon. It rather means that we should find a place for that universe and for the particular disciplines devoted to its exploration within the larger horizon of an inhabited human world. It will then no longer be the case that psychologists, sociologists and anthropologists feel compelled to search for a "legitimate" place for the lived and inhabited human world within the abstract universe of natural science. They will instead develop a different conception of the human sciences by seeking a viable, appropriate place for the modern natural scientific universe *within* the wider and more encompassing cosmic horizon of *homo habitans.*

About the Meaning of the Greek Kosmos

We should also explore the different ways we come to understand unity and order as these apply to a natural universe and a human cosmos. The unity of a natural universe is so absolute that it cannot support ontological distinction between an inside and an outside, or between a self and another. Yet, the unity of a cosmos is based entirely on such a distinction since its order issues from a threshold between neighbors. The unity of a natural universe constitutes an inalterable and literal fact that cannot be modified or destroyed by human actions. By contrast, the unity of a cosmos is the fruit of human and divine interactions that, like love and friendship, must be maintained in order to endure.

When T.S. Eliot in "The Wasteland" quotes the famous line of Yeats, "Things fall apart, the center cannot hold", he is not describing a natural event but refers to a human, "cosmic" failure. The center that holds represents the cultural labor of an entire generation just as it's falling apart testifies to the debacle of an entire civilization. It would appear, therefore, that the most important cultural and spiritual task of *homo habitans* is not the conquest of a natural and material universe, but concerns the preservation and strengthening of an inhabitable cosmos.

It is for this reason that our Greek ancestors thought of their political and social arrangements as *kosmoumena*, that is, as belonging to and conforming to the order of the cosmos. It is in the same sense that they spoke of public decorum and propriety as *kosmiotes*, that is, as reflecting the order of an inhabited world or cosmos. In the ancient world the idea of a cosmic order stood in direct opposition to the disorder of chaos, in the same way that a pleasing and welcoming human world represented the converse of an uninhabitable and disorderly one.

The Greek verb *kosmeoo* can be generally translated by verbs such as "to order", "to line up", "to array", or "to beautify" that are understood here within the context of festive and revealing human and divine encounters. The verb was used to describe the actions of a general "arraying" "ordering" or "lining up" his troops so as to bring them into readiness for a parade or for an encounter with the enemy. The Greeks thought of combat and competition as a revealing activity that could bring out the beauty, the force and the exemplary character of an individual. Homer's poetry concentrates almost exclusively on what combat and the struggle against adversity reveals about a human and divine world.

The verb *kosmeoo* was also used to describe the activities of a host or hostess as they busied themselves getting their house in the proper order to receive their friends. If we follow these indications we come to think of the cosmos (*kosmos*) as a place that is ordered (*kosmeoo*) in such a way that festive and meaningful encounters can take place there. Such "cosmic ordering" extended also into the personal realm of bathing, grooming and embellishing, all understood here as ways to prepare oneself for festive and revealing encounters. Hesiod (1959, pp. 72-76) used the verb when he described how Pallas Athena groomed and outfitted Pandora for her meeting with Epimetheus:

> The goddess grey-eyed Athena dressed and arrayed her;
> the Graces,
> who are goddesses, put necklaces of gold upon her body, while the Seasons,
> with glorious tresses,
> put upon her head a coronal of spring flowers,
> and Pallas Athena put all décor upon her body.

To this day we still use the word "cosmetics" for grooming aids, thereby unconsciously repeating the ancient idea that to embellish and to beautify oneself means to ready oneself for a festive encounter with family, friends and neighbors. Such beautifying invokes a specifically *cosmic* order in which heaven and earth, self and other, native and stranger are brought together so that they may reveal themselves to each other and thereby strengthen and embellish a specifically human or cosmic world. It remains ever possible to subvert the cosmological meaning of beautification and to use it instead as a way of masking rather than revealing oneself. This allows us to speak of "cosmetic" changes in the way we speak of "massaging" the truth. But we think in a more positive sense of showering, dressing and grooming as being preparations for a festive encounter. We think here of Socrates as he is described by Apollodorus at the beginning of *The Banquet* in Plato's *Symposium*:

> I met Socrates looking very spruce after his bath, with a pair of nice shoes on although, as you know, he generally goes barefoot. So I asked him where he was going, cutting such a dash. "I am going to dinner with Agathon," he said. (p. 528)

Within this ancient sphere of thought the idea of ordering and embellishing cannot be detached from the idea that human and divine encounters create the bonds by which a cosmic world is held together. Beauty in this instance is not a merely ephemeral moment that answers to superfluous aesthetic sensibilities. It answers to the fundamental order of a human world understood as a place of revealing human and divine encounters. Beauty forms an essential aspect of an inhabitable, cosmic world.

This ancient order of the Greek cosmos continues to manifest itself in certain common expressions that are still in use today. We still commonly speak of "getting our house in order" when we clean and tidy up our living quarters to receive our guests. Such "ordering" does not refer to the abstract natural order of a material universe, but evokes instead that of an inhabitable human and divine world. Such cleaning and ordering can be understood as "creating cosmos", if we understand by "cosmos" a place of meeting whose beauty and order inspire hosts and guests to open their hearts and minds to one another. House cleaning and ordering literally transform an unattractive, uninhabitable place, where the guests would withdraw defensively within their own selves, into an inviting and festive site that inspires open conversation and revealing insights.

The creation of such a festive place of meeting reminds us of ancient cosmogonic myths, such as told in the *Theognis* of Hesiod or in our own *Genesis*, that tell of the divine transformation of an uninhabitable chaos into a welcoming cosmos.

Something similar occurs when we "order" or "array" (*kosmeoo*) our thoughts and ideas while writing an essay or preparing for a public lecture. Beginning such a task always places us before a chaotic tangle of half-understood, confused and mutually incompatible images and ideas that must be disentangled and properly arrayed before we can find a place for them within the "cosmic" whole of a lucid essay or speech. This labor of tidying, ordering and embellishing serves the purpose of making our thought accessible to our readers or listeners, who enter our text or speech the way our guests enter a properly ordered and welcoming home. Writing or speaking in an intelligible and orderly fashion can thus be understood as a creative, welcoming act that derives its ultimate inspiration from creation myths that tell of the "ordering" and the coming into being of a human world.

We should note here that the cleaning of an office building or a factory floor constitutes a fundamentally different task from ordering, cleaning and beautifying a home in preparation for a feast. We clean an industrial building to promote the health and safety of the workers. We put obstacles out of the way to prevent accidents and to assure that the ongoing industrial, commercial or scientific work that takes place there can proceed without undue interruptions. It is within this same framework that we clean our garage or tool shed with the resolve to put it in readiness for future use. A purely functional space encourages us to confront a natural and universal world and to transform it by our labor. A welcoming and festive space, on the other hands, encourages us to cease our labors and to open ourselves to our surroundings. It invites us to reflect on what surrounds us while it encourages us to bond with others and thereby to create a more coherent cosmos. For us moderns work has become an unrelenting struggle with a natural universe while the effort to create cosmos has become devalued as mere entertainment or relaxation.

When we clean and embellish a place to make it ready for a festive meeting we participate in the order of the ancient cosmos. But when we clean and rationalize a space allotted to workaday, commercial, industrial or scientific pursuits we invoke the very different, abstract rational and functional order of a modern universe. We might characterize the order of the cosmos as fundamentally a *festive* order, understood here as an order that creates a time and space for meeting friends and neighbors. By contrast, we come to understand the order of a scientific and technical universe as a *workaday order* that permits us to interact fruitfully with a natural and material world.

We want to conclude this meditation on the meaning of *kosmos* with a fragment by the pre-Socratic philosopher Gorgias. Wheelwright (1966, p. 249) translates the keyword *kosmos* by "bright jewel":

> The bright jewel (*kosmos*) of a city is courage;
> of a human body it is beauty,
> of the soul, wisdom,
> of human action, virtue.

For contemporary readers the connection between civic order and a bright jewel is not immediately evident. We think of civic order in functional, workaday terms rather than in those associated with a festive order. We consider a well-run state or city to be one in which jewels can be effective produced, bought and sold, not one in which they are well displayed or worn. Civic order makes us think of sound government, of fair and equitable law, of disease control and sanitary conditions. All these are of prime importance to us because together they form the basis of a sound economy that is able to support a prosperous population. To our modern sensibilities civic order is akin to the order of a natural universe, understood as the ultimate, rational and material basis for all life on earth.

But Gorgias is thinking about the very different underlying order of a cosmos that makes possible human encounters and festive gatherings. At such gatherings jewels are worn and displayed rather than made, bought and sold. Jewels fulfill their ultimate purpose in radiating outward and illuminating a festive world. Such a world finds its ultimate meaning in revealing encounters, radiant beauty and sparkling conversation. Here even inanimate things come alive and are endowed with speech. As they speak, jewels do not proclaim their own beauty but sing the praises of the women who wear them and of the festive occasions that give meaning to a human world.

We cannot know exactly what Gorgias meant by courage, but we know that Plato in the *Republic* thought of it in terms of a steadfast rejection of corruption. He described it as "the universal, saving power of true opinion in conformity with the law" (Jowett, 1970, p. 143). If we lend this thought to Gorgias, we would conclude that the most appealing quality of a city, and one that would attract the admiring glances of its neighbors, would be that of lawfulness and resistance to corruption.

Again, it is easy to misunderstand Gorgias as recommending these virtues on the basis of their utility and their positive effects on commerce and industry. But the poetry of Gorgias is not concerned in this instance with an instrumental or universal order but addresses a specifically cosmic, jewel-like, festive order that brings people together and encourages them to shine. In this context, civic virtue also serves the cause of festive disclosure and not solely that of a sound economy. The jewel-like courage resists corruption, subterfuge and double-dealing because these hide the truth and darken the world and thereby harm the festive human encounters that hold the city together.

Can a Modern Natural Universe Replace the Ancient Cosmos?

We have maintained that the most pressing tasks faced by the arts, the humanities and the human sciences is to find a fitting place for the modern natural scientific universe within the larger context of an inhabited, human and divine cosmos. Modernity is particularly marked by its disastrous attempt to disconnect itself from its Greco-Roman, Jewish and Christian heritage and to replace the ancient cosmos with a modern naturalistic and materialist universe. It ceased at the same time to think of cultural activity as maintaining and building a cosmos and sought to redefine it as a progressive conquest of a natural universe.

As we have pointed out, the hospitable threshold constitutes the founding principle of a mortal, human world. This threshold lays down the essential conditions for human life predicated upon festive and revealing encounters between neighbors. Humanity can prosper only within a time and place that allows for fruitful exchanges between heaven and earth, man and woman, mother and child, native and stranger.

A fundamental trait of the modern, material universe is its radical "universal" unity that permits no reference to neighboring worlds and that cannot make place for cosmic thresholds or for human and divine encounters. Had we succeeded in fully actualizing this modernist project and had we been able to completely replace our festive and inhabitable cosmos with a natural scientific universe, we would have made both heaven and earth uninhabitable and made *homo habitans* an extinct species.

We cannot turn back from this disastrous modernist project and return to an earlier way of inhabiting our cosmos. There is no way back from lost innocence and we can therefore not escape the daunting cultural task of integrating the powerful modernist conception of a natural and material universe within the larger whole of an inhabitable cosmic world.

We have understood the threshold to be the founding principle of the cosmos and of all inhabited places, including the home, the temple and the city. It is the principle that limits and separates neighbors at the same time that it permits them to interact in ways that are specifically and uniquely human. A hut or a home separates and unites families, a temple holds separate and unites heaven and earth, a gravestone traces a threshold between the living and the dead. It is in the same way that the gates that lead towards and away from the city all at once separate and bind together an intramural and an extramural world.

A fundamental and irreducible aspect of an inhabited, cosmic world is that it permits the formation of pathways that lead from one threshold to another. This permits us to visit neighbors, to undertake pilgrimages, to transact commerce and to explore and discover neighboring worlds. Such visits and journeys inaugurate an entirely novel dynamic of leave-taking and home-coming that mobilizes all facets of our cultural life. In reflecting on our personal and communal life we should not lose sight of the fact that of all the creatures that live on earth, *homo habitans* is the only one able to cross thresholds and thereby link together various domains of an inhabitable world.

The primordial dual dynamic initiated by the threshold is reflected in various cultural activities that accord prominence to either leave-taking or homecoming. We think here of the practices of natural sciences as essentially leave-taken or *progressive* practices, while art, music, literature and thought can be understood as essentially conserving and homebound practices.

To hunt for game or to look for treasure we must leave the comforts of a familiar world and be willing to enter unwelcoming and hostile territories. The same is true when we engage in combat or seek to explore and conquer part of a natural universe. We may think of the hunter, the warrior, the scientist, together with the adventurer and the revolutionary, as masters in the art of saying goodbye to what is familiar and eager to take up the challenges of the road. To leave the homestead we must be willing to fight fatigue, to suffer heat and cold, hunger and thirst, and to forge ahead despite many drawbacks and defeats. In preparing for the outbound journey the warrior sharpens his sword or cleans his guns, the explorer trains his body so as to be able to climb mountains and cross rivers. The hunter practices the art of setting traps, of stalking and shooting, while the scientist rehearses the research strategies that will advance his explorations of the natural universe. All of these outbound adventurers hone their skills and train their minds and bodies so as to be able to subdue the natural world and make it yield its hidden treasures. The homebound journey serves here only to safely transport the conquered treasures: the hunter brings home his quarry, the adventurer his gold, the merchant his cash or his bartered goods, the warrior his bounty. The scientist brings home a treasure trove of mathematically elaborated observations that thereafter become a rich source for technological and material progress. The ultimate object of all these progressive, outbound journeys is to materially enrich and to physically empower the homestead and the city.

We conclude that the journeys of warfare, hunting, science and commerce all are marked by an active outbound phase in which the requisite skills and defining attitudes are employed and during which the essential purpose of the journey is achieved. It is during this outbound phase of the journey that the warrior pursues his enemy, the hunter his quarry and the scientist makes his objective observations. The homebound journey appears here as less eventful and demanding since it serves only to safely transport the treasures that were won during the outbound journey.

The journey of the poet, the artist, the thinker and the priest is quite differently construed. The most crucial phase of their travel concerns not the outbound but the homebound journey at the time when they compose their songs, formulate their thoughts and clarify the images inspired by the journey. They do so in anticipation of their return home when they hope to regale their family, friends and neighbors with stories and images that recount their journey. During this phase of the voyage they seek out forceful metaphors, effective gestures, strong images and evocative songs and stories that build a bridge between the hometown and the far ends of the world. By building this cultural bridge the adventurers of the human spirit strengthen the cosmos by situating their own world in respect to other worlds.

The power and wealth of the city increase by the outbound journeys of the hunter, the warrior and the scientist. But the city's cultural identity and the richness of its cultural life is determined by the homebound journeys of poets, musicians, painters, actors, priests and thinkers who situate their communities within the larger landscape of the cosmos. It is they who instill purpose and content into communal life while placing it under the expanding horizon of the cosmos. It is perhaps for this reason that artistic and musical performances appear to reenact a ritual of welcome that is extended to the hero as he returns home from his journeys abroad. That ritual casts the actor, the musician or the poet in the role of the returning hero and the admiring, applauding audience in the role of the hometown crowd that has come to welcome him back home.

We have noted that works of art, literature and poetry serve as a threshold that enable two different and distinct worlds to enter into a fruitful dialogue with one another. Such a dialogue can take place only within a festive atmosphere in which the participants fully open their hearts and minds to each other. By contrast, we see the spoils of war, of the hunt and of natural scientific explorations as forming part of a distinctly workaday world where *homo habitans* confronts obstacles and seeks victory over resisting natural objects and forces.

We may think of a place of dwelling as a harbor from which we set sail to foreign lands and to which we return bearing the material and spiritual fruits of our journeys. Without such a harbor there can be no journeys and without journeys there can be no human place of dwelling. Only a world in which we are truly anchored and have found our home can stir in us the spirit of adventure. Only a deeply beloved home and country can move us to explore a cosmos or a universe and awaken in us the thirst for outbound and homebound journeys.

The world of *homo habitans* presents us with a strange paradox that links mortality and human limits to human freedom. The paradox tells us that it is only by committing our life to a particular place and time that we gain the freedom to explore and understand our world. The cosmos does not reveal itself to a universal or abstract humanity or to human beings as they appear from within the perspectives of the natural sciences. The cosmos reveals itself only to incarnate human beings who have learned to dwell. It would appear therefore that our emotional, intellectual and spiritual life can come to fruition only by a loyal, loving attachment to particular places and particular persons. We can gain access to the cosmos only by entrusting our life to what is fleeting and mortal.

On the other hand, we gain access to a natural universe only by temporarily detaching ourselves from the persons and things we love and by donning masks and removing all identifying marks and signs from our person. We advance here in stealth upon a nature that we have come to confront, to conquer and to bend to our will. It is for this reason that we inhabit, explore, love and understand a cosmos, but can only calculate and mathematically infer the qualities and attributes of a natural universe.

The academic psychologist who studies human beings insofar as they form part and parcel of a natural universe must place himself at the same disciplinary distance from his subject as does the astronomer who calculates and measures heavenly bodies, or the biologist who observes the natural processes of animate bodies. There is no doubt that such a distancing, calculating and measuring perspective permits us to discover useful and interesting facts about human and animal life. There is also no doubt that this scientific and technological perspective has greatly enhanced the material quality of our life. But it is also true that this approach can reveal our humanity only as a natural thing among other natural things.

Moreover, such a revelation completely obscures for us the place or the standpoint *from which* it is possible to observe, measure and calculate a natural universe. That standpoint, understood as the very source from which springs natural science, is located, not in a natural universe, but in the human and divine cosmos that is the home of *homo habitans*.

References

Adam, C et Tanneny, P. (Eds.). (1913). *Œuvres de Descartes*. Paris: Cerf.
Eliade, M. (1965) *Le sacré et le profane*. Paris: Gallimard.
Hesiod. (1959). *Hesiod* (R. Lattimore, Trans.). Ann Arbor, Michigan: University of Michigan Press.
Jowett, B. (Trans.) (1970). *Plato's Republic* (IV, 430 a). New York: Vintage Press.
Klein, E. (1971). *A Comprehensive Etymological dictionary of the English Language*. Amsterdam: Elsevier. [See under "universal" and "catholic."]
Koyré, A. (1973). *Études d'histoire de la pensée scientifique*. Paris: Gallimard.
Plato. (1961). *Symposion* (174 a). In E. Hamilton & E. Cairns (Eds.). *The collected dialogues of Plato* (M. Joyce, Trans.).
Wheelwright, P. (1966). *The Pre-Socratics*, Odyssey Press, New York.

THE EPOCHÉ IS DEMANDED BY THE OTHER IN LEVINAS' "PHENOMENOLOGY OF ACTION"

George Kunz, Ph.D.

Seattle University
United States

Abstract

Amedeo Giorgi inspired his students to insist that their students reflect on the approach, as well as on the method and content of psychology. This has been my every class-opening for over 40 years. As a challenge to the reductionism and objectivism of mainstream psychology, Giorgi presented a mediation of the phenomenology of Edmund Husserl and that of Maurice Merleau-Ponty for the advancement of psychology. Such a psychology demands a special epoché, *a resistance from one's own efforts to the deep and destructive prejudices of modern science. Teaching this revolutionary psychology as infused with the dialogal phenomenology of Emmanuel Levinas, a student of Husserl, it is proposed that Levinas' major distinctions between totality and infinity, need and desire, self-initiated/self-directed and invested freedom, and between the «there is» and the «face», offer us further clarity to understand: a) the «enshrined characteristics» of science; b) the «problems of its method» for human study; and c) the needed «ethical adjustments» to make our science of the psyche even more scientific than that of the mainstream. This proposal resonates to Giorgi's claim in private conversation that Levinas was a "philosopher of action" and not a challenge to Husserl, the "philosopher of experience". Specifically, the importance of Levinas for phenomenological psychology lies in his assertion that the Other calls me out of myself to be empirical, to search for intentional meanings rather than "causes", and to go beyond value neutrality to act for the good of the Other. The goodness and neediness of the Other call me to a responsible* epoché *to attend to her/him who is always more than my phenomena, to shame my egocentrism, and to serve with simplicity, humility, and patience.*

> We will do, and we will be obedient.
> – Exodus 24: 7:

What's with the *epoché*? Why? Whence the mandate or inspiration? What's to be bracketed and *about* what are we to more lucidly attend? We've responded to these questions of *why* and *what* with the answer something like, "to get a closer and clearer understanding of the phenomenon, the «meaning that shows itself» existing behind the blinders of prejudice and embedded in horizons of contextual meanings to be held back enough to disclose its essence". Amedeo Giorgi taught us the power of the *epoché* to better guarantee the validity of our psychological understanding for empirical research and therapy. Not a one-time clean-up; we must be repeatedly challenged to purify our intentions to explicate the psychological. So, *who* makes this demand and about *whom* are we charged to *respect*? Is the *epoché* the independent initiative and sincere effort of the *observer* to understand the *observed*; or is it in response to the command by the Other to be understood in her/his world? Is the psychologist a self-legitimated voyeur? Seeking understanding peeking through the blinds with neither invitation nor permission? Or do they command *understanding* with respect by our *standing under* them with responsibility? Emmanuel Levinas helps us with his descriptions of the ethical command to respect the Other before the self (1961/1969; 1974/1981) and to escape from the burden of ego-centrism in order to serve the other (1982/2003).

In the sixties, seventies, and early eighties at Duquesne University, Giorgi taught Edmund Husserl's phenomenological philosophy, sharpened by the thought of Maurice Merleau-Ponty, as the foundational method for psychology as a human science. Fortunate to have been his student and research assistant from 1967 to 1971. I have been teaching psychology as a human science at Seattle University ever since. In conversations with Giorgi intermittently over the years and by reading his articles, I have sharpened my classroom discussions of psychology. He has remained the teacher of my students' teacher, even with our slight difference about Husserl and Levinas for psychology.

In the 1980's I deepened my understanding of the phenomenological *epoché* as I read the philosophy of Levinas. In 2007, Giorgi sent me a 1970 article by Levinas appearing in English in 1994, with his attached note about how he saw the difference between Husserl and Levinas. This article and Giorgi's note further deepened my understanding of the *epoché*, and sorted out our differences. Giorgi pointed out that Husserl's is a phenomenology of consciousness, while Levinas' is a phenomenology of action. With this distinction, I think Levinas has much to offer psychology with a way out of philosophy, especially for our work as therapists, researchers, and educators.

It is widely known that when only 23, Levinas studied under Husserl and Heidegger. It is not widely known that seven years later he, with Gabrielle Peiffer, translated into French *The Cartesian Meditations* (1936). Sartre credits Levinas with bringing phenomenology from Germany to France where it thrived as a philosophical movement. After WWII, he broke from Heidegger's thinking, whose *Being and Time* he had greatly admired. He rejected Heidegger's ontology as well as his politics; he found Heidegger's philosophical Dasein too like his political Überman. Besides the translation of *The Cartesian Meditations*, he wrote *The Theory of Intuition in Husserl's Phenomenology* (1963), gave lectures stretching from 1929 to 1977, collected by Cohen and Smith in 1998 under *Discovering Existence with Husserl*, and offered many other descriptions of Husserl's phenomenology which I find as clear as any. For example, he wrote, "The Phenomenological method permits consciousness to understand its own preoccupations, to reflect upon itself and thus discover all the hidden or neglected horizons of its intentionality", (1986, p. 14). He added, however, "Husserl's approach was always more abstract and ponderous – one really had to have one's ears cocked if one wished to understand his lectures!" (*ibid*, p. 15). He moved beyond Husserl while remaining loyal to *Husserlian* phenomenology. The title of his second major book expresses his difference from both Heidegger and Husserl, *Otherwise than being; or beyond essence* (1974/1981).

I begin my courses discussing Dr. Giorgi's claim in *Psychology as a Human Science* (1970) that every science has three parts: *approach*, *method*, and *content*. With these we review the mostly unchallenged presuppositions of mainstream psychology, then challenge them from a phenomenological *approach*, and offer a clear alternative. Our discussions returns to the six perennial questions first raised by the Greeks. Giorgi introduced me to MacLeod's book, *The Perennial Questions for Psychology*, (1975). Before discussing *method* and *content* we review this challenging but essential prerequisite work about *approach*. We take up these centuries old philosophical questions to see how they survive and change, especially when used to support the science of psychology. Overcoming initial resistance to reflection, students come to like arguing these perennial issues. They like Levinas' inspiration for a radical alternative to psychology: *a psychology for the Other*.

A First Look at Approach

With a *Husserlian-Giorgian* phenomenology and Levinas' further radicalizing, we look for problems in psychology with:

> The first question: what is the *ontological* nature of the human? Mind or body? Unique or common? Able to transcend or immanently trapped in nature?
>
> Second, the *epistemological* question: what about knowing? Sense or reason? Self-knowable or self-deceived? The psyche empirically visible or invisible?
>
> Third, the *ethical* question: responsible or caused by nature? Morals from society or self? The good for self-interest or for others?
>
> Fourth, the *aesthetic* question: What about beauty? Relative to each universal standards? More valuable, useless art or useful tools?

Fifth, the *political* question: whence authority and citizenship? Distribution of power and weakness? More fundamental, equality or inequality?

Finally, the *religious* question: bonded by independent choice or passive creation?

Bracketing beliefs in dependency we ask how we are *bonded* to others, family, ancestors, descendents, neighbors, everyone, even a Deity. Hint: the etymological root of re-ligion is from the Latin *religare* meaning to *re-* (again and again) + *legare* (to firmly bind). The enigma of religion: we *bind* ourselves to whom we are already *bound*.

Husserl challenged psychology by defining the psyche not as an object but as *consciousness intentionality* directed outside itself. Levinas challenges psychology by placing the self not at the center of the self, but in the Other. Classical phenomenology describes consciousness directing itself toward the world. Levinas agrees consciousness is directed, but aroused by the neediness and otherness of the Other. For both, "consciousness is consciousness of something other than consciousness itself". It can be seduced toward goods to fill self needs, or called to give for the needs of others. Husserl recognized the radical inter-subjectivity of subjectivity, that we associate and communicate with other conscious subjects. But he did not recognize that inter-subjective relationships are founded on responsibility to and for others; nor that objects become objective (transcendent) only when detached from the self to give to Others. Levinas radicalizes Husserl's radicality. His radicalizing of relationships provides necessary insights for psychology.

Fulfilling self-interest brings satisfaction, but inadequately – the morrow returns needs (1961/1969, pp. 143-144), and their fulfillment keeps the self trapped in itself leaving "nothing other than our powerlessness to take leave of our own presence" (1982/2003, p. 68). He writes "[…] indifference to all responsibility (for others) turns into monotony, anonymity, insignificance […]" (1974/1981, p. 163). The self can only escape its own malaise when centering itself in the Other (1974/1981). The very identity of the self is passively given. "The ipseity, in the passivity without *arche* characteristic of identity, is a hostage. The word *I* means *here I am,* answering for everything and for everyone" (1974/1981, p. 114). Down a paragraph he eases our anxiety from this extravagant language. "What can it be but a substitution of me for the others? It is, however not an alienation, because the other in the same is my substitution for the other through responsibility, for which I am summoned as someone irreplaceable. I exist through the other and for the other, but without this being alienation. I am inspired. This inspiration is the psyche." (p. 114)

Levinas describes what we all experience about the meaninglessness of consciousness attending only to the world of things for ourselves. In his early little book, *De l'évasion* (1935), translated *On escape* (2003), he offers the profound description of enchainment appearing in the form of suffering and hauntingly motivating the isolated subjectivity to escape – "[...] escape is the need to get out of oneself, that is *to break that most radical and unalterably binding of chains, the fact that the I (moi) is oneself (soi-même)*" (p. 55, his italics). Despite the inescapability from one's skin especially by an attempt to escape through pleasure or knowledge that turns out to be "an escape that fails" (p. 62) through disappointment and deceit, hope is not lost for the subject.

The self is offered escape from itself by the face of the Other jolting it out of self-centeredness. Levinas calls this jolting "traumatic" (1974/1981). The Other shows herself to be the most real of all reality, her call to be inescapable, fulfilling her needs to be the self's responsibility, her traumatic de-centering of the self, not by brute force but by an ethical imperative, and opened to be re-centered in the Other. Can I avoid the call? No! Can I turn away? Yes. Can I sabotage my own escape? This is the paradox. The Other gives me my identity by attracting my perceptual gaze, awakening consciousness, shaking up thinking, stimulating motives and emotions, investing freedom, and commanding service – which I can disobey. For Levinas conscience precedes consciousness. I am responsible before I am aware of my responsibility. The other person provokes conscience to arouse intentionality of consciousness: to perceive, to reason, to imagine, to remember, to feel. This provocation does not diminish but offers hope for goodness. Goodness reveals itself as coming from the Other.

A Return to Approach

Inspired by this de-centering of self and re-centering in the Other, we take a deeper look at the six *perennial* questions. Although Levinas places ethics as first philosophy, let's take them in the traditional order. *Ontology* asks about mind/body, unique/common, transcendent/immanent. For Levinas, ontological existence of the human is *embodied responsibility*. Humans are incarnate with eyes, ears, nose, mouth, skin to touch, arms to hold, voice to speak, lips to kiss, hands to feed, all to attend to the other (1974/1981, p. 67). "The trope of the body animated by the soul, psyche in the form of a hand that gives even the bread taken from its own mouth. Here the psyche is the maternal body" (p. 67). The psyche is the body offering goods from its comfortable sufficiency to give to the Other. The mother's womb and breast are the clearest example. Giving is the response to the command to give of oneself. It is not giving token left-overs or commodities exchanged for re-payment. The unique identity of each is not primarily because of self-consciousness and self-freedom, but because each is identified as irreplaceably the one at this place and in this time "backed up in its own skin" (1974/1981), designated as the one to be conscious of the Other's needs and invested with the freedom to be responsible for the Other. The self cannot escape itself by itself, but can be liberated.

The human is responsible before it is free. The neediness of others challenges complacent independence and establishes identity as the one called to transcend one's own bodily needs to offer its body to serve. On its own the self enjoys living from its hungers and happily filling them, but it is not fully human until it escapes, not by its own choice but by the pull from self-centeredness to the center of the others.

Natural Science Psychology has no center at all; well, maybe the organism. Obsessed with methodology, it has abandoned the psyche and subjectivity altogether in its reduction of behavior and experience to objectivity. Humanistic Psychology in its marvelous correction tends to be ego-centered. Existential-Phenomenological Psychology tries to liberate us from both but cannot offer psychology a way out of philosophy. Philosophy is reductionist and violent. Bernet points out that Levinas concludes both Husserl and Heidegger never got out of an ego-centered philosophy. "[…] Levinas essentially shares neither the epistemological preoccupation of Husserl nor the ontological preoccupation of Heidegger" (2002, p. 86). Psychology for the Other where the psyche is "ontologically" responsible can legitimate a radical psychology for therapy, research, and education.

Levinas' de-centered *epistemology* shows that we know by sense and reason: sensibility is the foundation of reason, not simply as the supplier of data, but as the provoker of reason, the origin of responsibility. Dermis and retina, eardrum and tongue and nostrils, all are the skin of the psyche knowing and being known. We can know and we can be deceive. An independent (objective) reality originates not from an independent intentional consciousness (subject) relating to the world in its horizons. Its subjectivity is *sensibly* shaken and commanded by the "proximity of the Other" (1974/1981, pp. 81-94) to figure out (*reason*) how to act responsibly.

Objects (food, blanket, kind word) to relieve needs can only be *objects* if they are detached from the self constituting of subjectivity. Objects for the self are constituted inside the subjectivity of the self; they are subjectized objects. To attain pure objectivity objects must be gratuitously given as gifts to those in need. Good old Dasein, "the being that in its being is concerned about its being" misses the point. He attaches objects to himself by his care; they are objects perceived as hand-able, as always already transformed by his subjective freedom.

But the threads of intentionality are thin when purely self-interested. They can break and lash back against the self. When these threads are thickened and toughened, the self refuses to give up its objects to others. Pathology is intentionality imprisoned in the chains of its thick and tough isolation. Health is when the Other's otherness and neediness loosen and soften the threads of intentionality to detach objects from the self's subjectivity and reattaches them to the Other making objects objective and the subject subjected. The transcendence of the object is fully achieved only as *gift*. The given objective world is a *gift* from others, to be *given* back to others. In the presence of the neediness of Others, the stuff of the world is not mine; its hers. Food from my table belongs to the needy other. Levinas goes so far to say, as we have already quoted, "[…] to take the food from my mouth for the Other" (1974/1981, p. 67). His image of the maternal psyche where the Other feeds off the self in the womb and suckles from the breast is a powerful metaphor articulated by Richard Cohen in his article, "The Maternal Psyche", in *Psychology for the Other* (2002).

This Other, whose neediness deposes me from the throne of my realm and claims my stuff, is ambiguously *visible* and *invisible*, *invisible* in her *visibility*. She is more real than any perceived object, more transcendent than any transcendental object, but I can't really see her. She commands my attention, but in her commanding reality, she is always beyond my perception. Levinas writes, "I do not know if one can speak of a «phenomenology» of the face, since phenomenology describes what appears. [But] access to the face is straightaway ethical. When one observes the color of the eyes one is not in social relationship with the Other. […] what is specifically the face is what cannot be reduced to that (the perceived)" (1982/1985, pp. 85-86). This foundation of the ethical *immanence* and *transcendence* of the Other for the self is both problematic for psychology and offers an alternative, a psychology for the Other.

It should be clear by now that Levinas puts *ethics* prior to both ontology and epistemology. The ordinary *proto-ethical* question of ethics is to ask if we are *free* or *determined* by nature. Then it asks if morals come from *society* or the *self*. Then if all motives are based on *self-interest* or can they be for the *good for others*? Recognizing the priority of the Other, Levinas gives us a *proto-ethics* where responsibility originates neither from *freedom* nor from determining *causes* in nature, but from the Other's command to be responsible. The Other says, without having to open her mouth, "do not do violence to me. Help my needs".

Levinas challenges "classical" phenomenology of Husserl and Heidegger founded on intentionality and freedom. He writes, "[My] book (*Time and the Other*) shows first some structures in the relationship with the Other which do not reduce to intentionality. It puts in doubt the Husserlian idea that intentionality represents the very spirituality of spirit" (Levinas, 1985, p. 61).

He continues this challenge by radicalizing their notion of temporality. "[...] the past, Husserl claims, is retained by the present, and the future is pre-contained in, or pro-tended by, the present. Time past and time future are modifications of the present" (1986, p. 26). In *Ethics and Infinity* he offers a phenomenological description of the experience of temporality, "Time [is] the relationship to unattainable alterity and thus, interruption of rhythm and its returns" (p. 61). Bernet, in his article, *Levinas's critique of Husserl* (2002), unpacks their difference when he writes that for Levinas:

> [...] the irreducible and irrecoverable alterity of the past should pave the way for a recognition of the other as the one who necessarily co-determines the meaning of my past. [...] (Levinas) attempts to establish that the past itself, in its most originary sense, is not my past but the other's past. The famous analyses of the "trace" and the immemorial do nothing else than establish the idea of past which, to use another famous formulation, "has never been present". The past, in this way testifies to the other's precedence over self-presence. (p. 89)

Therapeutic psychology can understand how the wounded past and the feared future can be made tolerable, meaningful, and even embraced in the present. The immemorial and irrecoverable past and the unanticipated and unpredictable future can be returned to the self by the other. How? By *forgiveness* of the past, *hope* for the future, *novelty* of the present, all gratuitous gifts from others.

Traditionally *aesthetics* asks if good taste is *relative* or conforming to *absolute* standards of beauty. It also weighs *useless* art against *useful* tools. With the priority of the Other, Levinas places *aesthetics* within responsibility. Beauty is enjoyed and sustains the self. Paraphrasing him, "we live from good art". The Other, however, can call us out of our aesthetic enjoyment to be for the Other. It is not a question simply of individuality or collectivity, but of the primacy of obligation. As far as I know, Levinas did not develop a specific aesthetics. He defined beauty as *unselfconscious splendor*, "perhaps the definition of beauty is the radiation as a splendor that spreads unbeknown to the radiating being" (1961/1969, p. 200). The flower is beautiful without consciousness of its splendor. The child shows her beauty as innocence. The other is always splendorously beautiful as the source of its own unselfconscious dignity and worth. The *cliché*, "everyone is beautiful" arises from this truth of unselfconscious splendor. Another *cliché*, "beauty is in the eye of the beholder", may hold some truth when applied to art. But it is seriously flawed when attending to the beauty of others. Everyone is splendorous when unselfconscious about their radiation. Ugliness comes when we sabotage our own splendor by self-initiated and self-directed attention for the deliberate exhibition of shape and form. The inherent beauty of the human person lies in their essential goodness. When irresponsible behavior contradicts this essential goodness it deceives those assuming this goodness, and lies about the radiating splendor of the person.

The *political* question asks about *inequality* and/or *equality* and the distribution of power and weakness. Levinas' priority of the Other over the self demands a *politics* of equality and justice already founded on inequality: the Other has rights over me (1981/1985, p 88). If there were only me and the Other, I would be ethically obligated to serve her without the right to demand a reciprocal consideration from her. Levinas writes, "I am responsible without waiting for reciprocity" (1982/1985, p. 98). Ethical relationships are not economic exchanges. When acts of goodness are initiated for the purpose of receiving a return, they are not ethical.

But what about the relationship between lovers? Certainly there is reciprocity there. Levinas has a section in *Totality and Infinity* (1961/1969) entitled, "Beyond the Face", devoted to the distinctive relationship between lovers. Its subsections, "The Ambiguity of Love", "The Phenomenology of Eros", and "Subjectivity of Eros", describe this relationship as both for-the-self and for-the-Other, or for-the-self by being for-the-other as ethical beyond ethical, the reciprocity here is beyond reciprocity. No love survives 50–50. "Love is not reducible to a knowledge (calculated sharing) mixed with affective elements which would open to it an unforeseen plane of being. It grasps nothing, issues in no concept, does not *issue*, has neither the subject-object structure nor the I-thou structure. [...] Its movement consists in going beyond the possible" (1961/1969, p. 261). The Other is beyond the other; she/he is the beloved.

Of course, I never find myself in a situation alone with the Other. My beloved and I hide in the "[...] night of the erotic, [...] the clandestine, the mysterious land of the virgin, simultaneously uncovered by *Eros* and refusing *Eros*" (1961/1969, p. 259). We try to exclude the third party, to remain intimate, dual solitude, closed society, the supremely non-public, but my beloved's others are implicitly present as are my own other others, her and my family, friends, associates. This is the beginning of the political. Levinas writes, "Everything that takes place here "between us" concerns everyone, the face that looks at me places itself in the full light of the public order" (1961, p. 212). "The third party looks at me in the eyes of the Other – language is justice" (*ibid*). Given the ever present "third" I have an obligation to those other Others as well as the immediate Other.

I do not have the freedom to be, or not be, responsible. This absence of freedom does not reduce me to impotence. I am called without choice, but must choose the manner to fulfill my responsibility. I can turn my back or give my life for another. I am not politically or socially obligated to give up my life or money to another when other Others, my family, my neighbors, any Others would suffer more. Equality is not the first principle for a democratic system; it is my inequality. The rights and justice I expect are derived from my inequality as obligated to Others. Justice founded on equality without unequal obligation of the self ends in conflict with everyone defending equal rights against the equal rights of others. Everyone would be an enemy.

The *religious* question asks how we are bonded to a creator and to "her" creation. The *proto-religious* question would ask if a supreme Creator knows and cares for each person. It asks if there is a bond established by *choice* or simply by being a creature of a Creator? Are we bonded to *others* or independently bound within ourselves responsible and answerable only to "number one"? Does the bond of *absolute dependency* enclose us in a unity with only the illusion of *independence*? For Levinas the religious experience is not primarily an allegiance and worship of God. He writes, "We propose to call "religion" the bond that is established between the same (self) and the other without constituting a totality" (1961/1969, p. 40). This description offers an unaccustomed way to consider religion. I ask students to bracket their beliefs about denominations, rituals, and dogmas and to reflect on the ambiguous but clear experience that the Other is both infinitely *close* in an inescapable bond and infinitely *far* away, beyond totalizing and being totalized. This raw religious experience of being simultaneously *close* and *far* from God is disturbing. The raw experience of being *close by* and *far away* from others disturbs even more. Our neighbor is more proximate. "[...] God reveals himself as absence rather than presence" (1986, p. 32). We are bonded to God not through a vertical conduit, but horizontally through love of neighbor. "Going towards God is meaningless unless seen in terms of my primary going towards the other person. I can only go towards God by being ethically concerned by and for the other person" (1986, p. 23). Religion, posed as belief in the mysterious *close* and *far*, rather than as an *either/or* bond to God is significant for psychology: we are both *alone* and *with* others. Are we singled out as responsible *for* others? This bond of responsibility defines us as a creature. This enigmatic "religious" experience that the good of the other is always our responsibility and yet always beyond reach, that the other is *immanently* here and *transcendently* beyond, that she is "in my face" and simultaneously impossible to "understand", is the haunting mystery that confounds psychology.

Ethical responsibility bonds us to those to whom we are already bonded. This bond is religious only if we can choose to re-bind, if we are not forced into a totality. We are bonded to others and to God without being swallowed up into a whole. Levinas says, "It is certainly a glory for the creator to have set up a being capable of atheism, a being which without having been *causa sui*, has an independent view and word and is at home with itself" (1961/1969, pp. 58-59). Ties to my family, tribe, ancestors, descendents, contemporaries near and far, even to God cannot be broken, yet I must choose to re-bind these unbreakable bonds. This is the mystery of religion. This is a psychological mystery: how to live lives paradoxically dependent and independent.

Levinas Distinctions

Before we return to review the characteristics of science Giorgi so carefully described with his phenomenological challenge, and before we begin rethinking these characteristics influenced by Levinas' description of the origin of the *epoché*, let us review seven of his distinctions: 1) totality and infinity; 2) need and desire; 3) activity and passivity; 4) self-freedom and invested freedom; 5) equality and inequality; 6) the said and saying; and 7) the there is and the face.

First, Levinas distinguishes *infinity* from *totality* (1961/1969). We totalize objects by cognitively grasping and manually using them. The hammer is *nothing more than* a tool to drive nails. We may try to totalize another person for our sake, reducing her to *nothing more than* a student, bus driver, beggar, or tycoon. But the other resists totalizing; she presents herself as *always more than* any label. And she is also *always less* than the characteristics of her public identity: the tycoon puts her pants on just like the beggar. From my perspective I totalize her, but from hers she is never reducible to my totalizing label. She introduces the experience of *infinity*: she is *always more than* whatever I know of her and try to reduce to a category and a use object. Given her infinite otherness, I cannot really reduce her. I may try, but she escapes my attempt to label her as "nothing more than..." I, in effect, reduce myself. She remains infinitely other. Her *ontological* existence is never simply another like an object is other than me. She is radically Other, infinitely Other. The origin of her otherness comes from her, not from my limitation. She is uniquely good, and I am uniquely responsible to respect her otherness, her uniqueness, her goodness. My freedom to categorize her is called into question; I am called to respect and serve the freedom of the Other. It is possible to exert my freedom from my center, and to "assign" her as *nothing more than* someone for me. But my freedom is fundamentally commanded by her infinite dignity to not reduce her, to not do violence, but to serve her needs.

Second, Levinas distinguishes *desire* from *need* (1961/1969). A *need* is a lack in the *self*. A *need* can be satiated when filled. Fulfilling a need for: 1) understanding (comprehension and certainty); 2) action (control); and 3) affectivity (consumption) are exercises of power. *Desire*, on the other hand, is the experience of the self «transcending» above itself toward the Other for the sake of the Other. While a *need* is satiable, *desire* is insatiable, not because it is too great a lack to be satisfied, but because "[...] desire desires beyond everything that can simply complete it. It is like goodness – the Desired does not fulfill it, but deepens it" (1961/1969, p. 24). It is insatiable on account of the character of its depth, not the extent of its depth, but the infinity of its depth. Desire is the response to the otherness and neediness of the Other; the origin of *desire* is from the Other. Not only is *desire* inspired by the *desired* but it has priority over *need*. The Other has priority over the self. Levinas sometimes uses the word «love» to signify *desire*. We experience love as placing the other before the self. However, he says, "I don't much like the word *love* which is worn out and debased" (In Robbins, 2001, p. 165). He reserves *love* for the specific relation between lovers (1961/1969, pp. 254 ff).

Third distinction: *radical passivity* has priority over *activity* (1974/1981). We *actively* initiate thoughts, actions, and feelings. But, we are *passive* to what is other than self, to the resistance and force of materiality, to the limits of our own body, to the rules and regulations of society, to the incessant flow of time, and especially to the interruptions of others. For those of us who consider ourselves in charge of our own lives, it is difficult to understand and accept our radical *passivity* to the revelation of the Other as infinitely Other, and our responsibility for *her or him* to be infinitely deep. We are more *passive* to the call to be responsible to the Other than any other *passivity*. We do not initiate responsibility. It is given before any choices. Although we can decide *how* to respond, and then act; obligation is given before choices and action. Responsibility is not a product of the self; responsibility is given by the *command* to *obey* the needs of others.

Levinas' fourth distinction is between *self-initiated/self-directed freedom* and *invested freedom* (1961/1969). Freedom is normally understood as «doing whatever one wants». But Levinas points out how this self-initiated and self-directed freedom is founded on a more radical freedom that is invested in the self by others. Freedom is not primarily capricious. It is responsible. While freedom is still freedom, it is to be used for good. It is invested in us by the other for the good of the Other. Freedom is *lent* to use as we want, but not against the good of the other. Using freedom invested in us by the other to violate the other is clearly unethical. We are allowed to use freedom for ourselves «by permission» from those for whom we are called to serve. We can neither squander this freedom nor use it to hurt the other. Self-initiated and self-directed freedom to enjoy life is wonderful. Mainstream psychology has tended to understand enjoyment only as reinforcement of behavior. Levinas has the richest description of the enjoyment of the nourishment from the things we live from (1961/1969, pp. 110-115). "Nourishment, as a means of invigoration, is the transmutation of the other into the same, which is the essence of enjoyment" (p. 111). He clearly and deeply reflects on enjoyment. He proclaims, "Life is the love of life" (1961/1969, p. 112). We live from good soup, good music, good conversation. However, when freedom enjoying itself violates others, it is unjustified. Our self-initiated freedom is called into question in the time and place the Other invests us with the freedom to be responsible.

Fifth, he distinguishes *social equality* and *ethical inequality* (1974/1981). Democratic *equality* is too often and easily considered our highest value. The violence of inequality when one person or group puts itself above others is condemned by all reasonable people. However, our own precious equality presupposes an ethical inequality where "*the Other has rights over me*" (1982/1985. p. 98). Unless we recognize this unequal, non-reciprocal responsibility for the Other, we cannot justifiably involve ourselves in the social, political and economic structures to fulfill our equal rights.

His sixth distinction is between *the said* and *the saying* (1974/1981). The *said* is information passed on. However, before this exchange of signification, the presence of the other *saying* "Here I am" is the first word. We are addressed before we address (Westphal, 2008). The Other's face with its independent dignity says this «first word» declaring its unavoidable presence before the self. This "here I am" is her declaration of independent existence and worthiness. It establishes the ground for whatever is *said*. This *saying* of the other is fundamental to any *said*. In return my *saying* is witnessing the truth of her revelation of presence. Responsibly facing the Other's facing, I say, "here I am. I am the one before you witnessing your saying *here I am*". The Other's *saying* is the revelation of her infinite otherness, her infinite dignity, her call for my responsibility. My facing her *saying* "here I am", affirms that I have «heard» her saying. *Saying* is the breaking through of the *Face*, the revelation of the Other. Levinas says, "The face speaks" (1961/1969, p. 66). This distinction is indispensible for «talking therapy».

His seventh distinction is between the *there is* and the *face* (1974/1981). The *there is* [...] is experienced as oppressive existence without any existent. It is the impersonal given like the threat of things in the dark without light to disclose. While existence is undeniable, no-thing shows itself in the *there is*. The easy but illusory escape from the horror of the *there is* [...] is through the world that provides light, sound, nourishment and enjoyment. But this haunting, rustling existence without any human existent, cannot bring escape. Isolation without any meaning from another brings horror. Stuff brings temporary respite but no escape from the there is... His best examples are when: "[I]n insomnia one can and one cannot say that there is an «I» which cannot manage to fall asleep. The impossibility of escaping wakefulness is something «objective», independent of my initiative. This impersonality absorbs my consciousness. I do not stay awake: «it» stays awake" (1982/1985, p. 49), and, "The indifference of neutrality turns into monotony, anonymity, insignificance, into an incessant buzzing that nothing can stop and which absorbs all signification" (1974/1981, p. 163). The schizophrenic receives impersonal voices and visions coming at him without sound and reflection of light, for which he must make sense. At one time or another all of us experience fear of «existence without existents». It is horror and panic, isolation, boredom, depression, the paranoia of being left alone. While Levinas describes it as neither *nothingness* nor *being*, he writes that it is "the phenomenon of being: *it*" (1982/1985, p. 48). There is an emptiness that is not nothingness, a terror without a terrible, an obsession without something obsessed, an awfulness without an existent awed.

The *face*, on the other hand, is the presence of another whose needs open the door for the ego haunted by the lonely rumbling of the *there is* to escape. The *face* of the other frees the self from oppressive existence by calling it out of the *there is* to responsibly respond. The uprightness of the *face*, its exposure, without defense calls the self out of its self-imposed night without the light of signification. The *face* signifies herself without context. While she always has a situation, a title, a location and status that the self knows as meaningful, she provides beyond and prior to these her own context. She is meaning all by itself. She is who she is without needing a context to designate her as «a someone». The face's meaning consists first in saying: "Here I am. Thou shalt not kill". This prohibition is a commandment whose authority comes from her independent and infinite worthiness yet vulnerability, her dignity in her destitution.

Each of these seven distinctions challenge those philosophical and psychological approaches founded on characteristics rooted in nature, as independent of others, and as only self-interested and self-affirming. The subject of natural science psychology is basically ego-centric. The subject of a Levinas inspired psychology is altero-centric. "[...] responsibility is the essential, primary and fundamental structure of (human) subjectivity. [...] responsibility is responsibility for the Other, thus as responsibility for what is not my deed, or for what does not even matter to me; or which precisely does matter to me, is met by me as face (1982/1985, p. 95).

Back to the Epoché

We can return to the topic of the origin of the *epoché*. Giorgi (1970) articulated the characteristics of the methods of science: "In essence, the approach of psychology conceived as a natural sciences is characterized as being *empirical*, *positivist*, *reductionist*, *genetic*, *deterministic*, *predictive*, and posits the idea of the *independent observer*" (pp. 61-62). He then identified the problems of each of these characteristics borrowed from natural science when adopted in a science of the human. He has offered a phenomenological adjustment of these characteristics for the epoché in psychology as a human science.

Levinas deepens the *epoché* for human science by recognizing an ethical imperative for *goodness* not just for *truth*. With this demand Levinas inspires us to make further adjustments to the characteristics of science by giving them an ethical foundation. Let's look at the five characteristics of science, phenomenologically challenge each, and describe Levinas' deepening contribution.

First, natural science is *empirical* defining itself as "relying on or derived from observation, experimentation, or measurement" (Tavris and Wade, 2001, p. 552). Experimentation under controlled conditions is generally considered the most reliable empirical method. Phenomenology warns us that the very act of controlling variables in a laboratory or observing events in the field does not allow the *meaning* of the phenomenon to be expressed independently of the observer's heavy handed control. Positing a hypothesis (predicting what will happen), controlling variables (disallowing the influence of meaningful conditions) and manipulating variables (applying an independent "cause" to change a dependent behavior rather than allowing meanings to be experienced), translating qualitative meanings into quantitative assessments (moving further away from the meanings naturally described by ordinary language) – all these characteristics of what has been required empirical guards are loaded with theoretical land-mines about the nature of the human that can sabotage the possibility of the psychological showing itself.

Levinas adds a dimension to the phenomenological understanding of empirical. Human Science defines *empirical* as allowing the phenomenon to show itself and describing it in language closest to the meaning without translation into theory or numbers. Levinas' insistence that the Other is the source of her own revelation of otherness and worthiness without the prejudgments of the observer reduces the traditional notion of empirical by showing how the other shows herself. The restraint on the observer to hold back prejudgments originates not from the human scientist's choice but from the ethical command of the observed to the observer to not do violence, to not impose significations, to not describe the other's phenomena with language other than that of the psychological participant.

The phenomenological observer observes and describes from her point of view, but that point of view is commanded to ethically accept the Other beyond the realm of the observer's perceptual observation. This is troublesome. How can one observe what is unobservable? Awakened from the dream of the self to attend, not to the essence of the other, but to responsibility; this is the origin of the *epoché*. This is the gift from the Other. This is the place where the command from the Other tells us to *know by not knowing*. This radical placing the relationship with the Other into the ethical realm and not from the ordinarily designated epistemological realm establishes the strongest form of the *epoché*.

The *epoché* from which all other "*epochés*" are modeled is from the trauma by the entrance of the Other onto the stage of my existence calling forth a radical self-skepticism. The *epoché* is the self-skepticism commanded by the Other. Here is another *existent* revealing meaning beyond mine. I am called into question. I am *epochéd*, if you will. Levinas' description of the infinite otherness of the Other beyond the knowing of the self strengthens the phenomenological argument against the narrow empiricism of mainstream research. To allow the "phenomena" of the Other to show themselves primarily by responsibility rather than knowledge recognizes her reality to be revealed by her before it is disclosed by the observer's cognitive efforts.

Natural Science does re-search: it searches again to verify what it has already hypothesized. Human Science discloses essences with its *epoché*: it illumines with its philosophy of the intentionality of consciousness. Psychology for the Other inspired by Levinas allows the Other to reveal herself by calling into question, by traumatizing, *epoché-ing*, the observer.

Second, natural science defines *objective*, the claim of positivism, as reality existing independently of subjectivity. Positivism assumes reality exists already within classes and subclasses and with properties distinguishing members from those of other classes. Science sets up controls and claims to observes what is there. It is basically taxonomy. Scientists observe specific members in their naturally given *objective* classes and describe their *objective* properties. Giorgi points out well that "[...] "objective" methods do not remove the presence of the researcher, they simply make him present in another way" (1970, p. 166). Phenomenology tells us that subject and object are not split. "The presence of the world cannot be independent of the knowing subject. The subject cannot know without a world to be known" (Husserl, *Ideas,* 1931, p. 35). Levinas adds to this subject/object relationship by showing that reality is only fully objective when it is detached from the subjectivity of the observer by the ethical command to responsibly release ownership of it in order to *give* it to the Other. All reality, all creation, is a gift from a Creator, but we experience it as given through Others to be given back to others to fill the needs of Others. Objectivity (disinterestedness) is not gotten by an epistemological mental strategy but by an interest detached from self-interest which is commanded by the Other's needs.

Third, natural science defines *reduction* as breaking the phenomenon down to its smallest parts and using the simplest explanation rather than one more complex. The law of parsimony demands an economy of assumptions in logical formulations. If the laws of cause and effect seem simpler than intentional meanings, if a biological explanation is simpler than a psychologically meaningful one, if an explanation of "why" is simpler than a description of "what", then parsimony tells us to disregard *meaning*, the *psyche*, and description of what shows itself. Natural Science reduction is nihilistic in the sense that it annihilates what it claims to value.

The phenomenological understanding of the *reduction* is a method to bracket any explanation to get to the essence of the phenomena. It tries to annihilate what gets in the way of the phenomenon revealing itself. It's like reducing carrots in a pan on low heat: boil off the moisture and impurities to get to the essence of carrot. Boil off the theories, the manipulative methods, and the false self-imposed disinterestedness to get to the essence of the phenomenon. Levinas goes further by describing how the observer cannot initiate any adequate reduction, but is reduced by the face of the Other. Not only are theories and explanations reduced, but the ethical place of the observer is unequal to the Other. The Other is radically allowed to reveal herself because she is above the observer. Levinas writes about "warped space", where the Other is experienced as higher than the self (1961/1969).

Fourth, natural science defines *determinism* as the theory based on facts of forces. All changes are a result of outside energy. Natural science psychology claims events of the self are determined by powers independent of the self. Human science, on the other hand, defines human determination as the *intentional meanings* of the self. Human events as human are based on "becauses" rather than on causes. Causes are found in nature; intentional meanings (becauses) are found supporting human behavior. Motives are not causes. They are the experienced meanings that provide the ground for choice while choices choose their meanings (Ricoeur, 1964). Hunger does not cause eating. It provides the basis (motive) to choose to eat. This choice chooses hunger over other competing meanings. There is not a lineal relation with the motive causing the behavior. It is a dialectical relation with the choice of behavior basing itself on the motive for its action, while the choice establishes this "because" the status of a real motive, the basis upon which it justifies itself. Motives provide the meaning *to motate* but do not cause. Only the meaning chosen is a motive (a mover). Other meanings may be wishes or urges; but until chosen, these meanings are not motives. Ricoeur makes no claim of any full awareness of these choices. But they are not mechanical causes. There is a dialectical relation between freedom and nature, the voluntary and involuntary, between choice and motives, between acceptance and facticity (Ricoeur, 1964). There is not a linear relation where one term is the cause and the other the effect.

For Levinas the "force" of responsibility can be stronger than either the causes of nature and the personal intentions of a subject. Psychological affairs are always interpersonal. The ethical imperative can weigh more heavily than natural laws. Of course humans can choose not to respond to the ethical call, and they act as if the self were the center of the self. The call or command for responsibility is not a physical force but a moral imperative.

Fifth, natural science claims it remains *neutral* with respect to *values* by constructing rigorous structures to detach the observer from the observed. We have already seen how the empirical methods of natural science are contaminated with the *disvalues* of "objectivism", "determining causes", and "reductionist" explanations. Human science defines *neutrality* by demanding the observer reflect on and bracket his/her personal and social values. The scientific method does not guarantee neutrality, does not demand or even ask the observer to become aware of the values influencing observation and to hold them in neutral. Levinas would locate the value of *neutrality* originating from the fundamental goodness of the observed. The other has her otherness and worth by being human, not by the judgment of the observer. The dignity and value of the other belongs to her. The infinite closeness and distance of the Other commands neutrality, the only remaining value is the inherent worth of the Other.

Finally

What a turn of events: an article by Levinas on Kant, sent to me by Giorgi, bridges a small difference between Giorgi and me over the contribution of Husserl and Levinas. The article points out how Kant insists pure reason must bow to practical reason. Pure reason is commanded by the practicality of action to act beyond reason. Levinas insists *reason* must bow to the command of the other to be *responsible*. The translator, Blake Billings (1994), of the short article Giorgi sent me summarizes the resonances between these two philosophers with the possibilities they can open up for psychology: "a morality beyond theory, a moral desire distinct from satiable need, the dignity or majesty of another person, an ethical giving without concern for repayment, religion as essentially moral" (1971/1994). From this article Giorgi sees Husserl's philosophy as a phenomenology of consciousness, and Levinas' as a phenomenology of action. We could never question Husserl's methodology; certainly Levinas did not. Husserl's wide and deep foundation for a psychology to release itself from scientism is one of the greatest philosophical contributions of the Twentieth Century. However, with this distinction, I think Levinas has as much to offer psychology by providing a way out of philosophy, especially for our work as therapists, researchers, and educators.

How So?

In research, the detachment required to produce faithful descriptions of revealed meanings must be founded on the ethical imperative to be responsible toward the participants before other scholars, readers, publishers. The other (participant) is infinitely *close*, closer to me than I am to myself, commanding my infinite responsibility to act for her good, and to suffer her because she suffers. Simultaneously the Other is infinitely *distanced*: her otherness is always beyond what I can know, her needs are always beyond what I can give, his suffering is always beyond what I can suffer.

In therapy the boundaries and detachment required by the therapist should not be for effective counseling technique designed to protect and take care of the therapist. The distance and closeness with the client should be founded on the ethical imperative for the therapist to be responsible. The therapist can never fully «understand» but can «stand under» her client.

For both research and therapy *simplicity*: *knowing by not knowing* is required. With my knowledge called into question by the infinite otherness and goodness of the Other, I can radically open myself to the revelation of the Other by not trying to interpret or disclose with my pre-knowledge.

Humility: to act by not acting is required. I must radically commit to the good of the Other with disinterested interest such that I do not act to achieve whatever good I think needed.

Patience: to suffer her suffering without trying to suffer her suffering is required. The Other's suffering is unique to her. I cannot reduce her suffering to what I claim I feel. I suffer because the Other, who does not deserve to suffer, suffers. I suffer my impotence to remove her suffering and take to myself.

Levinas' *phenomenology of action* gives priority to responsibility over knowledge. He writes, "Ethical testimony is a revelation which is not a knowledge" (1982/1985, p. 108). Certainly the call to do commands to know: but this command demands openness to the other before knowing. In the face of the other, "I must act before I know". This challenges the Greek tradition, "I must know before I act" and "know thyself". The Jewish tradition says I must be present to the Other, which is an act before action, before I know myself capable of responding, and before I know what will be asked what to do. I must say, "Here I am. I am testifying before I know about what I am testifying. Here I am, I am responsible before the other reveals her need. I am responsible for the Other's responsibility before I know what my responsibility will be and if my action will be appropriate to the need. Here I am, ready to obey before I know toward whom and for what I am here". The word, *obey* comes from the Latin *oboedire* «to listen to»: *ob* to + *audire* to hear. This is the non-intentional «listening» that precedes what is said by the other.

Exodus 24: 7: "We will do, and we will be obedient". Levinas refers to the tradition of the Talmudic scholars on this passage (1982/1994, p. 146).

> All that the Lord has spoken we will do, and we will be obedient (we will listen to it)". The term evoking obedience here ("we will do") is anterior to that which expresses understanding ("we will listen")... This obedience cannot be reduced to a categorical imperative in which a universality is suddenly able to direct a will. It is an obedience, rather, which can be traced back to the love of one's neighbor: a love without eros, without self-complacency and, in this sense, a love that is obeyed, the responsibility for one's neighbor, the taking upon oneself of the other's destiny, or fraternity. The relation with the other person is placed at the beginning!

References

Bernet, R. (2002). Levinas's critique of Husserl. In *The Cambridge Companion To Levinas,* (Simon Critchley and Robert Bernasconi, Eds.). Cambridge, UK: Cambridge University Press.

Cohen, R. (2002). The Maternal Psyche. In *Psychology for the Other: Levinas, ethics and the practice of psychology.* (Gantt and Williams, eds.) Pittsburg: Duquesne University.

Giorgi, A. (1970) *Psychology as a human science: A phenomenologically based approach.* New York, NY: Harper & Rowe.

Husserl, E. (1950). *Idea pertaining to a pure phenomenology and to a phenomenological philosophy.* Originally published in 1913 as *Ideen zu einer reinen Phänomenologie und phänomenologischen Philosophie. Erstes Buch: Allgemeine Einführung in die reine Phänomenologie.*

Kunz, G. (1998). *The Paradox of Power and Weakness.* Albany: New York State University Press.

Levinas, E. & Peiffer, G. (1936). Translation into French of *The Cartesian Meditation,* Edmund Husserl.

Levinas, E. (1969). *Totality and Infinity: An essay on exteriority.* Trans. Alphonso Lingis. Pittsburgh, PA: Duquesne University Press. (Originally in French in 1961).

Levinas, E. (1981). *Otherwise than being or beyond essence.* Trans. Alphonso Lingis. Boston: Martinus Nijhoff Publishers. (Originally in French in 1974).

Levinas, E. (1985). *Ethics and infinity: Conversations with Philippe Nemo.* Trans. Richard A. Cohen Pittsburgh, PA: Duquesne University Press. (Originally in French in 1982)

Levinas, E. (1986). Dialogue with Emmanuel Levinas. In *Face to Face with Levinas.* Ed. Richard A. Cohen. Albany: State University of New York Press.

Levinas E. (1994). The primacy of pure practical reason. Trans. Blake Billings in *Man and World.* Vol. 27: pp. 445-454. Netherlands: Kluwer Academic Publishers. (Originally as "Het primaat van de zuivere praktische rede", in *Wijsgerig Perspectief op Maatschappij en Wetenschap,* 1970-1971 Vol. 11, pp. 178-186). Article sent by Amedeo Giorgi to George Kunz.

Levinas, E. (1994). *Beyond the Verse: Talmudic Readings and Lectures.* Trans. Gary D. Mole). Bloomington, IN: University of Indiana Press. (Originally in French as *L' Au-Dela du Verset;* in 1982).

Levinas, E. (2003). *On Escape.* Trans. Bettina Bergo. Stanford, California: Stanford University Press. Published in French in1982 as *De l'evasion,* for Fata Morgana, edited by Jacques Rolland. (Originally published in 1935 in *Recherches Philosophiques*).

MacLeod, R. (1975). *The persistent problems of psychology.* Pittsburgh, PA: Duquesne University Press.

Ricoeur, P. (1966). *Freedom and Nature: The Voluntary and the Involuntary.* Tans. Erazim V. Kohak. Chicago: Northwestern University Press. (Originally in French in 1950.)

Robbins, J. (2001). *Is It Righteous to Be: Interviews with Emmanuel Levinas.* Stanford, CA.: Stanford University Press.

Tavris, C. and Carole Wade, (2001). *Psychology in Perspective.* (Third Edition) Upper Saddle River: New Jersey.

Westphal, M. (2008). *Levinas and Kierkegaard in dialogue.* Bloomington, IN: Indiana University Press.

HERMENEUTIC PHENOMENOLOGY AND PSYCHOTHERAPY

Bertha Mook, Ph.D.

University of Ottawa
Canada

Abstract

The field of psychotherapy has recently seen many technical advances. Yet it remains fragmented on a theoretical level and its philosophical foundations tend to be overlooked. Today, most of psychotherapy is founded on a natural science paradigm or alternatively, on social constructionism. In this chapter, I have critiqued these dominant paradigms and proposed instead a hermeneutic phenomenological foundation for psychotherapy as a human science. I explored the interface between hermeneutic phenomenology and psychotherapy in general. This is followed by Gadamer's concepts of play and its relevance for play therapy with children. Ricoeur's theory of narrative structure is applied to narratives in psychotherapy and in particular, to family therapy. The key concepts of understanding and of interpretation are also addressed from a philosophical point of view and in turn applied to the theory and practice of psychotherapy. The role and meaning of play in child psychotherapy was illustrated by means of a brief clinical case vignette.

Today, the field of psychotherapy is characterized by a multiplicity of diverse theoretical approaches and mini-theories. Above all, it is dominated by an ever-growing array of techniques to be used for specific therapeutic interventions. With their eyes focused on practice, modern day therapists show little interest in the theories of psychotherapy and even less in their philosophical foundations. Yet these very philosophical grounds determine how we view reality and the human being. They implicitly underlie our theories of psychotherapy and even our formulation of techniques. It is of vital importance that the philosophical foundations, which underlie various therapeutic theories be made explicit.

Introduction

In the theory of science, Kuhn (1962) pointed out that most scientists accept a specific viewpoint or paradigm regarding their subject matter which guides their research and determines what will be studied and how. In the course of its development, psychotherapy drew on different philosophical viewpoints including empiricism, rationalism and existential phenomenology which all contributed to the main schools of therapeutic theory and practice. Although a diversity of viewpoints continue to be embraced in psychotherapy today, we find that the empirical natural science paradigm has the greatest influence and remains the most dominant one. This is exemplified in the widespread appeal and application of cognitive behavioral therapy in individual therapy with children and with adults. It has produced successful evidence-based research and rightly pressures other models of therapeutic theory and practice to demonstrate their effectiveness as well.

Giorgi (1970) argued that psychology should not be conceived as a natural science but as a human science in order to do justice to its subject matter, i.e., the experiencing and behaving person. This is particularly true for the field of psychotherapy, which deals with the understanding, interpretation and healing of human suffering. We could say that psychotherapy is a human science par excellence. Within a human science paradigm, Giorgi (1985) found that the phenomenological method is the most suitable for the description and the analysis of the meaning of human phenomena as experienced by its subjects. In his innovative and productive career, he became the leading expert in the phenomenological method and its applications to psychological phenomena in various fields, including psychotherapy. I am indebted to him for his inspiration in my own phenomenological research in psychotherapy (Mook, 1985, 1987, 2003).

In the mid-twentieth century, existential phenomenology was the dominant philosophy in Western Europe and became a leading force in the field of psychotherapy with adults, children and families. For example, the existential phenomenology of Heidegger inspired both Binswanger (1963) and Boss (1963) to develop a new form of individual adult therapy called Daseinsanalysis although each one established his own following. In child psychotherapy, Langeveld (1955) and his co-workers initiated a phenomenological approach called imagery-communication specifically for work with children where they could express themselves through play, art and other creative media. Existential phenomenology was also used as a philosophical foundation for Laing and Esterson (1964) in their development of a new phenomenological school of family therapy. Although no longer so extensively a force, existential phenomenological approaches to psychotherapy continue to be practiced today.

Besides phenomenology, which seeks to understand and explicate the meaning structures of lived phenomena, psychotherapy as a human science also calls for hermeneutics. Hermeneutics deals with language and meaning and focuses on the understanding and the interpretation of spoken and written texts. Ricoeur (1981) defined hermeneutics succinctly as the science of the interpretation of texts. Gadamer (1982) extended the object of hermeneutic understanding to the broader field of human communication including play, art and verbal communication. In psychotherapy, we encounter complex narratives, dreams, art, play and other texts of patients, which need to be deciphered and interpreted.

The door to a philosophically grounded hermeneutic approach to psychotherapy was opened by Ricoeur's (1970) critical reading of Freud's psychoanalysis. He recommended that we replace Freud's mechanistic metapsychology by a narrativist approach based on human agency. Schafer (1981) was the first to initiate a narrative approach to psychoanalysis, which he called hermeneutic and formulated as the telling and retelling of patients' stories. However, by rejecting any philosophical foundation and holding that every person must choose his own narrative version, he fell into a radical form of relativism (Guignon, 1998). In the late eighties, Lubbers (1988) initiated a hermeneutic approach to child psychotherapy based on the philosophy of Gadamer (1982) in which he incorporated the phenomenologically based imagery communication. The work of Langeveld and Lubbers had a major influence on my own development of a hermeneutic phenomenological approach to child psychotherapy. Despite the obvious relevance of hermeneutics and the hermeneutic method for psychotherapy, its influence has remained sporadic and limited.

In the late eighties and early nineties, a challenging new paradigm emerged in the form of social constructionism, which brought about a significant shift in mainstream therapeutic thought. It was open to hermeneutics and placed a new emphasis on the importance of language and meaning in psychotherapy. This in turn led to the birth of narrative therapy in work with families (White and Epston, 1990). Narrative therapy was enthusiastically embraced by a wide range of family therapists and found to be particularly suitable to the practice of working with the troubled lives of postmodern families. It was also applied to work with individual adults and to a lesser extent with children.

In this chapter, I propose that psychotherapy is a human science which can be philosophically grounded in hermeneutic phenomenology as introduced by Heidegger (1962) and Merleau-Ponty (1962), and developed further by Gadamer (1982) and Ricoeur (1981). I will first briefly address and critique the leading natural science and social constructionist paradigms in psychotherapy before elaborating on a hermeneutic phenomenological approach as a possible philosophical foundation.

The Natural Science Paradigm in Psychotherapy

The modernist natural science paradigm, which is based on a Cartesian epistemology, continues to dominate the contemporary field of psychotherapy in theory, practice and research. It posits a dualistic relationship between person and world and adheres to a linear explanatory model of causality. A natural science approach assumes that there are causal mechanisms below surface phenomena and aims at providing causal explanations of human intentions and actions. In this viewpoint, the person is seen as an object amongst objects in the world whose characteristics can be analyzed, measured and explained by applying the leading methodological principles of the natural sciences. It is well known to phenomenologist and has been widely criticized in phenomenological circles (Giorgi, 1970, 1985). The natural science viewpoint is critiqued for not doing justice to human agency and for overlooking the uniquely human traits of freedom, transcendence, creativity, relatedness to self and others and attributing meaning to one's lived experience. In therapeutic practice, it is of vital importance that the therapist, who aims to alleviate his client's suffering, sees his client as a whole person with unique human characteristics and as an agent in his own right.

When family therapy was born in the mid fifties, it rejected the Cartesian natural science paradigm with its linear model of causality as unsuitable for conceptualizing family structures and functioning. Family therapists instead turned to the relatively new system and cybernetic theories, which reflected a different natural science approach based on an epistemology of pattern. Systems theory and cybernetic theory with their regulatory homoeostatic principles and their orderly notions of boundaries were found to be suitable and fruitful for thinking about and working with families. The leading structural and strategic family therapy models were problem-focused and called for objective descriptions of family behaviors and processes. Therapeutic change was brought about by specific techniques of breaking dysfunctional structures or repetitive interactive cycles of behavior within the family system.

The application of systems theory to family therapy was initially found to be liberating and made a unique contribution to the study of human communication and interaction. However, by the late eighties, some leaders in family therapy began to see the limitations of system theory and felt it had outlived its usefulness (Goolishian & Anderson, 1987). It had also been criticized from a phenomenological point of view for overlooking subjective and inter-subjective experience and the uniquely human dimension of meaning in family systems (Mook, 1985, 1987).

The Social Constructionist Paradigm In Family Therapy

Under the influence of postmodernist writings, feminist studies, the philosophies of constructionism and hermeneutics, some family therapists aimed to develop a broader view of family functioning. They began to focus on larger cultural systems and became aware of the power of history, the present social cultural context and the importance of language and meaning in the shaping of peoples' lives. Together these influences led to a paradigmatic shift from the earlier system theory to a narrative therapeutic approach based on social constructionism.

Proponents of constructionism argue that objective descriptions of family processes are impossible as reality itself is a social construction. They hold that the beliefs, values, institutions, customs and laws, which are reflected in our social realities, are constructed by the members of a specific culture as they interact with each other on a daily basis. Society in turn constructs the «lenses» through which their members interpret their world (Hoffman, 1990). A new family therapy approach based on social constructionism led to an emphasis on the importance of language, dialogue and narratives. In a constructionist viewpoint, narratives are seen as free creations, free of any factual accounts and not concerned with the discovery of the truth of a person's story (Guignon, 1998). The aim of psychotherapy is to come up with a good, coherent and useful narrative. A singular advantage of this narrative approach was that it liberated family therapy from the narrow confines of system theory as therapists moved away from being behavioral engineers and became «conversational artists» (McNamee, S. & Gergen, K. J., 1992). In a narrative approach, the therapist joins the family as a partner in dialogue. The focus on narrative discourse frees both the therapist and the family members from adhering to fixed categories of health and illness as they together generate and construct stories that are more relevant to the family's reality. The family therapist needs to stimulate the members' imagination by asking questions that spark curiosity and lead to alternative ideas in their joint effort towards a re-authoring of the family's life and relationships. At the heart of a narrative approach to psychotherapy lies the belief in the profound effects of language, conversation and stories for both the client(s) and the therapist (White and Epston, 1990).

The Influence of Hermeneutics

Anderson and Goolishian (1992) were the first family therapists to express dissatisfaction with a sole emphasis on a constructionist paradigm in family therapy. With their interest in the role of language and meaning, they moved instead towards a more interpretative and hermeneutic position. Influenced by both social constructionism and hermeneutics, Goolishian and Anderson (1987) pointed out that human beings are language-generating and meaning-generating systems and that the therapeutic system itself is linguistic in nature.

The authors' hermeneutic leaning was also present in their novel concept of therapeutic "not-knowing", by which they meant that the therapist should not let himself be influenced by his previous knowledge and experience. When the therapist joins the family, he should remain open-minded, create space and facilitate dialogue through therapeutic questioning (Anderson and Goolishian, 1992). The therapist becomes part of a linguistic system and a therapeutic conversation wherein the therapist and the family together explore the family's problems through dialogue. Anderson and Goolishian's constructionist stance remained evident in their assertion, that individuals in conversation with each other socially construct narratives.

In general, narrative therapists share with hermeneuticists an emphasis on the importance of language, meaning and narrative. Yet their adherence to social constructionism offers a questionable philosophical ground. From a phenomenological hermeneutic point of view, constructionism is a relativist philosophy, which holds that every person creates his own truth and his own reality based on his individual perceptions and thoughts. Constructionism overemphasizes cognition and language and neglects the person's relationship to the world in which he lives. Merleau-Ponty (1962) emphasized that the person and his world are intimately interrelated and that truth and reality does not reside in the mind. In his words: "Man is in the world, and only in the world does he know himself" (p. XI). Hermeneutic phenomenology critiques social constructionism for its one-sided focus on individual perception and cognition and its neglect of the person in his world-relatedness.

Hermeneutic Phenomenology and Psychotherapy

In contrast to the natural science and the social constructionist paradigms, Heidegger (1962), Merleau-Ponty (1962), Gadamer (1982) and Ricoeur (1981) claimed that hermeneutic phenomenology is an ideal philosophical foundation for the human sciences. Starting with Heidegger (1962), hermeneutic phenomenology aimed to move beyond both the natural science and social constructionist paradigms by presenting a different ontological account of human existence. Rather than assuming separation of person and world, this viewpoint held that the human being is an embodied subject-in-the-world who is conscious, engaged in his relationships to self and others, linguistic, meaning-giving and always seeking to understand and interpret himself and his world. Heidegger pointed out that human action has a dynamic temporal structure in which future direction gives shape to the past, and undertakings in the past gives sense to actions in the present. Life as a whole has a distinctive temporal structure and action gains it's meaning from the agent's entire life story (Guignon, 1998).

Hermeneutic phenomenology and psychotherapy are of course distinctly different disciplines with different origins, goals and applications. Yet beyond the surface they reveal some striking commonalities. As a philosophy, hermeneutic phenomenology aims to understand and interpret the meanings of lived experience as revealed and expressed in spoken or written texts (Gadamer 1982, Ricoeur 1981). In comparison, psychotherapy is concerned with the understanding and interpretation of the problematic life experiences of clients as expressed in their incomplete and often incoherent and obscure narratives. As a practical discipline, its goal is problem-solving and healing in the context of a therapeutic relationship. At heart, both disciplines are language-based and share a common and central interest in understanding and interpreting the meanings of complex texts or narratives as expressions of lived experience (Mook, 1991).

Hermeneutic phenomenology has provided some foundational contributions, which are of great significance to the field of psychotherapy. In his ground-breaking work, *Truth and Method*, Gadamer (1982) explicated the fundamental historicity of human existence and the pervasive nature of tradition and prejudices which needs to be taken into account in our attempts to understand a person's life. He helped us to see that people's life stories are always pre-shaped by the traditions of a shared life-world and emphasized that, whether we realize it or not, the effects of history are involved in all understanding. Gadamer threw a new light on the nature of understanding, dialogue and conversation, all of which are directly relevant to the work of psychotherapy. His hermeneutic philosophy also offered a new insight into the foundational nature of play and art, which in turn has implications for imagery-communication and play therapy with children.

In his oeuvre, Ricoeur recognized anew the importance of language and illuminated the meaning of metaphor and symbolism in human life. He offered us a complex theory of the interpretation of written or spoken texts, which can also be applied to psychotherapy (1976). Ricoeur is further known for his novel explication of the nature of narratives and its relationship to the temporality of lived experience (1984). In psychotherapy, the individual client or the family's expressions of their lived experiences can be viewed as narratives or texts, which the therapist and the client aim to understand and interpret within the context of a therapeutic relationship. In narrative terms, therapists together with the client or family aim to identify pathological narratives and work towards a re-writing of their lives in ways that are more congruent with their lived reality.

Despite the central role of play, narrative, understanding and interpretation in psychotherapy, little attention has been paid in mainstream therapeutic literature to the foundational meaning of these basic concepts. Hermeneutic phenomenology's explication of their basic character contributes indirectly to a philosophical foundation and a deeper understanding of the theory and practice of psychotherapy. In this chapter, we will address Gadamer's concept of play and its implications for the imaginative play in therapy with children.

This will be followed by a brief outline of Ricoeur's theory of narrative and its significance for child and particularly for family therapy. We will then turn to the therapeutic relevance of their hermeneutic theories of understanding and of interpretation.

Gadamer's Concept of Play

The imaginative play of children is a fascinating yet elusive concept, which has been reflected upon in philosophy, psychology, education, and in other human science disciplines. Various authors have pointed out that play is a primary and foundational phenomenon which underlies all expressions of art, language and culture. In this light, Gadamer (1982) began his *Truth and Method* with a description of the hermeneutic experience of art and the ontological significance of play. Children's play has a function of exhibition and presentation, which precedes language and calls it forth. Phenomenological studies of imaginative play have revealed that the child typically surrenders to the appeal of its play objects and becomes immersed in a different world with its own space and time, its own inner tensions, surprises and excitements, its own scenes, configurations and emerging themes. Referring to tragedy as a proto-typical form of play, Gadamer went further by asserting that play is an autonomous phenomenon with its own structure, a meaningful whole, which moves beyond the subjective world of the player and is revelatory in its own right. He posits the primacy of play over the player and holds that the true subject of play is not the subjectivity of the player but play itself. It is play that draws the player into its spell and its sole purpose is to represent itself. He wrote: "In the representation of play, what *is* emerges. In it is produced and brought to light what otherwise is constantly hidden and withdrawn" (p.101). The player in turn appropriates the meaning of his play to himself, which heightens his self-awareness and self-presentation.

Gadamer's novel concept of play reveals its power and its foundational character in human life. In psychotherapy, it throws a new light on the role and the meaning of play in play therapy with children. In view of the primacy of the play over the player, Gadamer has effected a figure-ground reversal with far reaching implications. Most of all, the meanings revealed in the child's imaginative play in therapy should not be reduced to subjective interpretations of the child's unconscious or his self as is typically done in play therapy. Play is an autonomous phenomenon in its own right which purpose is to represent itself. The therapist and the child should therefore first of all look and listen to what the play itself reveals and only subsequently appropriate these possible meanings to the child's life-world (Mook, 1999).

A Case Illustration in Play Therapy

The following case presents a relatively simple illustration of the role, the meaning and the healing power of play and creative expressions in imagery-communication therapy with children.

Mark was a soft and affectionate eight years old boy who suffered from overwhelming fears. He was afraid to be alone, afraid of the dark and above all, afraid of monsters who threatened him at night. These fears emerged after a traumatizing experience a few months earlier during which he witnessed a violent physical attack on his parents by outside intruders. On a verbal level, he forcefully refused to talk about these painful experiences.

Mark was drawn to a large sandbox with small toys, and created a village populated with human and animal figures whom he described as either all good or all bad. Set apart from the others was a monster family consisting of a father, a mother and a small child. Mark conveyed that they were the powerful rulers of the village but that they were unaware of their monster status and believed themselves to be good creatures. Mark was intensely drawn to these complex monsters. As this play image seemed central to his own problems, the therapist led him to make a monster family out of clay in order to concretize them, which in turn deepened his emotional involvement and participation. The child was eager to do this and, with the help of his therapist, he became deeply involved in the process of molding and shaping the figures of a monster family. They were immediately introduced in his play and became the central figures in his story, which unfolded over a few sessions. At first the monsters terrorized both the good and the bad people and animals in the village every single night. Gradually, their rage focused on targeting only the bad people. When Mark was ready and his feelings and thoughts became more differentiated in his play, he made another figure out of raw materials. He identified strongly with his new creation and called him Mr. Unique. This figure was given the important mission to unmask the monster family and to reveal their true identity to villagers and to themselves. Protected by Mr. Unique, the villagers rose up against the monster family and defeated them. Once this was accomplished in the play, Mark discarded them. As his fears of monsters were expressed and conquered through play, they gradually dissipated in reality.

This brief clinical example illustrates how Mark surrendered to the appeal of his play objects and how he became immersed in his play-world. In the light of Gadamer, we could say that the play rose above Mark's inner subjective world and represented its own meaning and its own truth. It exhibited and represented his view of a divided world and his overwhelming fear of monsters which even in play needed to be masked as benevolent before an exceptional and stronger figure emerged to reveal their true identity. His imaginative play provided him with a protective shield to face his fears indirectly and to master them through playing them out.

In subsequent plays, Mark became increasingly able through play figures to express and to face up to aggressive and hostile feelings and actions. Soon afterwards, he started to talk directly to his therapist about his frightening experiences and could express his rage at the intruders, who had violently attacked his beloved parents, first through painting and subsequently through words. Communicating through play and art in the context of play therapy gradually enabled Mark to solve his problems in more realistic ways.

The imaginative play of a child in play therapy can be very complex with multiple levels of meaning which demands therapeutic understanding and interpretation. It always involves a narrative dimension, which unfolds in time and reveals its own narrative structure. As we have seen, narratives are typically encountered in family therapy. This brings us first to Ricoeur's theory of narrative and its implications for the field of child and family therapy before turning to the problem of understanding and interpretation.

Ricoeur's Theory of Narrative and Psychotherapy

In his hermeneutic analysis of narrative, Ricoeur took the literary model of tragedy as his point of departure. In *Time and Narrative* (1984) he explored his basic hypothesis, i.e., that the activity of narrating a story and the temporal character of human experience are interrelated. In his analysis, he demonstrated that temporality and narrativity form a reciprocal relationship that reinforces each other in a dialectical fashion. He captured the integral interrelatedness of time, narrative and experience as follows: "Time becomes human time to the extent that it is organized after the manner of a narrative; narrative in turn, is meaningful to the extent that it portrays the features of temporal experience" (p. 3). By drawing on the Aristotelian concepts of *mimesis* or the active process of imitating, and *mythos* or emplotment, Ricoeur studied the mediating operations between lived human experience and narrative discourse. His detailed analysis led him to the important conclusion that in real life, our temporal experiences and actions do not yet have a narrative character but are instead structured in a *pre-narrative* fashion. Narrative itself goes beyond everyday concrete life experience as it calls for a semantic innovation and the invention of a plot. In his theory of narrative structure, Ricoeur explicated convincingly how a narrative text is pre-figured in the practical field of human actions and experience, how events and themes are configured through imaginative variations and emplotment and how the plot is in turn received and re-figured by the reader.

From a hermeneutic phenomenological point of view, Ricoeur's theory of narrative structure can be seen as foundational to narrative therapy in work with families and also to play narratives in therapy with children. Ricoeur revealed that our life experiences as lived are not random but have already a temporal pre-narrative character and they wait to be narrated. Applied to families, narrative structures are not formal or external nor are they cognitively constructed as held by constructionist theory. Narrative structures are instead seen as rooted and pre-figured in the everyday experiences and actions of people who in turn take up the pre-narrative structures in configuring and narrating their stories to each other. The act of linguistically narrating our real life experiences brings order, coherence and intelligibility to our lives.

In the practice of family therapy, the dysfunctional story of the family needs to be dismantled and rewritten by the joint effort of the therapist and the family members in the process of psychotherapy. The family usually presents a problematic surface story in which one member is seen as the identified patient. This presented narrative has a defensive and a protective function in which one member is victimized and seen as in need of treatment. The family therapist needs to break into this problematic surface structure to reveal the deeper lying problems, which need to be brought to the surface in the course of treatment. For example, in the Smith family with two parents and two elementary school children, John and Hanna, John was the identified patient. He was described as hyperactive, attention-seeking, destructive and always disrupting the family's activities. He was seen as the source of their constant sense of frustration and unhappiness. As the therapist listened carefully to the stories and the perspective of each family member and raised new questions, the presenting problem was diffused and other family problems were brought to the surface. The couple acknowledged that they had become estranged from each other and Hanna revealed that she had her own difficulties, which had been totally overlooked. Gradually, the family members came to see another reality and created together with the therapist a new narrative which was more in tune with their lives as lived.

In play therapy, the child's imaginative play stories also reveal a narrative structure. They are rooted and pre-figured in the child's life-world and creatively configured as the child in his play carries out imaginative variations on his own perceived reality. In the process, he becomes indirectly more aware of his problems and seeks alternative solutions through play, which are re-figured by both the child and his therapist. In the process of play therapy, these play stories need to be expressed, understood, questioned and challenged to enable the child to move forward towards healing and transformation.

The concept of narrative structure as developed by Ricoeur belongs to the human order (Merleau-Ponty, 1963a) as it is profoundly human, creative, evolving and transforming in nature. Only the human order has the unique power of transcendence, which allows us to create images and symbols. Merleau-Ponty saw this act of transcendence, that is, orienting ourselves by means of the possible and moving beyond existing structures to create new ones, as the essence of being human. In psychotherapy, narrative structures are created by the child or by the family members themselves and are in principle transformed by new experiences, actions and narrations. In revealing the pre-narrative character of lived experience and the integral interrelationship between narration, temporality and human experience, Ricoeur contributed in principle to a philosophical foundation for a narrative hermeneutic approach to family, adult or child psychotherapy.

In *Oneself as Another*, Ricoeur (1992) went a step further and applied his narrative theory to the concept of personal identity or the constitution of self. He came to the conclusion that personal identity has a narrative dimension which needs to be taken into account. His analysis showed that personal identity is characterized by the dialectic of sameness or *idem* and selfhood or *ipse*. Identity as sameness has been recognized in the literature and reflects permanence in time. However, identity as selfhood, which is variable in its manifestations, has been mostly overlooked. This dialectic between sameness and selfhood is seen as the major contribution of narrative theory to the constitution of self.

A narrative theory of personal identity reflects the connections between plot and character and between action and agent. In following Aristotle, action is seen as a connection of incident and facts, which reflect an initial narrative configuration. The identity of the person or character in the plot is submitted to imaginative variations and the interconnectedness of these variations, as events are constituted by emplotment. This in turn allows us to integrate the dialectic of sameness and selfhood where sameness is reflected in permanence in time and selfhood in diversity, variability, disconnectedness, etc.

Applied to psychotherapy, we can think of the client as a character in the plot of his personal narratives, which constitute his personal identity. The client's personal identity as sameness and selfhood is reflected in his personal narratives, which are problematic and often incoherent and unintelligible. Especially in psychotherapy, the troubled client's selfhood may reflect his fragility, vulnerability, brokenness and disconnection. We can also conceive of both therapist and client as characters in the plot of an unfolding therapeutic narrative where both are agents who perform actions. In the work of therapy, the client and the therapist work towards a revealing and a clarification of the client's troubled self and towards a re-authoring of his life.

The family or the individual client's new emerging narrative involves a new temporal order as selected problematic past experiences are relived and reintegrated in the present and shaped into a new future. Here Ricoeur's (1984) statement is relevant to the therapeutic process: "By reading the end in the beginning and the beginning in the end, we learn also to read time itself backward, as the recapitulation of the initial conditions of a course of action in its temporal consequences" (p.154). In therapy, this temporal re-ordering of the family or client's troubled experiences in a new narrative is called for in order to provide coherence and intelligibility.

In revealing not only the temporal pre-narrative structure of experience but also the structure of narratives and of personal identity, Ricoeur made a unique contribution to a hermeneutic phenomenological foundation for a narrative conception of self and of psychotherapy which can in principle be applied to family, adult and play therapy with children. Through therapeutic reflections and interventions, the therapist and the client can draw upon pre-narrative structures of past and present experiences and work together towards a narrative which endows events with a new temporal order and a new meaning in view of an overarching goal towards well-being.

The meanings revealed in the narratives of families, adults and children call for therapeutic understanding and interpretation. In psychotherapy, the processes of understanding and interpreting meanings expressed by clients through play, art, dreams, narratives and other forms of expression are poorly understood yet lie at the heart of therapy itself. In practice, a child's imaginative play story, for example, can be very complex with multiple levels of meaning (Mook, 1999, 2003). The same is true for other problematic client or family's narratives or texts in the multiple forms of stories, dreams, art or play. In their hermeneutic phenomenology, Gadamer's concept of understanding and Ricoeur's theory of interpretation are relevant to the theory of psychotherapy and throw a new light on these central therapeutic interventions.

Gadamer's Concept of Understanding

In *Truth and Method*, Gadamer's (1982) explicated his philosophical hermeneutic concept of understanding. Following Heidegger, he asserted that an immediate understanding of other people is impossible as all understanding is based on a pre-understanding, which is rooted in history, tradition and prejudice. Through his detailed analysis, he showed us that understanding is a profoundly historical, linguistic and dialogical process. From a position of pre-understanding, partners in dialogue listen to each other in an attempt to grasp what the other is saying. Their dialogue takes the form of a conversation in which both partners offer their perspective on a topic or theme. Understanding is born when an agreement is reached during which the horizon of the one fuses with the horizon of the other.

In this fusion of horizons the perspectives of the individual partners are transcended into a broader and new perspective.

Communicating understanding plays a central role in psychotherapy and is seen as the main therapeutic intervention in humanistic, client-centered and existential approaches. In the light of Gadamer's contribution, understanding in psychotherapy is not a just an intervention of the therapist during which he empathically reflect the client's thoughts and feelings, as claimed for instance in client-centered therapy. To the contrary, understanding is always dialogical and circular in character and involves both the therapist and the client. It is furthermore rooted in the pre-understanding of both therapist and client and reflects their respective history, tradition and prejudices. In order to understand the client, the therapist has to be open-minded and listen with wide attention to the client who in turn aims to grasp what the therapist is communicating. Both therapist and client's need to let their respective viewpoints of the problematic world of the client be shaped and modified by what they learn from each other. When they reach an agreement in their therapeutic dialogue, their horizons will fuse and a new understanding will be born. Understanding therefore is not reproductive but productive in character as it leads to a broader and new perspective of the client's world (Mook, 2003). For most of psychotherapy, this type of active understanding is sufficient to move the therapeutic process forward.

For Gadamer, the processes of understanding and interpretation are interwoven and inseparable from each other. Interpretation is not seen as the application of an abstract theory as is often done in psychotherapy. Rather, the process of interpretation constitutes a concrete application of understanding to the specific circumstances of an individual case. In the context of psychotherapy, a good interpretation is attuned to the concrete specific circumstances of a particular client. Its validity lies not in theory but with the client for only he can endorse it as congruent with his lived experiential reality (Mook, 1991).

Ricoeur's Theory of Interpretation

Ricoeur (1976) endorsed Gadamer's theory of understanding and incorporated it into his novel theory of interpretation, which also includes the concept of explanation. Ricoeur reminded us that in Dilthey's hermeneutics, understanding and explanation were seen as dichotomous and irreducible modes of intelligibility. This conviction led Dilthey (1977) to make a fundamental epistemological distinction between the natural sciences and the human sciences with two opposing methodologies in which explanation belonged to the natural sciences and understanding to the human sciences. This distinction had far reaching consequences and is still upheld by most scientists today.

Ricoeur argued that a dichotomy between understanding and explanation is untenable as both processes are present in any dialogical situation. We explain something to someone so that he can understand. In Ricoeur's (1976) words: "[...] in explanation we explicate or unfold the range of propositions and meanings, whereas in understanding we comprehend or grasp as a whole the chain of partial meanings in one act of synthesis" (p.72). For him, the concept of interpretation applies to the whole dialectical process, which encompasses both understanding and explanation. As such, the processes of understanding, explanation and interpretation are inseparably interrelated.

In describing the process of interpretation, Ricoeur used the metaphor of the reader and the text. The reader enters into a hermeneutic circular dialogue with the text and lets himself be grasped by its possible meanings. Within the hermeneutic circle, repeated readings of the text lead to a first level of interpretation, which he referred to as a *naïve* understanding. This level of interpretation is sufficient to grasp the meaning of most texts. When the text is multi-layered and complex, a more *comprehensive* understanding is called for. This is particularly true for the interpretation of dreams, imaginative play or other symbolic texts. Here the reader may need to draw on an explanatory theory such as psychoanalysis in order to raise tentative hypotheses for interpretation, which may open up new horizons of understanding. A hypothesis needs in turn to be submitted to the hermeneutic circle to verify if it does justice to the meaning of the text as a whole. In the process of interpretation, the interpreter must differentiate between the presented meaning of the text itself and its possible reference to the reality of the person's life. This is an important dialectical distinction, which is often overlooked.

In the practice of psychotherapy, the application of Ricoeur's first phase of interpretation referred to as *naïve* understanding is sufficient in most cases. However, in complex therapeutic texts, a comprehensive or second phase of interpretation is called for. Here the interpreter needs to take the dialectic of sense and reference into account, which is especially relevant to symbolic texts like dreams or imaginative play. For example, an adult client may have a dream in which a person unknown to him is attacked and dies. Who does the dream refer to and what does the attack and death mean to the client? The multiple possible meanings of such a dream fragment poses a question of interpretation. Alternatively, in the imaginative play narrative of an emotionally disturbed child, the family house may catch fire and the father figure may be kidnapped or imprisoned. What does this reveal about the child's real life? It is a work of interpretation for both the therapist and the client, in which the possible meanings of the fragment need to be contextualized in and verified with the text as a whole by applying the method of the hermeneutic circle. A hermeneutic reading searches for the most probable interpretation, which will be consistent with and do justice to the text as a whole.

In general, a hermeneutic phenomenological interpretation needs to abide by the text-in-context principle where partial and single narratives are seen in the context of the larger narrative, which unfolds in the process of psychotherapy and in the context of the client's history and present life-world.

Conclusion

In the context of the continuing dominance of the natural science paradigm in psychotherapy and the leading role of social constructionism in narrative family therapy, I have argued in this paper that psychotherapy is a human science and that hermeneutic phenomenology can serve as an alternative philosophical foundation for it. Hermeneutic phenomenology offers a perspective on what it means to be a human being in a world steeped in language, history and tradition. It shares vital domains of interest with psychotherapy in its philosophical explication of basic concepts such as play, narrative, understanding and interpretation.

Despite many phenomenological studies on therapeutic phenomena, much work remains to be done in exploring and demonstrating the relevance of hermeneutic phenomenology for psychotherapy. For example, a hermeneutic phenomenological approach to personality and to psychopathology which takes the role and the meaning of language, history and culture into account will be needed in order to bridge the gap between philosophical foundations and therapeutic theory and practice. An application of the phenomenological and hermeneutic methods to a systematic analysis of therapeutic narratives in child, adult and family therapy will contribute empirical evidence for the effectiveness of psychotherapy as a human science.

References

Anderson, H. & Goolishian, H. The client is the expert: A not-knowing approach to therapy. In: McNamee, S. & Gergen, K. J. (1992). *Therapy as Social Construction.* London: Sage.

Binswanger, L. (1963). *Being in the World.* (Translated by Jacob Needleman). New York: Basic Books.

Boss, M. (1963). *Psychoanalysis and Daseinsanalysis.* New York: Basic Books (Translated by L. B. Levebre).

Dilthey, W. (1977). *Descriptive Psychology and historical Understanding.* The Hague: Martinus Nijhoff.

Gadamer, H. G. (1982). *Truth and Method.* New York: Crossroads.

Giorgi, A. (1970). *Psychology as a Human Science.* New York: Harper & Row.

Giorgi, A. (Ed.). (1985). *Phenomenology and Psychological Research.* Pittsburgh: Duquesne University Press.

Goolishian, H. & Anderson, H. (1987). Language systems and therapy: An involving idea. *Journal of Psychotherapy*, 24, 529-538.

Heidegger, M. (1962). *Being and Time.* New York: Harper & Row.

Hoffman, L. (1990).Constructing realities: An Art of Lenses. *Family Process*, 29, (1), 1-12.

Kuhn, T. (1962). *The Structure of Scientific Revolutions.* Chicago: The University of Chicago Press.

Merleau-Ponty, M. (1963a). *The Structure of Behavior.* Boston: Beacon Press.

Merleau-Ponty, M. (1962). *The Phenomenology of Perception.* London: Routledge & Kegan Paul.

Laing, R. D. & Esterson, A. (1964). *Sanity, madness and the Family.* London: Penguin Books.

Langeveld, M. J. (1955). Bevrijding door Beeldcommunicatie. *Nederlandsche Tijdschrift van de Psychologie,* 2, 443-455.

Lubbers, R. (1988). *Psychotherapie door Beeld en Begripsvorming.* Nijmegen: Dekker & Van der Vegt.

McNamee, S. & Gergen, K. J. (1992). *Therapy as Social Construction.* London: Sage.

Mook, B (1985). Phenomenology, system theory and family therapy. *Journal of Phenomenological Psychology*, 16, 1-12.

Mook, B. (1987). Phenomenology and Family Therapy. In: Van Zuuren, F., Wertz, F., &

Mook, B. (Eds.). *Advances in Qualitative Research in Psychology.* Lisse: Swets & Zeitlinger.

Mook, B. (1989). Intersubjectivity and narrative structure in family therapy. *The Humanist Psychologist,* 17 (3), 251-264.

Mook, B. (1991). The significance of hermeneutics to child psychotherapy. *Journal of Psychiatry and Neuroscience,* 16 (3), 182-187.

Mook, B. (1999). Interpreting imaginative play in child psychotherapy: Towards a phenomenological hermeneutic approach. *The Humanist Psychologist,* 27, (2), 173-186.

Mook, B. (2003). Phenomenological play therapy. In C. E. Schaefer (Ed.). *Foundations of Play Therapy.* New York : Wiley & Sons, 260-280.

Ricoeur, P. (1970). *Freud and Philosophy.* (Translated by Denis Savage). New Haven: Yale University Press.

Ricoeur, P. (1976). *Interpretation Theory: Discourse and the Surplus of Meaning.* Fort Worth: The Texas Christian University press.

Ricoeur, P. (1981). *Hermeneutics and the Human Sciences.* New York: Cambridge University Press.

Ricoeur, P. (1984). *Time and Narrative.* Chicago: University of Chicago Press.

Ricoeur, P. (1992). *Oneself as Another.* Chicago: University of Chicago Press.

White, M. & Epston, D. (1990). *Narrative Means to Therapeutic Ends.* New York: Norton.

IT'S ALWAYS ABOUT THE EPOCHÉ

James Morley, Ph.D.

Ramapo College of New Jersey
United States

Abstract

To honor Giorgi's contributions to psychological research methodology, this essay strives to elucidate a key component of phenomenological methodology (the epoché*), which is too often taken for granted, misunderstood, or neglected in qualitative research and the secondary literature. It calls for a renewed appreciation of the* epoché *and the phenomenological reduction in light of current scholarship that restores Husserl's understanding of transcendental subjectivity as always an embodied subjectivity adhered to the lifeworld – not at all a transcendentalism. Furthermore the essay comments on how mundane versions of the epoché permeate everyday life and how the methodological* epoché *shares elements in common with contemplative meditation traditions across cultures. The essay concludes with an affirmation of the* epoché *as more than an intellectual operation, but as an action involving the entirety of the person in the manner of an* ethos.

> [...] the psychologist does not know what he is dealing with.
>
> – Merleau-Ponty, *Texts and Dialogues.*

Amedeo Giorgi's project to renew psychology as a human science calls the question of methodology. Many psychologists had discussed the inadequacy of a natural science based psychology but none, until Giorgi, actually developed alternative methodologies to those of naturalist experimentalism. Humanistic psychologists would criticize the reductionism of mainstream psychology while simultaneously defaulting into that very same reductionism when it came to doing research. Giorgi was the first to actually apply the insight that the trinity of *theoretical approach*, *subject matter* and *methodology* are always already a synthetic unity – each part influencing the other. He articulated how the methodology one chooses will circumscribe the limits of one's subject matter and this limitation in turn drives theory. It is ineffective at best and absurd at worst to proclaim "theoretical" opposition to reductionism while conducting reductionist methodologies in one's research. Giorgi pointed out how this failure to develop an alternative methodology to experimentalism sapped the energy out of the humanistic and existential movements in psychology and subverted their efforts. It is to Giorgi's lasting credit that of all the critics of reductionism in psychology, he is the one who actually took effective action by delving into Husserl's works and establishing an authentically phenomenologically-based methodology that enabled psychological researchers to explore phenomena hitherto "off limits" to experimental methods.

This trinity of "approach, content and method" works in the other ways as well. Since Giorgi's 1970 text, several other non-phenomenological "qualitative" methods have emerged. But because of this understanding that method, theory, and subject matter are always a gestalt totality, Giorgi's methodology is distinct from other forms of qualitative research. A qualitative method alone, without an accompanying theoretical context or overall worldview is continuously at risk of falling back into naturalistic thinking. In other words, without a fully spelled out epistemology (or theoretical approach), non-phenomenological qualitative researchers too often interpret their research results within the physically based assumptions of mainstream naturalist psychology and, again, subvert their own well-intended efforts. In contrast to these other "mixed" or confused paradigms, Giorgi's method is situated within the paradigmatic theoretical approach that is Husserl's transcendental phenomenology. Supported by Husserl's fuller and more comprehensive approach to empirical science, Giorgi's phenomenological psychology cannot default back into naturalistic paradigms – as so many qualitative methods unwittingly do. Through Giorgi's work, phenomenological psychology can stand on its own feet as a discipline distinct from that of experimentalism.

Retrieving the Epoché

The animating inspiration behind Giorgi's penetrating criticism of mainstream psychology and his positive methodological alternative is Husserl's own attempt to re-found the sciences on empirical phenomenological grounds. To honor Giorgi's vision of a truly human based science, this brief essay shall strive to elucidate a key component of Husserlian phenomenological methodology (the *epoché*), which I believe is too often taken for granted, misunderstood, undervalued, and underused in much qualitative research and even sometimes in phenomenological research itself.[1] In short, I wish to call for a refreshed appreciation of this central element of phenomenological research methodology at the core of Giorgi's life work.

Perhaps Husserl's greatest discovery, the *epoché* was achieved though his insight that objectivity itself is an "experienced" objectivity with structures that can themselves be elucidated and understood. While never denying that there is a real world surrounding us and to which we adhere, Husserl's work with mathematics showed him how this world is "sustained" through our experience of it. The most wondrous thing about how we sustain the objectivity (or sense of reality) of the world is that this is accomplished by a concurrent forgetfulness, which, like an unconscious process, descends upon us as we live our ordinary relations with the objects of the world. This "blind spot" that seems to overshadow all of our conscious interactions with the world is named by Husserl as the thesis of the natural attitude. It is important to reiterate that the thesis of the natural attitude "hides itself" within the process of human experience in the manner of a fundamental belief, not unlike a religious or political conviction, that is almost axiomatic or pre-categorical. In the manner of the Freudian unconscious, or a strongly felt conviction, this natural attitude or belief in the reality of the "objective" world cannot be elucidated through ordinary rational discourse alone. Rationality is a necessary but insufficient condition for the elucidation of the natural attitude. Something much more potent than reason alone was needed to loosen the intentional threads[29] that bind our awareness to the belief (or natural attitude) that the world is independent of our consciousness of it. It is in this context that Husserl developed the methodological *epoché*. The *epoché* is the means through which Husserl discovered the blind spot of the natural attitude and well as the "method" for overcoming its limitations and rediscovering the world in the manner of an explorer encountering a vast new continent.

Again, the full power of the *epoché* is too often taken for granted by qualitative researchers and even sometimes by those of us professing to be phenomenologists. We too often assume it is a simple matter to suspend judgments, hold back our prejudices, or become aware of our assumptions. But what Husserl meant by the *epoché* is much more radical than we often recognize. To hold back our existential commitment to the very existence of the world, i.e. the reality positing power at the very core of consciousness itself, is a profoundly challenging and painfully difficult undertaking. It would be incorrect to treat the *epoché* as a simple mental technique or "professional" procedure that could be easily taught in an institutionalized manner as one would instruct a simple craft or practical skill. For the *epoché* is an action that involves one's total existential position toward the world and is thus profoundly personal. In other words, the *epoché* is not a merely intellectual operation. It is often likened to a type of a conversion experience that can be a shock to one's previously held convictions. Furthermore, achieving the intellectual flexibility that permits one to stand back at a distance from the natural attitude involves an extended preparation and intellectual familiarization with phenomenological literature. While the reflexive discipline of phenomenology is thus best promoted through access to Husserl's own philosophical reflections, it is most importantly through the *practice* of the *epoché* that one comes to understand it, i.e. through the experience of the *epoché*. It does not come easy. This is why Merleau-Ponty writes: "There is probably no question over which Husserl spent more time – and to which he more often returned, since the "problematic of reduction" occupies an important place in his unpublished work" (1962, p. IX).

Epoché *and Reduction*

In light of the difficulty of undertaking the *epoché*, let me review some issues regarding terminology that have led to some misunderstandings. Firstly, Husserl had a remarkably open-ended and non-dogmatic approach to his work and was always revising his own thought and technical terminology, which can be very confusing to any reader. There is an ongoing ambiguity in Husserl as well as in the commentary literature on the concept of the *epoché*. Firstly, the terms *epoché* and phenomenological "reduction" are often used interchangeably or with subtle differences. When used in a manner distinct from one another the *epoché* more commonly refers to the initial process that uncovers the role of the natural attitude while the reduction more often refers to the advanced and more specific types of *epochés* undertaken after having first achieved the initial *epoché*. In other words, a reduction is what I do after having first already suspended the natural attitude.

Eidetic Reduction

Another feature of the "reduction" is what Husserl often called the "eidetic reduction" where I suspend existential assumptions about a particular phenomenon, or I view it only within a particular frame of interest or disciplinary domain. Relevant here, of course, is the psychological reduction where I put out of play all phenomena that are not psychologically relevant. What may be confusing is that there can be a multitude of eidetic reductions. To risk simplification again, one could best understand any eidetic reduction as the domain of the fictive or imaginary. One of the most radical implications of the *epoché* (or reduction) is that once I suspend my natural attitude assumptions of a Cartesian split between my consciousness of the world and the "external" world itself, an entirely new relationship is established between the imaginary and the non-imaginary. Within this standpoint, one can begin to see how all objects exist in time as gestalt composites of both imagination and perception and that these two aspects are always co-present as apperception (Husserl, 1964). So it is the task of eidetic reduction to explore this new apperceptive domain and to methodologically engage imagination to vary and interrogate the objects one is striving to understand. A synonymous term here is imaginary variation where I apply imagination to behold as many viewpoints of the phenomenon that are possible to arrive at what is essential to all possible perspectives. Thus, the eidetic reduction is contingent on the domain or discipline within which one is working as well s the particular phenomenon being studied. This is the domain most directly relevant to Giorgi's concrete phenomenological methodology.

The Transcendental Reduction

The next term I wish to clarify is the "transcendental reduction" which is the most debated and perhaps misunderstood feature of Husserl's methodology. An admittedly overly simple rendering is that the "transcendental reduction" is where I suspend my own ordinary standpoint as a particular existence. In other words, I step back from my own assumed subjectivity and take a new standpoint as a witness to the streaming of my own subjectivity. In Merleau-Ponty's terminology, we could call this a kind of "hyper-reflection". Poststructuralists and Postmodernists of the past few decades have reacted against the idea of a transcendental reduction as they misunderstood it to imply an absolute standpoint that was itself another variation of the foundationalism (or metaphysics of presence) of scientism on the one hand or romantic idealism on the other. Perhaps the term "transcendental" opened Husserl to these misconceptions, and it is true that his earlier publications may have offered this impression. But these dismissals of Husserl's thought are outdated misconceptions that recent scholarship is setting right (Zahavi, 2003; Weldon, 2003). When we take up his corpus in its entirety, another light is cast on this matter.

Unfortunately, there are historical circumstances that explain why the entirety of his manuscripts has been off limits to researchers for so long. Husserl's Jewish heritage made his scholarship vulnerable to the Nazi government's racial laws. The mass of his manuscripts written across an enormously productive career had to be hidden and remained tragically unpublished for decades. The failure of post war continental scholarship to put right this ongoing legacy of Nazi suppression is hard to defend. Fortunately, scholars such as Dan Zahavi (2003) have been demonstrating how, across the entire span of his career, Husserl always saw subjectivity as adhered to the world and our relations to others in an embodied and incarnate manner. His seminal text, *Ideas II,* though written in 1928 was only published in German in 1951 and translated into English as late as 1989. This material demonstrates Husserl's deep concern with the experiential body as the ultimate point of contact between consciousness and nature – which he calls "constitution". For Husserl, within the transcendental reduction, all possible experiences, perceived or imagined, appear as a spatio-temporal orientation to the perceiver's living body. Only through one's living-body can the experienced world become constituted. In Husserl's words, "[...] all that is thingly real in the surrounding world of the ego has its relation to the body" (1989, p. 61). He continues to say:

> Furthermore, obviously connected with this is the distinction the body acquires as the bearer of the zero point (*null punct*) of orientation, the

> bearer of the here and now, out of which the pure ego intuits space and the whole world of the senses. Thus each thing that appears has *eo ipso* an orienting relation to the body, and this refers not only to what actually appears but to each thing that is supposed [imagined] to be able to appear. (*idem*)

Thus, for Husserl, the entire spectrum of possible experiences, perceptual or imaginary, is rooted to this corporeal zero point which is the bearer of the here and now. From this we can see how Husserl's notion of the transcendental does not entail an isolated disembodied ego extended at a distance above the lived world of perceptual experience, as implied in the postwar literature, instead, corporeal experience is *itself*, for Husserl, the transcendental ground. This spatial zero point of the body coincides with Husserl's understanding of a temporal zero point, namely the impenetrable upsurge of the now point that perpetually slips from reflective articulation. All consciousness is, for Husserl, immersed in the ongoing temporal stream, but unlike abstract linear time independent of consciousness as experienced within the natural attitude, the transcendental reduction reveals how subjectivity *is* the upsurge of temporality itself. For Husserl the living present, which is the carnal presence of the body, is a spontaneously self-generated act, it:

> [...] is the absolute beginning [...] the primal source, that from which all others are continuously generated. In itself, however, it is not generated; it does not come into existence as that which is generated but through spontaneous generation. It does not grow up (it has no seed): it is primal creation. (1964, p 131)

So, again, we can see that the transcendental reduction is never a removal from the life world into another ideal world or into some absolute position of certainty. To the contrary, the further one engages in phenomenological interrogation the more one comes to see the deeper dimensions of our adherence in the world through our profound belief structures – or what Merleau-Ponty calls our perceptual faith.

Husserl's works are consistently taken up with the issue of the upsurge of meaning (or constitution) that is the continuous contact point between subjectivity and the surrounding life world. One of the most misquoted "critiques" of Husserl's methodology is taken from Merleau-Ponty's statement: "The most important lesson which the reduction teaches is the impossibility of a *complete* reduction" (1962, p. XIV). But Merleau-Ponty's careful use of the word "complete" does not indicate a rejection of the reduction at all. His is, in fact, a clarification and defense of its necessarily ambiguous character. Merleau-Ponty, who had access to Husserl's unpublished writings, goes on to paraphrase

Husserl's understanding of the reduction (or *epoché*) as the attitude of a perpetual *commencement* (p. XIV) or beginning. In this regard, the postmodern criticisms of Husserl's work as a kind of "metaphysics of presence" are quite inaccurate. It is ironic to note that in Merleau-Ponty's philosophy which was itself interpreted by many postmodernists as a proto-postmodernism, one can see the profound influence of Husserl's epoché across the entirety of his last and most significant work *The visible and the Invisible* from beginning to end. Finally, it was Derrida (1974), the seminal figure of postmodern thought who penned the critical notion of a "metaphysics of presence" who contributed to this misrepresentation of the transcendental reduction as "logocentric". While this was certainly a suitable critique of the naïvely materialist assumptions of naturalistic psychology, this concept was actually preceded by Husserl's own analysis (1964) of the temporal "now point" as perpetually slipping from the grasp of conscious experience. That this Derridian notion may have been used against Husserl is a matter of great irony.

The transcendental reduction is a "problematic" that one "enters into" in the consideration of it. There is no final goal, end point, or position to the transcendental reduction. It is as fluid and ambiguous as is the life-world itself. The so-called "ego" (or "I") that is the unique standpoint achieved through the transcendental reduction is best expressed in Husserl's own words: "But though the transcendental I is not my psychological I, it must not be considered as if it were a second I, for it is no more separated from my psychological I in the conventional sense of separation, than it is joined to it in the conventional sense of being joined" (1927, p. 702). So the mundane or psychological ego and the transcendental standpoint are really two "aspects" of a common subjectivity – one constructed as a natural object in the world and the other as a standpoint upon that objectified self. They are not "separated". Commenting on the same passage Zahavi remarks:

> The relation between the transcendental subject and the empirical subject is not a relation between two different subjects, but between two different self-apprehensions, a primary and a secondary. The transcendental subject is the subject in its primary constitutive function. The empirical subject is the same subject, but now apprehended and interpreted as an object in the world, that is, as a constituted and mundanized entity. (2003, p. 49)

It can be argued that a psychologist need not take recourse to the deeper "philosophical" dimension entailed by the transcendental reduction. It could be that the psychologist need only work within the disciplinary domain of the eidetic "psychological reduction" that confine itself to the strictly psychological phenomena. I must say, however, that I find it hard to understand how one could mindfully apply the psychological reduction without first grasping it's full context from within the hyper-reflective position of transcendental reduction. Once one enters the *epoché* and can stand apart from the natural attitude, why would one limit oneself to only one dimension of reflection? In this light, Davison and Cosgrove (1991, 2002) make forceful and detailed arguments for the necessity of the phenomenological psychologist to first achieve the transcendental standpoint in order to "return" to a more fully cognizant psychological standpoint. Also, while the disciplinary distinction between philosophy and psychology is appropriate, within the phenomenological standpoint these boundaries are considerably more porous and take on new meanings that require fuller explication.

The Epoché *of the Natural Attitude*

Alfred Schutz, a student of Husserl's who also had access to the unpublished manuscripts, best elucidates another aspect of the *epoché*, which is too often overlooked in the literature. Schutz's contributions were focused on the mundane multiple *epochés* that exist across the spectrum of everyday social life. He argues that the ordinary world of the natural attitude is itself is composed of many unreflective variations of the *epoché* and how, like figure and ground, we are always already within some variation of the epoché. Schutz describes how for the ordinary person, it is not *belief* in the world that is suspended, as in the disciplined phenomenological reduction, but that in the mundane course of everyday living the ordinary person is unwittingly always already performing an epoché of *doubt*. He does not suspend belief in the outer world and it's objects, but on the contrary, he suspends doubt in its existence. What he puts in brackets is doubt that the world and its objects might be otherwise that it appears to him (Schutz p. 229). For example: watching a good movie, reading a novel, or even in ordinary daydreaming I maintain my imaginary world because of my power to not only suspend my belief in the mundane non-fictive world surrounding me, but, most crucially, my ability to suspend any *doubt* in the fictional world I am temporally inhabiting. Daydreaming is particularly illustrative of this *epoché* of the natural attitude. Daydreamers can articulate how their fantasies are sustained so long as they can hold-off doubt in this fictive world (Morley, 1999). This is also the goal of any filmmaker or playwright – to allow an audience to postpone doubt in the fiction they are experiencing.

But there are further dimensions to this suspension of doubt. Schutz shows how it is an essential feature of the natural attitude itself to put in abeyance any contradiction to the naïve realism of the everyday assumptions of ordinary life. Phenomena anomalous to the assumptions of the natural attitude are put aside. It tellingly exhibits intolerance to the strange, the weird, or the uncanny, as much as it suspends the reality of personal death, or sexuality, or even certain social phenomena such as the pervasive economic injustice that surrounds us.

Furthermore, Schutz shows how the *epoché* of the natural attitude sustains multiple worlds, or "finite provinces of meaning" each one distinguished from one another through a sort of amnesiac barrier that is the natural attitude. Like soap bubbles each region of meaning is self-contained until contact with another region pops one bubble into another. There is the world of aggressive office politics that bursts when one enters a place of religious worship, a world of fantasy or daydreaming that ceases when I am forced to attend to the car I am driving, or the world of night-dreaming that explodes upon me at the sound of my alarm clock in the morning. Schutz describes how passage from each province to another is experienced, like any *epoché*, as a psychic jolt or "shock" as in a gestalt switch from figure to ground, but never gradual.

But distinctions must be made. The mundane *epoché* is an unfocused unreflective *epoché* that constrains experience and drives our awareness within the limitations of the natural attitude. In contrast, the phenomenological *epoché* is a focused, self-reflective, and disciplined *epoché* that offers options and possibilities for our understanding of the world in a manner best described as liberating. Nonetheless, this insight into this other aspect of the *epoché* could not only contribute to much empirical phenomenological research and open new avenues for methodology, but it could also support new pedagogical approaches to instructing students in the practice of the *epoché*.

The Epoché *and Contemplative Practice*

Husserl often used the term "meditation", in the sense of a mental discipline, to describe his methodology. Yet, as phenomenology was instituted as a rigorous response to 20th century natural science one hesitates at the use of this term as it is conventionally associated with religious practices. If one assumes meditation to be an inherently religious practice then his hesitation would be justified. But historical precedent indicates that this is not the case. There are many "meditation traditions" across culture and history that maintain an agnostic or even secular standpoint and meditation practice is not the sole property of any particular religious tradition. The Greco-Roman cynics and skeptics, from whom we actually take the word *epoché*, were famously secular. Chinese Taoism, Indian Samkya-yoga and the Buddhist mindfulness traditions are also secular or agnostic in matters of theology. And even those religiously monastic institutions that practice contemplative or meditative techniques are rarely religiously orthodox in the literal sense of the word as "right belief". I make this point to argue that phenomenologists need not fear any drift into mystical occultism should we engage in dialogue with other traditions of "mental discipline". And I suspect that there is much to learn from these traditions without risk of losing our own secular identity within the Western academy and sciences. Furthermore, it is a testimony to its validity to acknowledge how culturally specific versions of the *epoché* have previously been articulated and practiced in other cultures separated from us by geography and history. For example, one of the clearest examples of this corroboration is in the classical yoga tradition where the technical Sanskrit term *nirodaha* corresponds almost exactly to the meaning of the Husserlian epoché (Morley, 2001, 2008). These centuries old meditation traditions may indeed exist outside of the academic and scientific context of phenomenological psychology, but they may contribute very concrete insights into the meditation *practice* that is the *epoché.* It would behoove phenomenologists to take advantage of these living traditions and their rich literature and practices.

Conclusion

In light of our discussion of the transcendental reduction, I wish to conclude with a reiteration of the thought that, as the *epoché* is a practice that involves the full existential engagement of the researcher as a whole person, the *epoché* is more than an intellectual operation or a professional technique. While it is a method, it is not just a technique or tool in the ordinary sense. The *epoché* and all the various forms of the reduction entail a type of disposition or attitude, a value system. One could even call it a way of living. While I would not go so far as to say that the *epoché* is an explicit morality or ethic, I would venture to call it an implicit *ethos.* It is a commitment to assume the position of perpetual beginner and a childlike yet disciplined openness to the world as an ongoing birth of meaning. It is a stance of wonder, astonishment, and what is essentially a *trust* in the truth of the world to reveal itself on its own terms – not the terms of the mundane ego of the natural attitude.

Finally, I hope this brief essay has made a small contribution toward a renewed appreciation of the importance of the *epoché* to our research endeavors. I have made no attempt to pretend to give any final word on this enigmatic practice that is at the heart of the phenomenological endeavor. I only ask that it receive a more sustained discussion and focus in our work together. Again, I give thanks to our teacher, Amedeo Giorgi. For, by conscientiously instituting an authentic phenomenologically based empirical psychological methodology Giorgi has built upon and has, in all practical ways, even surpassed Husserl in this particular disciplinary domain. Because of Amedeo Giorgi the next generation of phenomenological psychologists have a very well worked soil from whence to grow and an infinity of tasks before us.

References

Davidson, L. & Cosgrove, L. A. (1991). Psychologism and phenomenological psychology revisited Part I: The liberation from naturalism, *Journal of Phenomenological Psychology*, 22 (2), pp. 87-108.

Davidson, L. & Cosgrove, L. A. (2002). Psychologism and phenomenological psychology revisited, Part II: The return to positivity. *Journal of Phenomenological Psychology*, 33 (2), pp. 141-177.

Derrida, J. (1974). *Of Grammatology*. (G. Spivak, Trans.). Baltimore: The Johns Hopkins University Press.

Finlay, L. (2008). A dance between reduction and reflexivity: Explicating the phenomenological psychological attitude. *The Journal of Phenomenological Psychology*, 39, pp 1-32.

Giorgi, A. (1970). Psychology as a human science: a phenomenologically based approach. New York: Harper and Row.

Husserl, E. (1951/1927). Phenomenology. In *Encyclopaedia Britannica*. Chicago, ILL: Encyclopedia Britannica Inc., p. 701.

Husserl, E. (1962). *Ideas I: general introduction to pure phenomenology*. (B. Gibson, Trans.). New York: Collier Books, section 69.

Husserl, E. (1989). *Ideas pertaining to a pure phenomenology and to a Phenomenological Philosophy, 2nd book: Studies in the phenomenology of constitution*. (R. Rojcewicz & A. Schuwer, Trans.). Dordrecht: Kluwer (original work written in 1928 and published in German posthumously in 1952).

Husserl, E. (1977). *Cartesian Meditations: an introduction to Phenomenology*. (D. Cairns, Trans). The Hague; Martinus Nijhoff.

Husserl E. (1964). *The phenomenology of internal time consciousness*. (J. S. Churchill, Trans.). Bloomington: Indiana University Press.

Husserl, E. (2001). *Analyses concerning passive and active synthesis: Lectures on transcendental logic*. (A. Steinbock, Trans.). Dordrecht: Springer.

Husserl, E. (2005). *Phantasy, image consciousness, and memory (1898-1925)*. (J. Brough, Trans.). Dordrecht: Springer.

Merleau-Ponty, M. (1962). *Phenomenology of Perception*. (C. Smith, Trans.). London: Routledge and Kegan Paul.

Merleau-Ponty, M. (1968). *The visible and the invisible*. (A. Lingis, Trans.) Evanston: Northwestern University Press.

Merleau-Ponty, (1992). *Texts and dialogues*. (H. Silverman & J. Barry, Eds). Atlantic Highlands: Humanities Press.

Morley, J. (1999). The private theatre: a phenomenological investigation of daydreaming. *The Journal of Phenomenological Psychology*, 29 (1).

Morley, J. (2001). Inspiration and expiration: yoga practice through Merleau-Ponty's phenomenology of embodiment. *Philosophy East and West*, 51 (1).

Morley, J. (2008). Embodied consciousness in tantric yoga and the phenomenology of Merleau-Ponty. *Religion and the Arts*, 12 (1-3).

Schutz, A., (1962). *Collected papers I: The problem of social reality.* (Ed. Maurice Natanson). The Hague: Martinus Nijhoff.

Weldon, D. (Ed.). (2003). *The new Husserl: a critical reader.* Bloomington: Indiana University Press.

Zahavi, D. (2003). *Husserl's Phenomenology.* Stanford: Stanford University Press.

Notes

1 Linda Finlay's (2008) recent publication offers a much more detailed exposition on the concrete practice of the epoché than is offered here. Finlay also calls for a more sustained focus on this issue and provides a remarkable example of how it is possible to explicate and teach the concrete *practice* of the epoché. Hers is one of the few concrete examples of how one actually performs the *epoche*' in psychological research. This essay is intended to be a compliment to hers – in every sense of the word.

2 In Husserl's words, this is an "inhibiting" or "putting out of play" of all positions taken toward the already-given objective world. Also a parenthesizing of the Objective world (*Cartesian Meditations,* pp 20-21). I think it best described in English through the expressions: suspension, holding in abeyance, and withholding of assent. It should never imply any sort of violent "cancelation", "cessation", "suppression" or "disregard" that would close off awareness. Regardless of terms, what matters is that the *epoché* is understood as an attitude of contemplative *openness.*

HUSSERL VERSUS DERRIDA

Richard Rojcewicz, Ph.D.

Duquesne University
United States

Abstract

At the end of his career, Husserl claimed to see spread out before him "the endlessly open plains of true philosophy," and he was cautiously optimistic that his followers could and would cultivate those plains by following consistently in his footsteps. Husserl's dream seems to have ended with the advent of deconstruction and especially with Derrida's direct criticism of the phenomenological theory of signs. In this paper I take up the cudgels against Derrida and try to show that his critique is eminently refutable. Yet to demonstrate that phenomenology is viable is not to prove that it is actually living. Derrida's critique, valid or not, has largely won the day. Why? I suggest an answer to that question by correlating deconstruction with Pop Art.

This paper takes up the cudgels against the Derridean critique of Edmund Husserl's theory of signs. That critique, in *La voix et le phénomène*, does not purport to affect merely one particular, tangential issue; instead, it is supposed to strike at the very heart of Husserl's philosophy. Thus what I offer here is a defense of phenomenology itself against deconstruction. I hope to show that phenomenology is not, *pace* Derrida, a philosophy of pure self-presence, a "metaphysics of presence". In the end I will ask why the Derridean critique, though eminently refutable, is nevertheless carrying the day.

Husserl's "Theory" of Signs

The context in Husserl's work is the first investigation of the *Logische Untersuchungen.* Husserl does not, however, actually present a theory of signs in general; he is for the most part concerned with distinguishing two kinds of signs, and indeed he is not even concerned so much with these two kinds for themselves but with showing they can function independently. Derrida, likewise, although his book is subtitled "An introduction to the problem of the sign in Husserl's phenomenology", is concerned primarily with showing that the two kinds are not independent, that one of them in particular cannot be "purified" from "contamination" by the other.

Regarding signs in general, Husserl uses no single term that would characterize their operation as such. He does not say they "signify" or "designate" or "stand for". He says only that every sign is a sign "of" something (*jedes Zeichen ist Zeichen für etwas*) (Husserl, 1913, p. 23). This means, presumably, that there is an intentionality or relationality about signs; they are essentially related to something or other. All signs possess this relationality, but Husserl sees two radically different ways the relating can be accomplished. On the one hand, the relation can be intrinsic, whereby the sign actually embodies that of which it is a sign. Or the relation can be extrinsic, such that the sign is merely a pointer. The first sort of sign is restricted to language and is called "expression" (*Ausdruck*). The other is wider in scope and is called "indication" (*Anzeichen*). It is wider because all expressions can also function as indications.

Linguistic signs are signs of meaning (*Bedeutung*) or sense (*Sinn*); i.e., these signs express a meaning, or, put differently, language expresses thoughts. Words do not merely point to a meaning but actually bear or embody it. There is no distance between the words and the meaning; to understand a word *is* to grasp its meaning. According to Husserl, the expression and the meaning unite, they are "phenomenally one" (1913, p. 31) in the consciousness of the person who utters, hears, or reads them.

Husserl does not say more about this unity and seems to take it for granted that the difference from external, indicational signs is obvious. He does not spell out the difference, but we might find a clue to it in his declaration that "indications do not harbor meaning in the pregnant sense [*im prägnanten Sinne*] of linguistic signs" (1913, p. 31). Perhaps we could then claim that what is distinctive about words as signs is precisely their being pregnant with their meaning. This not only implies an intimate relation between expression and meaning but also suggests that expressions *give birth* to their meaning. That is, without words there would be no conceptual meaning, no thought. There is no pre-expressed thought. Prior to being expressed, thoughts are no more than gropings in a haze.

For Husserl, as for all phenomenologists, words are not merely an outer packaging of already constituted interior thoughts, enabling those thoughts to be communicated to other people. On the contrary, we need words just in order to have definite thoughts. Our thoughts do not lead a previous existence apart from the expressions which crystallize them. Words allow thought to precipitate out of the haze just as, in Merleau-Ponty's analogy, the earth did out of its planetary nebula (1945, p. 374).

Husserl's own philosophical work is a prime illustration of this languishing of thought in words. Husserl was a graphomaniac, and his voluminous manuscripts have been preserved. What is most evident about these assorted scraps of paper, apart from the fact that they are written in shorthand, is the intense struggle going on there, as is evident by all the crossing out and reworking. This could hardly be a mere struggle to find words in order to clothe thoughts that were already clear in his mind. It is a struggle aimed at finding the thoughts themselves, e.g., the thought of the reduction. According to Merleau-Ponty, "There is certainly no question which required of Husserl a greater expenditure of time in order to clarify – i.e., to clarify *for himself* –and no question to which he returned more often, as is evident by the important place the "problematic of the reduction" occupies in his unpublished manuscripts" (1945, p. v).

If words are signs in the pregnant sense and thus are, so to speak, feminine, then other signs do not give birth and are masculine. Thereby the adage is confirmed: *parole femine, fatti maschii.* Consider smoke as a sign of fire. Smoke does not bear fire, for there can be fire without smoke. Likewise, there can be a country without a flag, and my cattle can be my property without displaying my brand. For Husserl, an indicative sign is one that merely motivates a conviction in the existence of that of which it is the sign. Indeed, we sometimes say fever "means" an infection is present, a salute "expresses" respect. Husserl, however, would consider this a loose way of speaking, and he himself is terminologically strict. He uses "meaning" and "expression" only for linguistic signs. All other signs are externally and presumptively related to that of which they are signs.

Perhaps the difference between the two sorts of signs is most visible in the fact that indicative signs can lie. The soldier saluting might actually harbor no respect at all. We can only presume she does, we are motivated to believe she does, but the respect remains extrinsic to the salute. The reason, according to Husserl, is that indication is "non-insightful", *nichteinsichtig* (1913, p. 24), *uneinsichtig* (p. 25). If, in contrast, linguistic expressions are accompanied with insight, then the dissimulation which always menaces the indicative sign is impossible with them. To understand the words is to grasp their meaning without any further ado. The words, "The door is locked", cannot possibly mean that the door is not locked.

Husserl is content here to paint with a broad brush, and Derrida does not challenge the general distinction between the two kinds of signs. His critique concerns the relation between the two kinds in the case of language. Husserl's position is that linguistic signs alone are meaningful, and indeed always function meaningfully, but they can also function indicatively. According to Husserl, however, only the expressive function, and not the indicative, is essential to language. The entire issue for Derrida is the intertwining, and possible separation, of these two functions of words.

In ordinary discourse, i.e., in communicative speech with others, words always both bear a meaning about some subject matter and indicate something about the speaker. If I tell my confederate that the door is locked, my words communicate to him a meaning, they bear a message about the door, but they are also a sign indicating to him how I feel about this state of affairs. From my tone of voice, for example, he might surmise that I am astonished, frustrated, or happy about the door being locked. At the very least, my words indicate to him that I am a rational living being, i.e., one possessing language (*zoon logon echon*), one that animates words with an intention to say something and does not just produce random vocalizations. In short, my words indicate that I am a human person with a conscious life, that I have a soul.

The particular sort of indication attaching to linguistic signs is called by Husserl "intimation" (*Kundgabe*), a term that connotes very well the lack of apodictic certainty. Every indication, according or Husserl, is only a motivation to believe in the existence of something which is not properly present. In the specific case of intimation, my own feelings and even the existence of my soul cannot be properly present to anyone but myself. To others, my soul is only apperceived, i.e., improperly given with a lesser degree of evidence, and to some extent is merely presumed.

I have privileged access to my own soul, which is to say that its existence is apodictically certain to me. But Husserl is not so foolish as to maintain that anyone has adequate knowledge of his or her own soul. Husserl uses "adequate" in the etymological sense of "equal to", "exhaustive". No one knows himself perfectly, and indeed for Husserl adequate knowledge of anything whatsoever is beyond the scope of us finite human beings. There is always more to know of even the simplest things, let alone something as recondite as the soul.

The crucial question is whether the indicative function, the intimation of the state of the soul, belongs essentially to the phenomenon of language. For Husserl, the way to an essential determination is through the method of free variation. That method is the attempt to find (in actuality or in imagination) an instance in which the reputedly essential factor is not included. If in that instance the phenomenon remains what it was, the factor is inessential. If its absence destroys the phenomenon, essential.

Suppose I say to a confederate that the door is locked. If he hears me and understands my words, we then share the same meaning. We possess the one meaning in common; it is commun-icated. This of course does not imply we are convinced the door is locked; it entails only that we are both entertaining in our minds the thought of the door as locked. Is the intimating function operative in both of us? Obviously not; only my confederate takes my words as external indications that I have a soul. I do not myself listen to the tone of my voice and from that tone draw the probable conclusion that I am surprised about the locked door. I already know I am surprised, because I am a conscious being: I know myself "along with" knowing things in the world. I do not need a roundabout way of arguing to the state of my soul. At the very least, I already know I have a soul, because it is properly, even if imperfectly, present to me; versus the souls of others, I do not need to "appresent" my own soul to myself and presume it exists.

Thus a variant can be found in which the meaning function of language goes on while the indicating function drops away. At its simplest, this is the variant in which I do not even utter words to anyone but, instead, pronounce them silently in my mind, in the solitary life of the soul (*im einsamen Seelenleben*). In this case, the words are still expressive, they bear the meaning they always bear, but they do not function as indications. It would be purposeless and indeed counterproductive for me to take my own words as indications of the existence of my own soul, since such indications would merely give me in a lesser way a knowledge I already possess in a more eminent way.

Indeed to have recourse to such indications would be pathological. It would be an instance of the abnormality that was first called "soul blindness" (*Seelenblindheit*) and later included under "aphasia". In the phenomenological literature, the most celebrated case of this disturbance is that of Schn., the brain-injured soldier investigated by Kurt Goldstein and referred to extensively by Merleau-Ponty.

"Soul blindness" exactly describes the condition of Schn., for he lost the normal contact a person has with himself. Schn. then had to resort to external signs by way of compensation. For instance, he lost the normal possession of his own body, and to know his posture he needed either to look at his body or to interpret certain signs. The pressure he felt on the soles of his feet was interpreted by him as an indication that he was standing.

The point is that such recourse to external signs is precisely pathological. For a person to take his own speech as an indication of the existence of his own soul would then be an extreme abnormality, a way of compensating for an extreme soul-blindness. It would be equivalent to someone checking the obituary column every day to see if he were still alive.

Derrida's Critique

Husserl's view of the inessentiality of the indicational function of words seems innocuous and sane, and yet Derrida contests it and believes he is thereby driving a stake through the very heart of phenomenology. According to Derrida, this issue has "unlimited consequences" (1967, p. 53) for Husserl's philosophy, and so his critique is a radical one and not merely a disagreement concerning one fine point.

The unlimited consequences actually derive from Derrida's own oppositional understanding of the distinction between expression and indication. For him, these oppositions are as follows: central/marginal, self/others, presence/absence, non-physical/physical, soul/body, voluntary /involuntary, inner/outer, spirit/nature, pure/contaminated, immediate/ mediate, certain/uncertain. Expression is associated with the first member of each opposition, indication with the second. Derrida would have it that Husserl, by maintaining the independence of expression, is excluding everything associated with indication. Thus Husserl's is a traditional, exclusionary philosophy which denigrates all that is other, foreign, and messy. Derrida himself stands with the impure and the marginalized, and thus arises his critique of Husserl's theory of signs.

Derrida always condemns binary, oppositional thinking, which he places at the core of the strategy of metaphysics. In my view, however, Derrida is the one who is here thinking oppositionally. Husserl does not distinguish expression and indication the way Derrida charges. Consequently, there is no need to bring back in all the elements associated with indication; they were never excluded by Husserl in the first place. Furthermore, Derrida's prescription to redress the exclusivity, namely, by way of indications, is misguided and indeed impossible.

I hope to make my case by reading very closely what I take to be the main argument in Derrida's book. It is a laborious, convoluted argument, which I shall try to make sense of by breaking down into five steps. According to Derrida, for Husserl:

1. Expression is, in general, a realm of purity.
2. Expression cannot be shared with others; i.e., meaning cannot be communicated.
3. Expression is exteriorization, namely, of something fully present prior to being expressed.
4. Expression is voluntary, and whatever resists the will, such as the body or nature, is excluded from expression.
5. Expression harbors concealment and so (in Derrida's view) must be supplemented by indicative signs.

The first four steps are premises of the fifth in the sense that they trace a path of ever greater exclusion which the last step is supposed to reverse.

1. *Expression as* purified *by excluding indication*:

Derrida belabors the fact that, for Husserl, words are able to function meaningfully in the absence of their indicative function, i.e., in the solitary life of the soul. But Derrida completely and conveniently neglects the fact that for Husserl words also function meaningfully in communicative dialogue, i.e., when the expressive and indicative functions exist side by side. Derrida emphasizes the meaning function in the former case to such an extent that he excludes the latter: he *identifies* meaning with the solitary life of the soul. Thus the title of the central chapter of his book is "Meaning as soliloquy", *Le vouloir-dire comme soliloque*.

Taken strictly, it makes no sense to speak of meaning as soliloquy. Meaning cannot *be* soliloquy, and Husserl never claims it is. The meaning function of words is not destroyed in soliloquy, that function goes on in soliloquy, but the function itself cannot be identified with the circumstance under which it is exercised. That would make no sense. Meaning cannot be equated with monologue any more than intimation can be equated with dialogue.

If Derrida is not to be taken here in the strict sense, then he is speaking loosely and is claiming that meaning occurs *par excellence* in soliloquy. The meaning function is at its highest in soliloquy – that, presumably, is what Derrida intends by repeating *ad nauseam* that meaning is "pure" in soliloquy, freed from "contamination" by the indicative function.

Yet Husserl himself never uses a term such as "pure" or "free" or "contaminate" in this context. In fact, he does not actually characterize the separation of the two functions at all. His one and only statement on the matter is this: "Expressions carry out their meaning function also in the solitary life of the soul, where they no longer operate as indications" (1913, p. 24). This is a completely neutral characterization of the separation of the two functions and certainly does not imply the meaning function is purified in the solitary life of the soul. Husserl merely says it is "also" in play there.

Husserl does characterize the conjunction of the two functions in dialogue, but it is not at all a matter of "contamination". Husserl first says that in dialogue the two functions exist "side by side" (*neben* each other, 1913, p. 23). He also says that in dialogue the meaning function is always "plaited" (*verflochten*, p. 24) to the indicative function. Finally, he speaks of the two functions as "linked" (*verbunden*, p. 36). These are all neutral terms for describing a concomitance and in no way imply the functions have any effect on each other, let alone the one of contamination. In fact, Husserl is explicit that the actual operation of the meaning function is indifferent to its circumstance of monologue or dialogue.

Husserl asserts this indifference twice. He says at the very beginning of his discussion that when words do not function indicatively, "this does not affect what makes expressions expressions. They possess, as before, their meanings and indeed the same meanings they had in dialogue" (1913, p. 35). Or again, he says that if we understand the words, "then they are expressive, and they express the same whether they are directed to someone or not" (p. 35). These statements show clearly enough that for Husserl the two functions, when they exist concomitantly, are *merely* "side by side." The link between them is an external one, and they remain independent in their actual functioning.

From all the evidence, then, the meaning function is not in its purest, highest state in soliloquy. The connection to the indicative function is not a contamination. Indeed that connection could be called with equal justification a complement, such that the meaning function would exist in a *deficient* state in soliloquy. A book on Husserl's theory of signs could then just as well include a chapter called "Meaning as dialogue".

Accordingly, Derrida's constant use of the term "pure" to characterize expressions in monologue is unwarranted. The meaning function is not pure there; at least it is no purer there than it is anywhere else. Now, this is not an inconsequential mistake on Derrida's part, nor is it an innocent one. Derrida has an ulterior motive, which is to accuse Husserl of taking the solitary life of the soul as a domain of pure self-presence. To be sure, for Husserl the intimating function is absent in monologue precisely because the soul already knows itself in a more eminent way than intimation allows. Derrida takes this to mean that expression is *purified* of intimation because the soul already knows itself *purely*, i.e., is completely self-present. But this exaggeration is unjustified, and all of Derrida's uses of the word "pure" with regard to Husserl are suspect.

2. *Expression as incommunicable*:

Derrida believes that for Husserl not only is expression purified of intimation, it is also purified of other people--in the sense that meaning is incommunicable. Expressions cannot be shared. Other people and communications with them belong entirely to the domain of indication. Husserl, according to Derrida, assigns the communicative operation of speech exclusively to the indicative function of words and denies it to the expressive function. Thus what is communicated is solely what can be intimated.

For Derrida, "communication or manifestation is by essence indication" (1967, p. 43). He also speaks of "communicating, informing, or manifesting, i.e., indicating" (1967, p. 53). (The word "manifest" is actually out of place in these phrases, for that is Derrida's translation of Husserl's *Kundgabe*, "intimation", and intimation is of course a kind of indication, it is indication by way of words.) In fact, however, communicative or informative speech (these terms, *kummunikativ* and *mitteilend*, are synonyms for Husserl) is not related in a simple way to the indicative function of words. Derrida is mistaken to identify communication with indication and to draw a strict line between "expression and indicative communication" (1967, p. 56). On Derrida's account, the meaning of expressions cannot be communicated, because communication is intimation, and intimation merely motivates the conviction in the *existence* of conscious acts but does not give information about their content or meaning.

Derrida is mistaken here, but the mistake is an understandable one. To a casual reading, it might indeed appear that Husserl equates linguistic communication with intimation. For example, with regard to expressions as they function communicatively, Husserl maintains that "this function rests essentially on the fact that expressions operate as indications" (1913, p. 35). This surely implies that expressions can be communicated inasmuch as they function indicatively, and therefore only what is intimated by an expression is communicated. Moreover, according to Husserl, "where the intimating function is linked to the meaning function, there thoughts are not merely to be expressed in the mode of a meaning but are also to be communicated through [*mittels*: "with the help of", "through the mediation of"] intimation" (1913, p. 36). Again we see a close connection between communication and intimation. Husserl seems to be saying communication takes place through intimation in the sense that the communicated and the intimated are one and the same. Finally, Husserl asserts that, in communicative speech, the meaning-conferring acts "indeed form the most essential core of intimation. To make the hearer aware of these acts – precisely that must be, before all else, the interest of the communicative intention" (1913, p. 39). This says that the communicative interest lies in the intimation of the existence of the meaning-conferring acts. Thus communication is equivalent to the intimation of these acts.

Yet a closer reading shows that Husserl does not identify communication with intimation. The relation between them is that communication "essentially rests on" intimation, or takes place "through" it, or has a prime "interest" in intimation. But they are not the same function and indeed are utterly separate.

For Husserl, communication is in fact *always* the communication of meaning; i.e., the content of a thought is precisely what is communicated. Expressions, supposedly pure in the solitary life of the soul, can be shared. Husserl even uses the term "communication" exclusively for a sharing of the meaning conferred by the meaning-conferring acts. Thus Derrida is exactly wrong, for the communication of the meaning of these acts and the intimation of their existence are not only distinct but even have nothing in common.

To be sure, the separate functions of communication and indication are connected. For Husserl, in order for a speaker to communicate a thought to a hearer, the latter must first apprehend the speaker as a speaker, as a *person* with a soul who is animating vocal sounds with an intention to say something. The apprehension of the intentional acts which confer meaning is a precondition for the grasp of the meaning. That is, in order to grasp the meaning, one must first surmise that a meaning is being expressed at all:

> [...] the speaker, in certain psychic acts, confers on the sounds a meaning, a meaning he wants to communicate to the hearer. But the communication is possible only if the hearer also understands the intention of the speaker. And he does so insofar as he apprehends the speaker as a person, one who is not producing mere sounds but *is speaking to him*, who thus is carrying out, along with the sounds, at the same time certain meaning-conferring acts, acts whose existence the person wants to intimate to the hearer, acts whose meaning the person wants to communicate to the hearer. (1913, p. 33)

Thus communication and indication are not identical; instead, the connection between them is that the latter makes the former possible. It does so by allowing the hearer to surmise that the speaker is a genuine speaker, i.e., a person with a soul, with the capacity for intentional, meaning-conferring acts. It is the existence of these acts that is intimated; the meaning conferred by the acts is what is communicated. Accordingly, the two functions are separate and have separate objects: on the one hand, the existence of thoughts in the soul of the speaker and, on the other hand, the content of those thoughts, the meaning to be shared. Yet the two functions are connected; the one is founded on the other.

It is this connection, and not an identity, Husserl is referring to when he says that communication "depends essentially on" intimation or takes place "through", i.e., "through the mediation of" intimation. It also explains the "interest" of communication in intimation. The interest derives from the fact that only if the hearer imputes meaning-conferring acts to the speaker does he understand what is said. That is, communication, the understanding of the speaker's meaning, has a vested interest in intimation, for without such intimation the speaker's meaning would not be conveyed to the hearer. Thus Husserl is not claiming intimation is the prime interest of communication in the sense of the *goal* of communication; it is only a precondition for the operation of communication. Intimation does not *carry out* communication but only paves its way.

Two comments are here in order. In the first place, Husserl's position would seem to involve him in a vicious circle. He maintains that a precondition for understanding someone is the imputation of meaning-conferring acts: only if I surmise that the speaker is actuated by a meaning-intention can I grasp his meaning. But does not the converse also hold? Only if I recognize that the speaker is making sense do I impute to him the intention to make sense. I doubt the rationality of someone who is just babbling. Put differently, the question is how I could know there are meaning-conferring acts present in the soul of the speaker unless I grasp that a meaning is actually being conferred on vocal sounds, i.e., unless I *already* grasp meaning. Therefore it would seem communication makes intimation possible just as much as the reverse.

Perhaps the easiest way out of this difficulty is to recognize that a person indicates his rationality in other ways besides speaking. Thus "indication" should not be restricted here to intimation. When a stranger approaches me, I am given many signs this is a human person, even before she begins to speak. These are all genuine indications in Husserl's sense, motivations to surmise the existence of certain conscious acts which are not properly present to me. But they are not intimations in the strict sense of linguistic indications. Therefore, in slight opposition to Husserl, intimation as such must merely be the *confirmation* of something already surmised from other signs. Yet, in support of Husserl, linguistic intimation may indeed provide the *best* indication of rationality.

The other comment is that Husserl does not deny the capacity of indications to make known many things about a person. He is not saying the meaning communicated is all that matters in dialogue or is necessarily more important than what is intimated. From indications, according to Husserl, other people "may indeed learn all sorts of things [*mancherlei*] about our inner thoughts and feelings" (1913, p. 31). This learning, however, is not a matter of communication and is subject to the non-apodicticity menacing every extrinsic sign. But it might be what the speaking is all about. For example, lovers whisper sweet nothings to each other. What matters to them is not the meaning of their words (indeed they whisper "nothing" or simply say "I love you" over and over in different ways); what matters is the sweet feeling with which the words are charged.

At the other extreme is the functional speech of those who are indifferent to each other, such as the seller and buyer of stamps at a window. All that matters in this case is the expression, the meaning of the words, namely, the price of the stamps, how many are required, etc. Yet, just as lovers make some sense and do not simply coo, so, conversely, in this case there is a minimum of intimation. I may be almost totally indifferent to the clerk as a person, but I still do not interact with her the way I would with a machine that dispenses stamps. Thus, as Husserl says, in communicative speech words *always* function indicatively.

3. *Expression as exteriorization*:

For Husserl, according to Derrida, the self-presence of the soul is so pure and immediate that this presence excludes intimation, excludes others from sharing in it, and even excludes language. Expression does not give birth to self-presence but, on the contrary, merely exteriorizes it. That is the force behind Derrida's claim that, for Husserl, expression (Derrida hyphenates: *l'ex-pression*) is sheer exteriorization (*l'extériorisation*): "It imprints in a certain outside a sense first found in a certain inside" (1967, p. 34).

Derrida is here translating a term Husserl does employ in this context, *Äußerung*. But Husserl does *not* apply it to expression as such. It refers to outward signs like the play of the features or the mien [*Mienenspiel*] and gestures, and these are precisely not expressions in Husserl's sense but, instead, are indications. Husserl also says that an expression can be exteriorized, which simply means it can be spoken aloud to another person. But expression itself is not exteriorization; on the contrary, it is something that can *be* exteriorized. Husserl certainly does not understand it in the sense of ex-pression, the mere outer imprint of an already constituted inner meaning. In fact, such an imprint would define indication; it would lack the pregnancy characteristic of linguistic signs.

Derrida is very careful to say that expression imprints in a *certain* outside something first found in a *certain* inside. Thus it is not a matter of an inside and outside in the usual sense, namely, *in* consciousness and *out* in the external world. For Derrida, the inside and outside of expression remain *within* consciousness: "This outside and inside are absolutely original: the outside is neither nature, nor the world, not a real exteriority in relation to consciousness" (1967, p. 34). I grant that the concepts of "inside" and "outside" have to be qualified in some way when referring to Husserl. My objection is that Derrida does not also qualify the word "sense" when he says it is exteriorized in expression.

What is this sense which precedes exteriorization? It cannot be what Husserl means by "sense", namely, "meaning". For, meaning does not precede expression; meaning is precisely what comes to birth through expression. Furthermore, if sense is constituted prior to expression, i.e., without language, then the work of words is already accomplished and there is no need to put thoughts into words. The thoughts have already crystallized. On the other hand, if expression does have something to accomplish, if it contributes to the birth of meaning, then what precedes it must lack sense, or at least must possess sense only in some qualified way.

The pre-expressive stratum must violate the principle of excluded middle and be neither sense nor non-sense. If it is sense, then expression is superfluous, for there would be no distinction between the expression and what precedes it.

If the pre-expressive stratum is sheer non-sense, then expression is impossible, for there would be no internal connection between expression and what precedes it. Derrida accuses phenomenology of taking up the former position: there is a pure, pre-expressive contact with the world and with the self, and this contact is simply mirrored or ex-pressed at the level of speech. But Derrida, in my view, occupies the opposite extreme. For him, there is *no* self-presence prior to language (and, if I understand him correctly, none afterwards either), and the pre-expressive stratum is empty.

In fact it is precisely phenomenology that avoids the extremes – by recognizing that, for the first position, pre-expressive consciousness is too rich for expression to be productive and, for the second, too poor for expression to be possible. The first position amounts to idealism and the second to realism, and Merleau-Ponty's critique of them applies in full. That critique is formulated in one way as follows:

> The consciousness that conditions language is merely a global and unarticulated grasp of the world, as is that of the child at its first breath or that of the drowning man who lunges out toward life. It is indeed true that all particular knowledge is founded on this first, global view of the world, but it is no less true that this view needs to be reconquered, fixed, and made explicit through perceptual exploration and speech. (1945, p. 463)

This says that the relation obtaining here is the dialectical one Husserl calls "founding". The pre-expressive, founding stratum is everything and nothing. Everything, because expression will simply bring out what is latent there and indeed will never exhaust it. Nothing, because it does not by itself lead to expression and without expression would never even manifest itself. Husserl's image of the pregnancy of linguistic signs says the same. To give birth is not to create out of nothing. On the contrary, it is to bring to fruition something that has already been implanted. Yet to bring to fruition is precisely to bring forth something *new* in relation to what was implanted.

Thus Husserl does not maintain or even suggest that expression is exteriorization, for he does not believe there is something further inward simply waiting to be ex-pressed. What is further inward is not sense, not a clear idea about myself which merely has to be clothed in words. The notion of a pre-expressive, pure self-presence is something Derrida foists onto Husserl.

Once again, it is Derrida who is thinking oppositionally. He sees only two alternatives: the pre-expressive must be either full sense or complete non-sense. Derrida qualifies everything except sense. He is thereby oblivious precisely to what is most proper to phenomenology, namely, an appreciation of phenomena, that peculiar realm where the principle of excluded middle is violated or, as Merleau-Ponty says, "where contradictions embrace" (1945, p. 12).

Inasmuch as violation of the principle of non-contradiction (= excluded middle) is the death of logic, phenomenology is not, *pace* Derrida, a logocentrism.

4. *Expression as voluntary:*

Derrida does qualify the concept of exteriorization, but in a way that removes it even further from Husserl. Derrida claims that for Husserl expression is *voluntary* exteriorization and the essential difference between expression and indication is that between the voluntary and involuntary. Furthermore, the latter difference is the one between the inner and the outer. Therefore Husserl is in complicity with a voluntaristic "metaphysics of presence" which denigrates the outer (body) in favor of the inner (soul).

According to Derrida, "expression is an exteriorization which is voluntary, decided, conscious through and through, intentional" (1967, p. 35). It is true that for Husserl vocal sounds, in order to be actual language and not simply comparable to the "rattle of machinery" (1913, p. 67), must be animated by an intention to mean something. But it is not the sheer fact that they are performed willfully that makes linguistic signs expressions. Other signs can be accompanied with just as much will, or with even more, and yet they remain indications. Instead, what is crucial is whether or not the signs are such as to unite with the intention or remain extrinsic to them.

Our actions, all of them, can be carried out with varying degrees of volition. We can choose our words deliberately and can also speak inadvertently, listlessly. We can gesticulate absent-mindedly and also with complete attentiveness, the way a mime or a choking person does. Yet this maximum of volition will not turn a gesture into an expression, whereas the minimum of volition will do so for words.

The reason is that not everything is equal in receiving, i.e., embodying, a meaning-intention. For Husserl it could be said that the distinction between expression and indication is a noematic not, with all due respect to Derrida, a noetic one. The mere intention is not what is decisive; that which receives the intention is equally so. There is something about linguistic signs – versus all other ones – that enables them to become pregnant with a meaning-intention. Thus what is decisive is not simply the will to impregnate but whether the sign *can* become pregnant.

Therefore Husserl's theory is not a voluntarism. What is decisive is not simply the will. Nor is Husserl denigrating the external, the bodily. According to Derrida, "In expression, the intention is absolutely explicit because it animates a voice which can remain completely interior" (1967, p. 35-6). It is true that words do not have to be spoken aloud. Inner speech, for Husserl, is still expression. But what Derrida is omitting is the plain fact that, for Husserl, words can also be external – spoken aloud or written. Indeed, for Husserl, it is a matter of complete indifference to the meaning function whether the words are silent or spoken. Words are not more meaningful in monologue and are not less meaningful in dialogue. Thus words do not need to be "purified" of everything bodily in order to be genuinely expressive words. What matters is not whether the sign is internal or external but, instead, what sort of sign it is, namely, a word or something else.

Derrida concludes his discussion of expression as exteriorization by saying that "the essence of language is its *telos*, and its *telos* is voluntary consciousness as [the act of] meaning" (1967, p. 38). I strongly suspect that we have here a slip of the tongue or a typographical error and that Derrida actually means the *arche* of language, not the *telos*. If volitional consciousness is indeed the end of language, then that would take back everything Derrida says about language as ex-pression. It would mean that to come to self-consciousness is the *result* of language (which I believe *is* a thesis of phenomenology), whereas Derrida accuses Husserl of positing a pure self-presence *prior* to expression.

If Derrida did mean to say volition is the *arche* of language, that would be consistent with his position, but it would still be unfaithful to Husserl. Volition is indeed one of the *archai* of language, but the will cannot by itself constitute expression. Words form another *arche* of language. And, of course, words can function meaningfully whether they are internal or external. Thus Husserl is not in complicity with a voluntaristic metaphysics that tries to exclude what is bodily.

5. *Expression as harboring concealment:*

Having supposedly shown the massive exclusions at work in Husserl's understanding of expression, Derrida proceeds to reintegrate the marginalized, i.e., the indicative. He begins: "It is indeed not enough to recognize oral discourse as the milieu of expressivity" (1967, p. 39). This statement already gives us pause, for oral discourse is not the milieu of expressivity. It is the milieu of intimation. Expression *can* take place in oral discourse, but Derrida does *not* recognize that; for him the proper milieu of expression is monologue, silent discourse.

Derrida proceeds: "Once we have excluded all the non-discursive signs (gestures, the mien, etc.) which present themselves immediately as exterior to speech, there still remains, this time interior to speech, a non-expressivity of considerable amplitude" (1967, p. 39-40). Presumably, what Derrida means here by "speech" (*la parole*) is expression, the meaning function of words, since we have excluded non-expressive signs. Then he is saying that once the indicative function of words is excluded as non-essential to expression, there still remains, within the meaning function, a non-expressivity. That is Derrida's claim, and we shall have to see if he makes good on it.

According to Derrida, "this non-expressivity is not merely due to the physical aspect of expression ([quoting Husserl] " the sensible sign, the articulated phonic complex, the sign written on paper ")" (1967, p. 40). This is a misleading statement, for the physical aspect of words is *not* excluded by Husserl as are non-discursive signs. It is only Derrida who maintains that the meaning-conferring acts need to animate inner, silent speech, what he calls the "phenomenological voice" (whence Derrida's accusation of phonocentrism). For Husserl, it is a matter of indifference to expression whether the signs that bear the meaning are silent or spoken out loud, i.e., whether they constitute the phenomenological voice or what Husserl might call the living voice, the full voice, the *vox viva*. (The title of Derrida's book is *The voice and the phenomenon*, but in my view he grasps neither one in Husserl's sense.)

Thus it is somewhat disingenuous of Derrida to quote Husserl in parentheses above and even more disingenuous to cite Husserl in support of the presumed non-expressivity of expression itself: "The mere distinction between the physical sign and the meaning-conferring lived experiences is altogether insufficient, especially for logical purposes" (1967, p. 40, quoting Husserl, 1913, p. 32).

Derrida does not pursue what Husserl means, which has to do with names. Husserl says that in every name there is a distinction between what is intimated (as always, the experiences in the soul of the one who speaks the name) and what is expressed. In turn, however, the latter can be distinguished into the meaning (or content) and the object named. This is Frege's distinction between sense and reference, or, in Husserl's terminology, between meaning and object. Husserl, a few pages later, devises this example: the two names "the victor at Jena" and "the vanquished at Waterloo" have different meanings, different content, but the same object, i.e., they name the same person (1913, p.47).

Does this demonstrate a non-expressivity within expression itself? Is the object named something that is not expressed, not meant? Husserl discusses various ways to split hairs on this issue, and he himself leaves the terms somewhat indefinite. But his conclusion is most definite: "These allusions may be enough for the time being; their purpose is simply to obviate the erroneous view that meaning-conferring acts could seriously be divided into two distinct sides, one of which would give the expression meaning while the other would give it directedness to a determinate object" (1913, p. 50).

Thus the meaning includes both functions of names (both non-indicative functions), and there is no distinction to be made here between an expressed meaning and a non-expressed object. The meaning and the object are simply moments of one complex expressivity. Therefore names as understood by Husserl do *not* supply evidence of what Derrida is claiming.

Evidently Derrida never intended to pursue the concept of names, for he now proposes evidence of a different sort, namely, the "metaphysical tenor" of Husserl's phenomenology, i.e., its exclusionary movement: "Considering the non-physical aspect of discourse (*le discours*), Husserl thus excludes from it, always under the label of indication, everything that pertains to the communication or intimation of lived experiences" (1967, p. 40). This states the obvious, for indications are composed solely of the physical aspect of discourse; thoughts cannot be communicated by ESP. So Derrida is simply saying that Husserl excludes the non-physical from the physical. That does have a metaphysical ring to it, one which Derrida exploits in this conclusion: "in the last analysis, what separates expression from indication is what could be called the immediate non-presence to self of the living present" (1967, p. 40).

This is Derrida at his hyperbolic best, but he simply means, I suppose, that through expression the speaker is immediately present (to himself) and that through indication he is only mediately present (to another). Thus the metaphysical tenor of Husserl is his privileging of expression over indication, i.e., of self-presence over presence to another. It is this privileging that Derrida challenges. But he does so in a typically deconstructive way. He does not argue, for instance in the manner of Scheler, that there is no privileging of self-presence since we can also be immediately present to one another. Instead, Derrida's view is that there is no privileging since we cannot even be immediately present to ourselves.

That is why Derrida is so intent on refuting Husserl's view that expression is essentially independent of indication. If expression cannot be purified of intimation, then self-presence is always contaminated with indication; i.e., self-presence is never pure and immediate but, instead, always partakes of the indirectness of intimation.

We come now to the core of Derrida's argument, and in my view everything hinges on an ambiguous term he introduces altogether arbitrarily. The term is "the signified" (*le signifié*). It is supposed to refer to the object of signs in general, including both expressive signs and indicative. It is not a Husserlian term, since Husserl always specifies: the correlate of an expressive sign is the expressed or the meaning, and the object of an indicative sign is the indicated. The ambiguity in the term "signified" is a dangerous one, because what is true of the expressed is not necessarily true of the indicated, and vice versa.

Derrida says: "Each time the immediate and full presence of the signified is concealed, the signifier will be of an indicative nature" (1967, p. 43). That statement is true, as long as "signified" means "indicated". It then says that whenever the existence of the soul of the speaker is not fully present – in the sense of apodictically given to the hearer – then the speaker's words will only be outward signs, indications, allowing the hearer to surmise the existence of the speaker's soul. But the statement is not true if "signified" means "expressed". For it then says that whenever the meaning is not fully present – in the sense of adequately given to the speaker himself – then the words are only indications of that meaning. It is not true, because meaning is never adequately given. Specifically, I do not know myself adequately, I am not fully present to myself. My thoughts about myself are not equal to myself. What these thoughts "signify" (i.e., express or mean, namely, myself) is somewhat concealed to me. But that does not make my own words indications of myself, outward signs by which I surmise the existence of my own soul. It simply means that my words are not adequate expressions. But they remain expressions. I could never express myself adequately, such that my words would capture everything there is to be expressed about myself. Likewise, I could never express any other thing adequately. But that merely demonstrates that my finite capacity to know is never equal to the infinite capacity of any thing to be known. It does not prove that the signs by which I speak of myself become indications to myself. Yet that is just what Derrida believes he is proving, having fallen victim (or taking unfair advantage of) the ambiguity in the term "signified".

Derrida says again: "All discourse, or rather, everything in discourse which does not restore the immediate presence of the signified content, is non-expressive" (1967, p. 43). Here too, the statement is true if "signified" means "indicated." But then it is also trivial, for it simply means that everything in discourse which is merely indicative is non-expressive. Derrida could hardly be saying something as trivial as that, and indeed he wants to suggest the statement applies to one's own self-presence. Then "signified" has to be taken in the sense of "expressed". Accordingly, the statement says that everything in discourse which does not make the speaker adequately present to himself is non-expressive. Understood in this way, the statement is false. Simply because an expression is not adequate to that which it wants to express does not make the expression an indication. That merely makes it an inadequate expression; but all expressions are inadequate, something Derrida refuses to acknowledge. Or else he is vastly shortchanging Husserl, as if the founder of phenomenology were oblivious to the limits of human knowledge.

Put differently, Derrida is unaware that the privilege of self-presence is, for Husserl, a privilege only in the order of apodicticity, not in the order of adequacy. I am more *certain* of myself than I am of others, but that does not mean I know myself more *perfectly* than I know others or than others know me.

Derrida is fond of asserting that Husserl posits a "full", "immediate" self-presence. These are not Husserl's own terms, but they do apply, provided they are taken in the correct sense. By no means may they be taken in the sense of "adequate" or "complete". "Full" must be taken in the sense of Husserl's "fulfilled", i.e., intuitively given. I do not intend myself "emptily", as if I knew myself only by hearsay. And "immediate" must here mean "not mediated through indications". But it does not mean "not mediated through language, through expressions". If expressions give birth to meaning, then my knowledge of myself *must* be couched in language. Husserl is well aware of the essential role of language in self-knowledge: "A great role is ordained to expression in the uncommunicative life of the soul [...] [There] thoughts must be expressed, in the mode of meanings" (1913, p. 35-6).

Thus it could just as well be said that Husserl posits a non-full (i.e., inadequate) and non-immediate (mediated through language) self-presence. Derrida has spilled a great deal of ink trying to establish what Husserl has already known.

Furthermore, Derrida has confused my concealment to others, which can be mediated through outward signs, and my concealment to myself, which cannot be mediated through indications. For, what could I hope to gain by taking my own words as indications? Besides the fact that it would be a pathological way to proceed, it is logically impossible. Derrida does not mention it, but perhaps the weakest feature of Husserl's theory of signs is that the intimative operation works by way of an "argument by analogy". I take another's speech as a sign that there exist meaning-conferring acts in his soul because I know my own speech arises from my own conscious acts. That is, my own experience of myself is the prime analogue, the basis of the analogy. If I had no knowledge of myself, the argument by analogy would have no foothold and could never begin. Now, if I am to take my own speech indicatively, I would reason that when others speak in such and such a way, they are having such and such experiences, and so my similar speech indicates those experiences are also present in me. But I could look in this way to the experience of others, i.e., make them the prime analogue, only if I had already surmised the existence of their experience by means of an earlier argument by analogy in which I myself was the prime analogue. Thus this appeal to intimation commits the logical fallacy of begging the question: it presupposes what it is trying to establish, namely, my own presence to myself. That is what drives intimation from the beginning; to make it the end of a complex chain of reasoning is merely to go a long way around to arrive at the starting point.

Conclusion

There can be no doubt that deconstruction almost completely overshadows phenomenology today. Yet it has not *refuted* phenomenology; Derrida's critique leaves Husserl unscathed – on the level of abstract argumentation. On a deeper level, however, deconstruction has touched a cord, just as phenomenology once did.

Merleau-Ponty remarks that there were portents of phenomenology everywhere and that it presented itself to people much less as a new philosophy than as "what they were waiting for" (1945, p. ii). To suggest a reason deconstruction found favor, I offer, painting in very broad strokes, what I believe is one portent of it, namely Pop Art.

This movement stems from the period of incubation of deconstruction, namely, the early 1960's. Perhaps the high point of Pop Art consists in the series of Andy Warhol's paintings of Campbell's Soup cans dating from 1962-68. What is most evident about these paintings (in opposition to impressionism, one of the portents of phenomenology) is their everydayness. They are everyday paintings of everyday objects by an everyday artist. In other words, they are marginal paintings of usually marginalized things. They are celebrations of the marginal. They are egalitarian.

It is here, I believe, that Derrida has struck a cord. Deconstruction is a philosophy of radical egalitarianism. In other words, what matters in Derrida's critique is not so much *what* Husserl has excluded (one sort of sign from another), but *that* he has excluded anything at all. I consider Derrida's an unsatisfying position, for it is *impossible* to include everything, even exclusionary thinking. But I can find nothing else on which the appeal of *La voix et le phénomène* could be based, since its actual argumentation is weak in the extreme.

References

Derrida, J. (1967). *La voix et le phénomène: Introduction au problème du signe dans la phénoménologie de Husserl.* Paris: PUF.

Husserl, E. (1913). *Logische Untersuchungen. 2. Bd. Untersuchungen zur Phänomenologie und Theorie der Erkenntnis.* (2. Auflage.) Tübingen: Max Niemeyer.

Merleau-Ponty, M. (1945). *Phénoménologie de la perception.* Paris: Gallimard.

A HISTORY OF AMEDEO P. GIORGI'S CONTRIBUTIONS TO THE PSYCHOLOGY DEPARTMENT AND PHENOMENOLOGY CENTER OF DUQUESNE UNIVERSITY IN HIS TWENTY-FOUR YEARS THERE

David L. Smith, C.S.Sp., Ph.D.
Duquesne University
United States

Abstract

With reference to "the signs of the times" (the cultural situation of the 1960's), this chapter first introduces brief histories of Amedeo Giorgi's family and educational background. It then proceeds to his early professional and academic history, which is his Duquesne University years, 1962-1986. The chapter details the recruitment of Giorgi to the University's Psychology Department, his academic schedule, and his direction of dissertations. Reference is made to his dialogue with the intellectual giants Erwin Straus, Aron Gurwitsch, and Stephen Strasser. Concurrent with this dialogue at the time was the evolution of the graduate psychology programs at Duquesne University and this is discussed. Giorgi's chairing of Duquesne's Psychology Department 1966 through 1969 and the evolution of his empirical phenomenological research methodology, as well as his founding of the Journal of Phenomenological Psychology (1970) and his publications and his pivotal role in the founding of the Simon Silverman Phenomenology Center, are presented at this point.

Man's reach should exceed his grasp or what is heaven for.

R. Browning.

When the 1960's first dawned upon the United States of America, the nation breathed a collective sigh of relief, content to bid farewell to the drab society of the "gray flannel suit" and a culture of the "lonely crowd". Everyone seemed to sense that there was a fresh spirit blowing throughout the land, a spirit of change and renewal, an authentic "Greening of America". Almost overnight, due in part to the influence of the new Humanistic psychology, such words as self-actualization, autonomy, creativity and self-transcendence became the coin of the realm. When good Pope John XXIII sat on the Chair of Saint Peter and John F. Kennedy occupied the Oval Office, the human future seemed opened to infinite possibilities. America was witnessing what Karl Jaspers would call an "axial age", a major shift in the tectonic foundations of the culture, when all basic assumptions about life and culture could be challenged and many of the old traditions would not survive close scrutiny.

In *The Feminine Mystique*, Betty Friedan (1963) advocated for women's rights; Martin Luther King marched for the civil liberties of Blacks; Mario Savio organized for students; and César Chávez picketed for the rights of immigrant field workers; and "Stonewall" became the icon of gay liberation. The country seemed to resound with the tocsin of the French revolution, "Liberty, Fraternity, Equality", for one and all. "The times they were a-changing" (Bob Dylan), and psychology would not escape the spirit of the new age. Nearly fifty years after joining the new doctoral program in existential-phenomenological psychology at Duquesne University in the Fall of 1962, Giorgi (in press) would recall the times.

> Perhaps it was the climate of the 60's, which were just beginning, but we were optimistic that a whole new and revolutionary approach to psychology could be implemented. We wanted to raise foundational questions, root psychology in a different philosophy, redefine it, and then show how the redefinition was superior to what was being practiced by mainstream psychologists. (p. 18)

These dreams of the Duquesne Group (the Faculty who created the original graduate program of a phenomenologically based Human Science psychology) for a new and better human psychology resonated with the hopes of Gordon Allport who had written as early as 1949 of his expectation of a "revolution of American psychological thinking" (as cited in C. Graumann, 1981, p.10). Giorgi (1970), among others, has delineated the historical alternatives to the American brand of natural science psychology. Among the European existential philosophers and psychiatrists, Karl Jaspers as early as 1930 dismissed the psychology of the day as "Entangled in a multitude of indifferent matters of infinitesimal importance [...]" and ending in "nothing more than the embryo of a science" (1951, p.166). Just a few years prior to the outbreak of the Second World War, Husserl, in a prophetic lecture delivered in Prague in 1935, wrote: "the reason for the downfall of a rational culture does not lie in the essence of rationalism itself, but only in its exteriorization, in its absorption in naturalism and objectivism" (1936/1965, p.161). This naturalistic objectivism has dominated scientific psychology from its inception in the laboratories of Wundt, Fechner, and Ebbinghaus. Without attributing malevolent motives to any one individual psychologist or psychiatrist, Aron Gurwitsch (1945/1984) has detected in this naturalistic philosophy seeds of the Nazi racial ideology. Whenever human beings are conceived as objects to be measured and controlled, they become vulnerable to use, abuse and ultimately to disposal.

Following upon the tragedy of the Second World War and the trauma of the Holocaust, Western civilization longed for a new humanism and psychology sought new paradigms to respect the full range of human phenomena. On the American scene, Gordon Allport (1955) pleaded the case for turning from the Lockean passive *homo naturae* to the study of human beings as free and active agents. In 1959, Viktor Frankl, survivor of Adolf Hitler's death camps and a Viennese psychiatrist, took the psychological world by storm with the publication of his book, *From Death Camp to Existentialism* (1959). Based upon his personal experience in the camps, he challenged Freud's theory of "frustrated sexuality" and Adler's "will to power" and insisted that the most profound human motivation is the human "will-to-meaning". Another typical example of the new psychology found expression in the publication of *Existence: A New Dimension in Psychiatry and Psychology* (1958). With this publication the American public was introduced to existential thought which Rollo May defined as:

> [...] the endeavor to understand man by cutting below the cleavage between subject and object which has bedeviled Western thought and science since shortly after the Renaissance. This cleavage Binswanger calls "the cancer of all psychology up to now [...] the cancer of the doctrine of the subject-object *cleavage* of the world. (p. 11)

Giorgi had made the correct diagnosis. It was certainly, at least in part, due to the climate of the 60's that the Duquesne Group could hope for a new age in the history of psychology.

Giorgi's Personal and Educational Background

Amedeo Peter Giorgi was born on July 9, 1931 in the borough of the Bronx, New York City. His parents, Paul and Palma were Italian immigrants and the family lived in an Italian ghetto, a working-class neighborhood with a large extended family nearby. He had one older brother, Louis, who would become a priest of the Archdiocese of Philadelphia and one older sister, Assunta. When he was one year old the family moved to Philadelphia to open a grocery store and his sister Elena was born there in 1940. The move from the Bronx to Philadelphia would inject some troubling changes into young Giorgi's life.

In a personal essay, *Professional Marginalization in Psychology: Choice or Destiny?* (In press), Giorgi wonders about how he came to be what he calls a "marginalizd person" and "marginalized psychologist". At some length, he considers to what degree his life and career were shaped by his own free choices and how much by the contingencies of his concrete existence. It seems that ethnic, cultural, religious, and language issues all played a role to set him apart from his peers and evoke a sense of being "different" and "other". His name, Amedeo, was foreign to his peers and even to his teachers. He tells us that "this feeling of being between worlds" continued throughout his education until the time of his doctoral studies.

When Giorgi began his college education in 1949 at St. Joseph's College in Philadelphia, a Jesuit institution, he first chose English as his major, primarily to fulfill a requirement, but also because he felt more inclined to the humanities than to the natural sciences. One day during his sophomore year he asked a fellow student what his major was and he replied "psychology". Giorgi asked him about a good psychology book to read. His response would set the course for the rest of Giorgi's life. "There's a guy named [William] James who wrote a good book on psychology. It should tell you all you want to know" (Giorgi, 1984, p.18). Giorgi scanned the *Principles of Psychology* and liked what he saw. There and then, he made the decision to major in psychology. Ironically, it seems that that would be the last time he would ever hear a substantive reference to James' work throughout his entire education.

The psychology major at St. Joseph College was the cookie-cutter type to be found at all colleges throughout the country at the time. It was basically a natural science approach with large doses of statistics, physiological psychology, scientific methodology and experimental findings. When he began his graduate studies in 1953 at Fordham University in New York City, another Jesuit school, he soon discovered that at the MA and Ph.D. levels the approach would be very similar to the undergraduate level, but now with an increased degree of specialization. Giorgi completed a dissertation on the psychophysics of vision and was awarded the doctorate in 1958.

In his personal memoir, Giorgi discusses at length how his persistent and profound dissatisfaction with his graduate education in psychology sensitized him to the basic concerns that would inspire his entire career. He confesses that throughout his graduate education he " did not experience a psychological center that was holding things together" (Giorgi, in press, p.9). More and more he reflected upon the fundamental questions confronting the science of psychology; "What is the meaning of psychology? What, after all, is the psyche? How does one delimit the field"? (pp. 8-9). Even to this day, Giorgi struggles to find adequate answers to these questions, while mainstream psychology continues on its merry way, too oblivious even to ask the questions. His experience then reflects the status of psychology still. "It was as though what was called psychology was 90% conglomeration of other fields and 10% psychology – but what was that 10 %?" (p. 9). In this state of disenchantment with psychology, Giorgi departed the halls of higher education. For the next few years, from 1957 to 1960, he worked as project director and research psychologist at Dunlap and Associates in Stamford, CT, engaged mostly in engineering projects related to military systems.

Teaching Career

During a brief tenure at Manhattan College, NYC, Giorgi reports that one day a student drew his attention to the fact that his teaching was a constant critique of his subject matter. Giorgi recognized the validity of the criticism and asked himself if he would continue in "eternal critique" or find a "constructive alternative?" (pp. 15-16). He recalls that about this time, one of his former classmates from Fordham days, Father Edward W. Hogan, C.S.Sp., wrote to him about a colleague at Duquesne University, a young Dutch priest by the name of Adrian van Kaam, C.S.Sp., who made many of the same criticisms of traditional psychology as Giorgi had made. To create an alternative psychology, he had turned to the philosophy and the psychology of the existential-phenomenologists. In their philosophy he had discovered an alternative vision of human being radically divergent from the positivistic philosophy that dominated the American psychology of the day. In 1959 van Kaam would launch a new Masters program in psychology at Duquesne University, a program inspired by the existential-phenomenological approach.

Following up on Hogan's initial news, Giorgi arranged to meet van Kaam in Waltham, Massachusetts, while van Kaam was substituting for Maslow at Brandeis University, who was on sabbatical. Giorgi reports that they talked for many long hours far into the night about phenomenology and psychology. Giorgi (in press) writes, "I asked him whom I should read, and out came another series of unknown names: Husserl, Heidegger, Merleau-Ponty, Sartre, Buytendijk, Gurwitsch, and so on" (p. 17). It was at this first meeting that van Kaam invited Giorgi to join the Duquesne Group to direct the research program based upon a phenomenological perspective. Giorgi was open to the invitation, especially when van Kaam assured him that one could be a phenomenological psychologist without being a clinician, but before formally accepting he needed the assurance that the department would initiate a doctoral program.

After this initial meeting with van Kaam, Giorgi began to read voraciously in the phenomenological literature and to take courses in phenomenology at the New School for Social Research in NYC. In particular, he was greatly impressed by Aron Gurwitsch, one of Hussserl's most loyal and distinguished students. At the time, one of the most important centers for phenomenological thought was the University of Utrecht in Holland where the great Buytendijk had held sway for many years. His successor, Johannes Linschoten, was a visiting professor at Duquesne University in the Spring semester of 1961 and when he went to Philadelphia to give a lecture, Giorgi arranged to meet with him. When Giorgi expressed interest in visiting at the University of Utrecht that summer, Linschoten readily welcomed him. When he arrived, much to his surprise and wonderment, he soon discovered that none of Linschoten's students, or the master himself, was actually engaged in doing phenomenological research. The long and the short of Giorgi's visit to Utrecht that summer of 1961 was his discovery that there did not seem even to exist an empirical research methodology (Letter to Rev. Henry Koren, 1999).

Giorgi's Duquesne Début *(1962-1986)*

Giorgi joined the Department of Psychology at Duquesne University in September 1962, the very year that the doctoral program in existential-phenomenology began. Within a few years he would enjoy the distinction of directing one of the first two dissertations of the new program, that of Frank Siroky, "The Modes of Awareness of the Other Person Implied in Perception of a Common Task" (1964). Already we can detect in the very title the introduction of the human and personal into empirical systematic research. It was for this very reason that the new program had been established. In the Proposal submitted by the Department to the University administration, the rationale for the new program reads "[…] the psychology specialties and courses have as their focus the human person, seen primarily as a whole" (Smith, 2002, p.36). Forty years after Giorgi's arrival at Duquesne, Smith would write of him that, "He would bring to the department a strength and emphasis for rigorous empirical research following a phenomenological approach and contribute substantially to a sharper focus of the department's program" (2002, p. 39).

Giorgi's Teaching Career

When Giorgi arrived at Duquesne, the doctoral program offered four different sequences from which a student could choose for a concentration: (1) the clinical-theoretical sequence; (2) the clinical-empirical sequence; (3) the empirical-theoretical sequence; and (4) the theoretical-empirical sequence (Smith, pp.37-38). It should come as no surprise that Giorgi's teaching would focus on the empirical-theoretical sequence, since, as he recalls, when first invited to teach at Duquesne, "It was intended that I should work out an integration of phenomenological principles and psychological research, which I finally realized was precisely what I wanted to do" (1984, p. 23).

When Giorgi began his teaching career at Duquesne in the fall semester of 1962, he lectured on the relationship between phenomenology and experimental psychology. The earliest extant record of his course schedule available unfortunately begins only in the 1971-1972 semester. It includes four graduate courses; Qualitative Research, Psychology of Merleau-Ponty, Psychology of Perception, and Integrational Seminar (Annual Report, p. 22). Among the core required courses at the time Giorgi joined the department there was one entitled, Phenomenological Psychology, described as "An introduction to the fundamentals of the phenomenological approach to psychology and its application to empirical research" (UB, 1962-1963, p. 99; Smith, 2002, p. 38). Based upon this description it is reasonable to assume that Giorgi would have taught this course.

In his various courses, Giorgi tried to work out "methods for doing psychological research along lines that would be consistent with phenomenological philosophical presuppositions" (Giorgi, 1984, p.24). Rather than employ the traditional term "experimental" psychology with its negative connotations of the manipulation and control of discrete variables in a laboratory situation, Giorgi opted to use the term "systematic" to describe his own work. While preserving some of the rigor of the traditional methods in which he had been trained, he wanted to approach his research based upon phenomenological analysis to study the classical issues of learning, sensation and perception, in particular the relationships among the fundamental human phenomena (1984, p. 24).

With these interests uppermost on his academic agenda, it comes as no surprise that Giorgi's course work from his earliest years at Duquesne would include the Graduate Research courses where he could work out the practical and concrete issues involved in the development of an empirical phenomenological methodology, as well as more speculative courses such as the psychology of Merleau-Ponty where more theoretical issues related to research could be explored. Unique to the Duquesne program at the time was a course in Qualitative Research, developed by Giorgi and regularly taught by him during his twenty-four year tenure at Duquesne.

When Giorgi became Head of the Department in 1968, the Duquesne Group created a distinctive process for the doctoral dissertation trajectory. The traditional comprehensive exams were eliminated and replaced with a comprehensive research seminar. In the second semester of their second year all doctoral students were required to write a "Qualifying Paper" for entry into an "Integrational Seminar", designed to demonstrate that each student had indeed selected a significant human phenomenon worthy of being researched for the dissertation. The student had to show how the phenomenon fit within the psychological tradition and how a phenomenological approach could enrich or correct the tradition. At the end of the seminar the student was required to write a "Mock Proposal", and upon approval by the Faculty, this became the student's dissertation proposal. Giorgi regularly conducted this Integrational

Seminar in tandem with another faculty member. It was during these early years of his teaching career at Duquesne that Giorgi (1984) discovered the history of an "alternative" or "dissenting" tradition in psychology (pp. 24-25), discussed at length in his book *Psychology as a Human Science* (1970).

In the fall semester of 1967, upon the sudden resignations for personal reasons of both the Chair and Associate Chair of the Department, Giorgi found himself catapulted into the Leadership of the Department overnight. In his first Annual Report as Chair, he described the Aims of the Department as follows:

> The aim of the graduate program [...] is essentially to prepare scholars for both academic and professional careers [...] It is not a pragmatic, professionally oriented program...Rather, it is academically oriented, stressing the importance of psychological theory and its philosophical assumptions [...] The department has the intention of continuing and strengthening the basis of its world-wide reputation, namely, its unique program in existential-phenomenological psychology (1967-1968, p. 16).

Giorgi continued as Chair until the spring of 1969 when he took his first sabbatical leave. He spent this sabbatical as a Visiting Resident Scholar at the Institute of Psychology, University of Aarhus, Denmark. During this sabbatical, Giorgi was disappointed to discover that he still could not discover anyone who was actually doing empirical phenomenological research. Faced with the lack of an empirical phenomenological methodology, upon his return to the United States, Giorgi determined to commit himself to remedy this situation. In the context of his course on Qualitative Research, he took upon himself the immense task of working out not only the concrete steps of a truly empirical methodology, but he also articulated a theoretical justification and rationale for it based upon phenomenological principles. This qualitative analysis method relied upon the demarcation or discrimination of meaning units culled from the descriptions of lived experiences provided by the subjects of the research to reveal the structure of the phenomenon. In the works of Husserl and Merleau-Ponty, Giorgi found the theoretical grounding for his original methodology and their insights would influence the form his methodology would take.

Giorgi's Major Duquesne Publications

Each of the following major Duquesne publications by Amedeo P. Giorgi are introduced by the respective title.

– *Psychology as a Human Science: A Phenomenologically Based Approach* (1970):

During his 1969 sabbatical in Aarhus, Denmark, Giorgi spent a considerable amount of time working on this book. It would be his seminal contribution to an "alternative" or "dissenting" approach to psychology. The title itself reflects his long-held conviction that a new direction was possible for psychology and that an alternative vision could enjoy a productive future. Giorgi would argue the case that to revision psychology, to liberate it from its thrall to a natural science approach, it was imperative to adopt a human science approach. By adopting the natural science approach, mainstream psychology had either distorted, or covered over, the original and basic experiencing of the primordial ground of our human existence, namely, what Husserl had called the *Lebenswelt* or Life-world.

It had now become the task of a human science psychology to reawaken the originating basic experience of the life-world to ground the new psychology. Only a descriptive approach could allow the phenomena to speak for themselves, but since every experience suggests more than what actually appears a rigorous interrogation of the phenomenon would be required to reveal what still remains in shadow. Giorgi's presentation of his concept of "approach" clarifies the most basic issue at stake in the development of a human science psychology. He writes,

> By approach is meant the fundamental viewpoint toward man and world that the scientist brings, or adopts, with respect to his work as a scientist, whether this viewpoint is made explicit or remains implicit (p. 126). [...] approach [...] is a place where psychological theorizing and the theorizing concerning metapsychological or even philosophical issues can take place. (p. 127)

As a human science psychologist, Giorgi fully grasped the significance of the basic phenomenological insight that there exists an essential mutual relationship between the human being and the human world, thus binding up the wounds inflicted by the Cartesian dichotomies. Applying this insight to empirical psychology, he wrote that "behavior must not be seen in the context of the movement of a "thing" or the "dynamics" of an object or even as the response of an organism, rather the primacy is with the behavior itself, i.e., the relation between man and world of which behavior is but an expression or manifestation" (p. 159). It was also in this book that Giorgi articulated the essential relationships of approach, method and content involved in all psychological research (p.125). In addition to this ground-breaking book, another fruit of Giorgi's 1969 sabbatical at the University of Aarhus was a trip to Sweden where he met Jan Bouman, a Dutch existential psychologist who directed an existential psychotherapy clinic in Stockholm. Giorgi would invite him to deliver a graduate course at Duquesne and some years later the executors of his estate would donate his personal library to the Simon Silverman Phenomenology Center at Duquesne University.

– *Duquesne Studies in Phenomenological Psychology*. A. Giorgi, C. Fischer & E. Murray. (Eds.). Vol. I (1971):

Under Giorgi's indefatigable leadership, the Department of Psychology launched this series to "communicate to our colleagues as well as to those who would study psychology something of the flavor of our orientation at Duquesne University" (p. V). The Duquesne Group was involved in an original project that was often misunderstood and at times even ridiculed as nothing more than armchair psychology. They understood their own project as rooted in honorable philosophical and psychological traditions, but involving a fresh synthesis of both. Situating their work in the historical context of the young department, the editors of this volume wrote,

> Through his [van Kaam's] singular effort the project to found psychology as a human science received its original conception as well as its initial impetus. However, the further development and articulation of the enterprise has been an expression of the entire department. (p. VI)

This first volume is a concrete expression of that common effort. It is, as well, a demonstration of Giorgi's prodigious productivity at this point in his career.

In addition to all the ordinary activities that occupy a university professor, such as teaching, committee meetings, researching, directing dissertations, Giorgi not only completed the book previously discussed, but he was also engaged in working out his new methodology, lecturing in the States and abroad, chairing the department and about to found a new journal, when he undertook to serve as the senior editor of this new series. Volume 1 contains four of his articles; (1) Phenomenology and Experimental Psychology I (1965); (2) Phenomenology and Experimental Psychology II (1966); (3) Experience of the Subject as a Source of Data in a Psychological Experiment (1967); and (4) A Phenomenological Approach to the Problem of Memory and Social Learning (1967). All four articles were originally published in the *Review of Existential Psychology and Psychiatry*, as indicated by the dates and they express some of Giorgi's early efforts to revision and redirect traditional psychology along the pathway of a human science. Giorgi's project was without doubt influenced by his personal contact with Stephan Strasser while he was a visiting professor at Duquesne University and his collaboration with him as Editor of the Psychological Series of the University Press which published a number of Strasser's books, including *Phenomenology and the human sciences* (1963).

It was also in 1971, following discussions between Dr. Giorgi and Father Edward L. Murray, C. S. Sp., the Chair of the Department at the time, that the Department initiated an original program known as the "mini-course". The "mini-course" was a one credit offering conducted over one weekend and taught by renowned scholars who supported the concept of psychology as a human science. The list of these "mini-course" professors over the years included Paul Ricoeur, Mircea Eliade, Peter Berger, Jay Lifton and Jan van den Berg. At this time, the Department also launched a program to invite distinguished scholars to offer three credit summer courses. This list over time would include such phenomenological luminaries as Johannes Linschoten, Erwin Straus, Stephan Strasser, Hubertus Tallenbach, and Viktor Frankl. Thanks to these two singular course offerings, the graduate students enjoyed the opportunity to learn from some of the most prominent phenomenological thinkers of the day.

– *Journal of Phenomenological Psychology: Studies in the Science of Human Experience and Behavior*, Vol. 1, No. 1 (1970):

At the time Giorgi began his academic career at Duquesne, 1962, van Kaam served as the editor of the *Review of Existential Psychology and Psychiatry*, an ideal forum for the publication of Giorgi's earliest phenomenological papers. With a change in the orientation of the Journal, van Kaam withdrew from the editorship and this forum ceased to be available. Faced with the reality that a journal no longer existed for the publication of scholarly articles in phenomenological psychology, Giorgi approached Simon Silverman, the owner of Humanities Press, and asked him if he would be willing to fund a new journal. Receiving an affirmative response, Giorgi began his planning just at the time he was planning to spend his 1969 sabbatical at the University of Aarhus.

During this sabbatical, he made every effort to meet as many European phenomenologists as possible, including Carl Graumann whom he had met on an earlier visit in 1961. Graumann was now the Chair of the Department of Psychology at the University of Heidelberg. When Giorgi invited him to serve as a coeditor, he readily agreed and proposed that the journal publish articles in French and German as well as English. Giorgi acceded to this proposal and then invited Georges Thines, the Chair of the Department of Psychology at the University of Louvain-la-neuve to cover the French flank. Upon the death of Simon Silverman in November of 1984, Giorgi became the sole editor and the Journal began to publish only in English (see Giorgi's article, "The Origins of the Journal of Phenomenological Psychology and Some Difficulties in Introducing Phenomenology into Scientific Psychology", 1988).

The first issue of the journal appeared in the Fall of 1970 and in the Editorial, Giorgi set forth its aims and policy.

> The journal is dedicated to the aim of approaching psychology in such a way that the entire range of experience and behavior of man as a human person may be properly studied. The priority is placed on the fidelity to the phenomenon of man as a whole and all aspects that are studied must be mindful of their human relatedness. (p. 5)

The first issue included a book review by Giorgi of Buytendijk's *Some Aspects of Touch*. Giorgi would continue to edit the journal for the next twenty-five years when he would turn over the editorship to Dr. Frederick Wertz of Fordham University. The journal remains to this day the flagship publication for phenomenological psychology and has served over the years as the major outlet for the scholarship of the graduates of Duquesne's program in phenomenological psychology.

– *Duquesne Papers in Phenomenological Psychology: Student Manuscripts*. E. Murray & A. Giorgi (Eds.). Vol. I (1974):

In his history of the graduate programs of the Department of Psychology at Duquesne University, Smith (2002) wrote that "Popularity is no guarantee of quality and statistics alone can never capture the true academic caliber of a graduate program. Still, they can suggest the status of its reputation and how it is evaluated by others" (p. 60). A mere eleven years after the inauguration of Duquesne's doctoral program, Misiak & Sexton (1973) had christened it "the capital of phenomenological psychology in the New World" (p. 62). In the year prior to the publication of these *Duquesne Papers*, the Department was swamped with over 1,500 inquires and almost 350 resulted in completed paid applications. Very often these applicants would inquire how they could learn more about the programs and educated non-professionals also expressed interest in existential-phenomenology. To respond to these two interests, Giorgi and Murray decided to publish a selection of graduate students' course work. Thus, there occurred the birth of the *Students Manuscripts*.

– *Duquesne studies in Phenomenological Psychology*. A. Giorgi, C. Fischer & E. Murray. (Eds.). Vol. II (1975):

This volume extends the intent of Duquesne's Department of Psychology to familiarize interested colleagues and students with the nature of its programs in existential-phenomenological psychology. In their Introduction, the editors ask the most urgent question for all of psychology, still unanswered by mainstream psychology to the present day. "What is it about being human that it is possible for psychological phenomena to appear to us as they do" (p. 10)? The key to the answer is, of course, to be found in Husserl's notion of the intentionality of consciousness. Along these lines, this volume holds a place of major significance in the history of empirical phenomenological psychology, containing as it does two groundbreaking articles by Giorgi. The first, "Convergence and Divergence of Quantitative and Qualitative Methods in Psychology" (pp. 72-81), presents for the first time in print his original empirical qualitative methodology (pp. 74-75). While demonstrating the distinctive features of his own methodology, he is still able to detect in the parallelisms between quantitative and qualitative methods the possibility of surpassing the prevalent bias in favor of exclusively quantitative analyses (p. 79).

In his second article, "An Application of Phenomenological Method in Psychology", Giorgi turns to the phenomenon of learning in everyday life to illustrate his methodology at work. The question of interest is what constitutes this type of learning? Leading into the actual description of the research project, he reminds us that what most interests the phenomenological researcher are the structures of consciousness. This observation reflects the fact that he had discovered in the works of Husserl and Merleau-Ponty the theoretical justification for the methodology. What makes the phenomenological approach so worthwhile is how it enables the researcher "to gain direct access to meaning by interrogating the qualitative aspects of phenomena" (p. 102).

– *Duquesne Studies in Phenomenological Psychology.* A. Giorgi, R. Knowles & D. Smith (Eds.). Vol. III (1979).

Following the design of the first two volumes, Vol. III organizes its contents into three parts. Part I, as in the previous volumes, explores theoretical issues in psychology, psychotherapy and psychological research. In this section there are two articles by Giorgi, "Phenomenology and Psychological Theory (pp. 60-80) and "The Relationship Among Level, Type, and Structure and Their Importance for Social Science Theorizing: A Dialogue with Schütz" (pp. 81-96). The articles in Part II present studies of psychological topics based upon data obtained from descriptions of the life-world, for example, qualitative studies of lived-space in early childhood and one on the experience of being criminally victimized. A distinctive feature of this volume is Part III, which for the first time in the series contains articles on hermeneutical phenomenology and psychology.

– *Duquesne Studies in Phenomenological Psychology.* A. Giorgi, A. Barton & C. Maes (Eds.). Vol. IV (1983).

Volume IV brings this series in human science psychology to a close. Like its predecessors, it is divided into three parts. Part I focuses on clinical and therapeutic issues, an area somewhat little addressed by the series until now. In Part II the authors explore themes related to the interface between hermeneutics and phenomenological psychology and in Part III a fresh heading appears, "Systematic Psychology". As mentioned earlier, this term was adopted by Giorgi to substitute for the traditional term, "Experimental", in order to bypass the negative connotations of manipulation and control. In addition to an article by Giorgi, "The Importance of the Phenomenological Attitude for Access to the Psychological Realm" (pp. 289-221), we also find articles based upon their dissertations by two of Giorgi's students. F. Wertz presents the results of his doctoral research in "Revolution in Psychology: A Base Study of the New Look School of Perception" (pp. 222-243), and C. Aanstoos presents his work in "A Phenomenological Study of Thinking" (pp. 244-256). In their Introduction to this volume the editors expressed their pride in what the Duquesne Group had accomplished over the past twenty-five years to develop and promote existential-phenomenological psychology and they reiterate the commitment of the Department to continue its efforts to refound psychology as a human science. In the fall semester of 1984, Giorgi was on sabbatical at the Institute of Pedagogy of the University of Goteberg, Sweden where he continued to work on his Merleau-Ponty book and deliver lectures and seminars.

– *Phenomenology and Psychological Research*. A. Giorgi (Ed.). Pittsburgh, PA: Duquesne University Press (1985):

In the Preface, Giorgi recapitulates in a few pages his long journey from his days as a graduate student in psychophysics and his struggle to transcend his dissatisfaction with the deficiencies of traditional psychology as a natural science. While expressing appreciation for its rigor and systematic strength, he laments its narrow worldview and incapacity to address adequately human phenomena. It was only in phenomenology, he reminds us, that he finally discovered "the foundational framework that would enable psychologists to study in a genuinely scientific way the complex processes of human psychological phenomena" (p. VIII).

There are two articles by Giorgi in this volume. "Sketch of a Phenomenological Method" (pp. 8-22), is a demonstration of his qualitative research methodology applied to the study of a concrete learning situation. In his second article, "The Phenomenological Psychology of Learning and the Verbal Learning Tradition" (pp. 23-85), he makes the case for his methodology as both scientific and phenomenological at the same time. It is a lengthy article, substantive and complex, at both the theoretical level and praxis levels, but it does lay out a clear and cogent scenario of where Giorgi's phenomenological journey had led him after twenty-four years of ground-breaking psychological work at Duquesne University. Even at this point in his pioneering career, Giorgi acknowledged with modesty the immensity of the task he had undertaken, when he wrote, "[...] it should be noted that much more work, both theoretical and practical, will have to be done before I feel fully satisfied and all the problems and complications have been worked out" (p. 1).

– *Qualitative Research in Psychology.* (1986). P. D. Ashworth, A. Giorgi & A. J. J. de Kooning (Eds.). Pittsburgh, PA: Duquesne University Press.

Obviously, this is the first publication we come across where Giorgi did not serve as the major editor. Even though, it still serves as a fine tribute to his lifelong work as the premier figure in the area of qualitative research. In his Introduction, the senior editor acknowledges Giorgi's trailblazing endeavors to develop and advance qualitative research in psychology. The book consists of the "Proceedings of the International Association for Qualitative Research" and includes one article by Giorgi, "Theoretical Justification for the Use of Descriptions in Psychological Research" (pp. 3-22). In this article Giorgi touches on the heart of the matter when he writes that "a phenomenologically grounded science uses a descriptive approach in order to obtain the facts of a given experience in order to clarify their meaning" (p. 8).

"Meaning" is a key word here. The human science researcher, employing a qualitative methodology, unlike the traditional psychologist, is not so much interested in discovering the "causes" of the experience or how to "explain" it, but rather wishes to elevate the experience to a higher level of clarification by the explication of its fuller meaning. Still, following the trail blazed by Husserl, Giorgi demonstrates that the qualitative researcher can be present to meanings "as directly as pointer-readings can reveal numbers" (p. 19). Beyond question, this article is required reading for anyone seriously interested in understanding qualitative research with a phenomenological orientation. It is rare, and perhaps unique, in the psychological literature to find one article where such topics as the "meaning of experience", "behavior", and the "psychological" itself are so richly explained.

The Simon Silverman Phenomenology Center at Duquesne University

Spiegelberg (1972) would write of him, "Without Straus, phenomenological psychiatry in America would have remained a "promissory" intention without live "fulfillment". In more than one sense he is today its most vital embodiment" (p. 262). Giorgi would have met Straus, probably for the first time, when he attended the First Lexington Conference organized by Straus and presented in 1963. In 1965 at the Third Lexington Conference on The Phenomenology of

Memory, Giorgi participated with Straus on a panel discussion. Due to these initial contacts with Giorgi and other Duquesne faculty members, Straus would be invited to Duquesne to teach a graduate course in the Fall of 1963 and the Spring of 1970. Over the coming years, the Duquesne University Press would publish all five volumes of the Lexington Conferences.

Given this rich association with the Duquesne Group, when word reached the Duquesne campus that Straus had died on March 20, 1975, Giorgi decided at once to attend his funeral. Straus would have been pleased with this decision for he also knew of Giorgi from personal correspondence with the great Dutch phenomenologist, F. J. J. Buytendijk. In a letter of July 1, 1969, Buytendijk had written to Straus of a visit from Giorgi, "a young psychologist very involved in phenomenology" (Struyker-Boudier, 1988, p. 87), and in a letter dated September 14, 1971, he informs Straus that he has received the first issue of the *Journal of Phenomenological Psychology* edited by Giorgi (p. 87).

After the funeral of Straus on May 22, Giorgi met with Mrs. Straus to express his sympathy and pay his respects. At this meeting she asked him if he would like some of her husband's books which she was distributing among his friends and colleagues. It seems like an inspired moment when Giorgi suggested that she might want to consider keeping his library intact and donating it to some university, perhaps Duquesne (A. Giorgi, personal communication, October 11, 1994).

Upon his return to Duquesne, Giorgi met with the University Librarian and was able to convince him to accept the library of Straus as a special collection. Giorgi then returned to Lexington with Fr. Edward Murray, C.S.Sp., Chair of the Department of Psychology at Duquesne, to seal the agreement with Mrs. Straus. Not only did she agree to donate the library, but her husband's manuscripts, personal files and manuscripts as well, and even his office furniture which he had been able to retrieve after his flight from Germany in 1938. After a follow-up meeting with the University Librarian and considerable private pondering over the matter, Giorgi decided, "Why not just make it a Phenomenological Center"?

Since the Philosophy Department as well as the Psychology Department enjoyed solid reputations in the area of phenomenology, Giorgi invited John Sallis, a renowned Heideggerian scholar at Duquesne, to work with him as the Co-director of the new Center (A. Giorgi, personal communication, November 11, 1994).

As Giorgi envisioned it, the purpose of the Center would be "to contain all the literature on phenomenology, in all of the original languages and wherever it infiltrated" (A. Giorgi, personal communication, May, 2002). From its beginning, Giorgi decided that the Center should be a "Live Center", not merely a repository of books, but an active sponsor of new publications, lectures and symposia.

The Administrative Council of the University officially established the Center at its regular meeting on April 29, 1980. Once the Straus library actually arrived at Duquesne in February of 1977, Giorgi faced the challenge of finding the funds to support the Center, especially its "Live" activities. He immediately thought of Simon Silverman, who had already proved to be a good friend in the past when Giorgi was seeking funds for his new journal. When asked, Silverman readily agreed to be the *bon ange*. As an expression of appreciation and gratitude, there was universal agreement that the Center be named in his honor, "The Simon Silverman Phenomenology Center". Giorgi worked tirelessly to promote the Center and singlehandedly acquired the Archives of E. Straus, A. Gurwitsch, and S. Strasser that now grace the Center, as well as the Jan Bouman Collection. With the able collaboration of Dr. Richard Rojcewicz, he initiated in 1983 the first Annual Spring Symposium of the Center.

At this point in its history, 2008, the Center holds in excess of 20,000 volumes, plus 2,000 filed and indexed articles related to existential-phenomenology, a complete set of the Husserl Archives, the Moser transcripts of Heidegger's Marburg lectures, and F. J. J. Buytendijk's *Pensée Repensée*. Thanks to the initial vision and action of Giorgi, the Center contains the largest collection of existential-phenomenological literature worldwide.

Retrospective

Giorgi's academic and scholarly career at Duquesne University from 1962 to 1986 amply demonstrates his monumental contributions to psychology as a human science. As a young academic, he had appeared on the American psychological scene at a moment in history when the science of psychology had lost its soul to Freudian instinct theory and its mind to the tyranny of Skinnerian S-R behaviorism. However, "the times they were achanging", and many psychologists perceived an urgent need for psychology to change with them.

Throughout his career, Giorgi would find himself always on the frontline and down in the trenches in this effort to revision psychology and direct it away from its naturalistic orientation toward a more human science future. From the outset, he faced two immense challenges. Erwin Straus (1952) once expressed the first task when he wrote, "To regain the genuine theme of experiencing we will have to remove the historical debris under which it is buried at present" (p. 315). Straus would clarify his meaning when he wrote "of the urgent task to rediscover once again the problem hidden through familiarity in the life world or obscured through scientific interpretation" (1974, p. 89). To respond to this challenge, in his early work, Giorgi engaged in a critique of the naturalistic approach that had shaped psychology from its birth. Beyond this critique, his primary goal from the beginning was to restore the "human to human" psychology, both at the theoretical and praxis level. This major goal flowed naturally from his long-held conviction that "When it came to genuinely human problems that had to be solved at a properly human level, psychology was no better than common sense" (1984, p. 21).

To promote his positive agenda for a renewed psychology, Giorgi would find strong support in the philosophy of Husserl, especially with his notion of the intentionality of consciousness. Here was the riposte to the psychologists so enchanted with the models of physics and chemistry. Today, we could add neurology and genetics. None of these can ever serve as adequate models for psychology, for as Giorgi (1984) points out, though they all involve materiality, only consciousness and experience, "while embedded in materiality, always transcend it" (p. 30). Sartre's notion of situated behavior and Merleau-Ponty's notion of structure also contributed mightily to Giorgi's project for a human science psychology. Influenced by their insights, he would write, so contrary to traditional psychology, that " it is not the organism itself that is the sufficient condition of constituting the proper object of psychology, but rather the organism in relation to a situation [...] the situation as it is for the organism"(1984, p. 21).

At the level of praxis, Giorgi's empirical qualitative research methodology has taken on the status of a holotype for all empirical phenomenological research. In addition to the actual concrete steps of the methodology, he made a major contribution to empirical research in psychology when he articulated the major co-constituents of the total research process, namely: "(1) The constitution of the research situation; (2) the constitution of the data; (3) the constitution of the data analysis procedures; and (4) the constitution of interpretive and communicative procedures" (1975, p. 74).

In the Introduction to her encyclopedic work, *Phenomenology World-Wide* (2002), Dr. Anna-Theresa Tymieniecka extolled "phenomenology as the inspirational force of our time" (p. 1). Giorgi would be the first to acknowledge the profound influence of that force in his own life and in his own work. In a previous quoted citation in this essay, Spiegelberg (1972) once said of Erwin Straus that without him, "phenomenological psychiatry in America would have remained mostly a promissory "intention" without live "fulfillment" [...] he is today its most vital embodiment" (p. 262). We can say with equal justice that without Giorgi, human science psychology and empirical-phenomenological research may well have remained only a promissory intention without live fulfillment. He remains their most vital embodiment to this day.

References

Allport, G. (1955). *Becoming: Basic considerations for a psychology of personality*. New Haven: Yale University Press.

Annual Report (1967-1968). Department of Psychology. Duquesne University, Pittsburgh, PA (unpublished).

Annual Report (1971-1972). Department of Psychology. Duquesne University, Pittsburgh, PA (unpublished).

Frankl, V. *From death camp to existentialism: A psychiatrist's path to a new therapy*. (I. Lasch, Trans.). Boston: Beacon Press.

Friedan, B. (1963). *The feminine mystique*. NY: W.W. Norton.

Giorgi, A. (1970a). *Psychology as a human science: a phenomenologically based approach*. New York: Harper and Row.

Giorgi, A. (1970b). Editorial: Journal aims and policy. *Journal of phenomenological psychology*, *1* (1), 5.

Giorgi, A. (1970c). Toward phenomenologically based research in psychology. *Journal of phenomenological psychology*. *1* (1), 75-98.

Giorgi, A. (1971a). Preface. In A. Giorgi, W. Fischer, & R. von Eckartsberg (Eds.). *Duquesne studies in phenomenological psychology I*, (pp. V-VII). Pittsburgh, PA: Duquesne University Press.

Giorgi, A. (1971b). Phenomenology and experimental psychology: I. In A. Giorgi, W. Fischer, & R. von Eckartsberg (Eds.). *Duquesne studies in phenomenological psychology I*, (pp. 6-16). Pittsburgh, PA: Duquesne University Press. (Reprinted from [The] *Review of existential psychology and psychiatry*, *7* (3), 1967).

Giorgi, A. (1971b). Phenomenology and experimental psychology: II. In A. Giorgi, W. Fischer, & R. von Eckartsberg (Eds.). *Duquesne studies in phenomenological psychology I*, (pp.17-29). Pittsburgh, PA: Duquesne University Press. (Reprinted from [The] *Review of existential psychology and psychology*, *6* (l), 1966).

Giorgi, A. (1971c). The experience of the subject as a source of data in a psychological experiment. In A. Giorgi, W. Fischer, & R. von Eckartsberg (Eds.). *Duquesne studies in phenomenological psychology I*, (pp. 50-57). Pittsburgh, PA: Duquesne University Press. (Reprinted from [The] *Review of existential psychology and psychiatry*,*7* (3), 1967).

Giorgi, A. (1975a). An application of phenomenological method in psychology. In A. Giorgi, C. Fischer, & E. Murray, (Eds.). *Duquesne studies in phenomenological Psychology I*, (pp. 82-103). Pittsburgh, PA: Duquesne University Press.

Giorgi, A. (1975b). Divergence of qualitative and quantitative methods in psychology. In Giorgi, A. C. Fischer, & E. Murray (Eds.). *Duquesne studies in phenomenological Psychology II*, (pp. 60-71), Pittsburgh, PA: Duquesne University Press.

Giorgi, A. (1979a). Phenomenology and psychological theory. In A. Giorgi, R. Knowles, & D. Smith (Eds.). *Duquesne Studies in phenomenological psychology III* (pp.60-80). Pittsburgh, PA: Duquesne University Press.

Giorgi, A. (1979b). The relationship among level, type, and structure and their importance for social science theorizing: A dialogue with Schütz. In A. Giorgi, R. Knowles, & D. Smith (Eds.). *Duquesne studies in phenomenological psychology III*, (pp.81-96). Pittsburgh, PA: Duquesne University Press.

Giorgi, A. (1983). The importance of the phenomenological attitude for access to the psychological realm. In *Duquesne studies in phenomenological psychology IV*. (pp. 209- 221). Pittsburgh, PA: Duquesne University Press.

Giorgi, A. (1984). The "unfinished business of psychology". In Rogers, D. P. (Ed.). *Foundations of psychology: Some personal views* (pp. 18-34). New York: Praeger.

Giorgi, A. (1985a). Editor's preface. In A. Giorgi, (Ed.). *Phenomenology and psychological research* (pp. VII-VIII), Pittsburgh, PA: Duquesne University Press.

Giorgi, A. (1985b). Sketch of a psychological phenomenological method. In A. Giorgi (Ed.). *Phenomenology and psychological research* (pp. 8-22). Pittsburgh, PA: Duquesne University Press.

Giorgi, A. (1985c). The phenomenological psychology of learning and the verbal learning tradition. In A. Giorgi (Ed.). *Phenomenology and psychological research* (pp.23-85). Pittsburgh, PA: Duquesne University Press.

Giorgi, A. (1986). Theoretical justification for the use of descriptions in psychological research. In P. Ashworth, A. Giorgi, & A. J. J. de Kooning (Eds.). *Qualitative research in psychology* (pp. 3-22). [*Proceedings of the international association for qualitative research*], Pittsburgh, PA: Duquesne University Press.

Giorgi, A. (1998). The origins of the journal of phenomenological psychology and some difficulties in introducing phenomenology into scientific psychology. *Journal of phenomenological psychology, 29*, 2, 161-176.

Giorgi, A. (in press). Professional marginalization in psychology: Choice or destiny? In L. Mos (Ed.). *History of psychology in autobiography.*

Graumann, C. (1981). Psychology: Humanistic or human? In J. Royce & L. Mos (Eds.). *Humanistic psychology: Concepts and criticisms.* (pp. 1-18). New York: Plenum.

Husserl, E. (1965). Philosophy and the crisis of European man. In *Phenomenology and the crisis of philosophy. (Q. Lauer, Trans.).* New York: Harper & Row.

Jaspers, K. (1951). *Man in the modern age.* (E. & C. Paul, Trans.). New York: Doubleday. (original work published 1931).

May, R. (1958). Introduction: The origins and significance of the existential movement in psychology. In R. May, E. Angel, & H. Ellenberger (Eds.). *Existence; A new dimension in psychology and psychiatry* (pp. 3-36). New York: Basic Books.

Misiak, H. & Sexton, V. (1973). *Phenomenological, existential, and humanistic psychologies: A historical survey.* New York: Grune & Stratton.

Murray, E. & Giorgi, A. (1974). Introduction. In E. Murray, & A. Giorgi (Eds.). *Duquesne papers in phenomenological psychology: Student manuscripts, 1* (pp. I-VII). Pittsburgh, PA: Department of Psychology, Duquesne University.

Smith, D. (2002). *Fearfully and wonderfully made: The history of Duquesne University's graduate psychology programs.* Pittsburgh, PA: Simon Silverman Phenomenology Center, Duquesne University.

Spiegelberg, H., (1972). *Phenomenology in psychiatry and psychology.* Evanston, IL: Northwestern University Press.

Straus, E. (1952). The sigh: An introduction to a theory of expression. *Tijdschrift voor Philosophie* 14, Jaargang, *4*, 298-315.

Straus, E. (1974). Sounds, words, sentences. In E. Straus (Ed.). *Languages and language disturbances. The Fifth Lexington Conference of Phenomenology Pure and Applied, 1972* (pp. 81-105). Pittsburgh, PA: Duquesne University Press.

Struyker-Boudier, H. (1988,Spring). Letters between F. J. J. Buytendijk & E. Straus. *Journal of phenomenological psychology, 19* (1), 79-92.

Tymieniecka, A. T. (2002). Introduction: Phenomenology as the inspirational force of our times. In A. T. Tymieniecka, (Ed.). *Phenomenology world-wide: Foundations, expanding dynamics, life engagements. A guide for study and research.* (pp. 1-8). London: Kluwer Academic Publishers.

BACK TO THE THINGS THEMSELVES: THE RELEVANCE OF EMBODIED UNDERSTANDING FOR CARING PRACTICES[1]

Les Todres, Ph.D.
Bournemouth University
United Kingdom

Abstract

Amedeo Giorgi has found in Edmund Husserl's writings a philosophically consistent way to articulate the illusions of reductionism. Giorgi, furthermore, has explored how Husserl's phenomenological philosophy could be modified to serve the practice of human science research through a phenomenological psychology. In the context of this phenomenological psychology and in the follow-through of Husserl's injunction, "Back to the things themselves", there is found a concrete, interrelated world of experience before self and world, mind and body, are differentiated from each other. Such an irreducible world of experience is in need of description if psychological knowledge is to be faithfully informed by an epistemological ground that gives experience its central place in psychology. This chapter explores how caring practices in applied disciplines such as psychotherapy or nursing benefit from a research approach that "goes back to the things themselves". It will particularly emphasize the importance of embodied knowing in both research and practice: how embodied openness to the "things themselves" through phenomenological research is also productive of a kind of embodied understanding that is crucial for caring practices. An embodied emphasis in phenomenological research is then shown to be adequate for a judgment-based care that requires sensitivity to transferable, intersubjective phenomena, as well as to unique persons, contexts, and practices that are always transcending rules and categories.

> [...] if language did not in some way express the non-linguistic, it would have fallen into disuse long ago.
> – Amedeo P. Giorgi, *Theoretical Justification for the Use of Descriptions in Psychological Research.*

> [...] clinicians have to meet humans and their problems as they find them and so require knowledge that is concrete, person-oriented, holistic and contextual.
>
> – Amedeo P. Giorgi, *Towards a New Paradigm for Psychology.*

These two quotations begin to say something about how Amedeo Giorgi has addressed both philosophical and pragmatic concerns that are relevant to the direction of the present essay: why phenomenologically-derived qualitative research findings offer the kind of knowledge that is particularly helpful to the practice of care in everyday life (be it psychotherapy, nursing, social work).

With this direction in mind, I would like to develop a view of a kind of understanding that I will refer to as "embodied relational understanding". I will consider why such understanding is important to healthcare practice, and how the findings of phenomenologically-derived qualitative research are particularly well suited for generating such practice-relevant understanding.

Figure 1:

Goodness of Fit

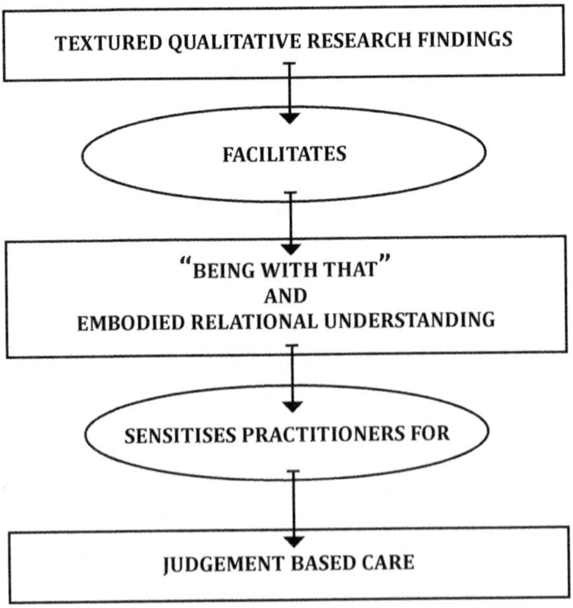

I wish to argue that there is a "goodness of fit" between "embodied relational understanding", the practice of care that is judgment-based, and an emphasis in phenomenological description that can better serve such concerns. I finally argue that phenomenologically-derived qualitative research findings can facilitate "embodied relational understanding" and judgment-based care by focusing more attention on the ways in which we express and disseminate our findings, and also by focusing more attention on the potential educative role that such findings may play in supporting the holistic development of the person of the practitioner engaged in caring practices. In order to argue this "goodness of fit", I will proceed in three steps:

1. To outline the particular view of practice that I wish to highlight: judgment-based caring practice.
2. To clarify the nature of "embodied relational understanding", drawing on the writings of Giorgi, Gadamer and Gendlin.
3. To champion a particular emphasis in phenomenologically-oriented qualitative research that could enhance "embodied relational understanding" by attending to:
   a. The way we present our findings.
   b. Their educative/transformational potential for the person of the practitioner of health and social care.

1. A consideration of judgment-based caring practice

In his book, Practice and the Human Sciences: the case for a judgment-based practice of care, Donald Polkinghorne (2004) offers a critique of a technical view of practicing care. He is concerned that this technical view is becoming unquestioned within the so called evidence-based care movement, and he wishes to offer what he believes is a more appropriate epistemological foundation for caring practice, which he calls judgment-based care. He goes back to Aristotle for help in clarifying the difference between the kinds of practices that are appropriate for the physical realm, where one is appropriately trying to make or control some aspect of the physical or natural world, and the kinds of practices that are more appropriate to the complex living situations of human beings who are seeking a life of worth and value. Within this spirit, he is critical of a narrow view of care that conceptualizes it as a technical resource to be controlled or mastered. For Polkinghorne, there is something about caring practice as a human activity in particular that needs judgment or practical wisdom and not abstract evidence. For him, everyday caring practice requires something qualitatively different than the application of technique, rules and standardized behaviors.

Max van Manen (2007) pursues the critique of a technical-rational view of practice in even stronger terms in that it: "[...] too easily involve(s) reifying what escapes re-ification, thematizing what cannot be thematized, and bringing practice within the reach of objectivist technological thought" (p. 18). He feels that this instrumental view of practice pressurizes us to accept "[...] overly simplistic ways of summarizing standards of practice, codes of ethics, and technological solutions to method that belie the tact of enquiry and the limits of control and technological procedures" (p. 19). He further notes how terms such as "excellence", "potential" and "quality" have lost their substantive meaning and have become quantitative concerns that "can be measured in terms of outcomes, observables and standards" (p. 19).

Polkinghorne (2004) sees judgment based care as requiring:

> [...] a kind of thought that can deal with complex and competing goals and take into account the timing and context of the action, as well as the unique and particular characteristics of the situation and person for whom the action is understandable. (p. 21)

Such thought focuses on interactions rather than things, requiring a consideration of multiple values that are sensitive to the intricacies of the human realm.

Polkinghorne (2004) clarifies these notions further. He declares that judgment-based care, "draws on all our human sensitivities including our emotions" (p. 77). Moreover, it "integrates background understandings, felt meanings of a situation, imaginative scenarios, prior experiences and perceptive awareness" (p. 84). Background understandings involve, "not a set of logically ordered rules about what to do and when to do it, but [are] a holistic web of understandings about how to go about and get things done in the world" (p. 113).

These arguments from Polkinghorne and Van Manen thus focus on the kind of knowing and understanding that is most appropriate for judgment-based practice. Eugene Gendlin (1974) also makes a point about the nature of practice in everyday life, and the kind of knowledge and understanding that can support such practice.

For Gendlin, everyday caring practice would benefit from various levels of knowledge, but he is worried that certain kinds of knowing can be too abstract and form what he calls a "thin pattern" which takes the place of a more detailed, "thinking further" into the "thickness of living", that is, the alive, changing, unique and context-bound circumstance of practice situations. To quote: "If we always listen beyond what we know, we will see in a step or two, both how different and how more detailed is the matter […]" (Gendlin, 1974, p. 3). Gendlin is cautioning against a reliance of knowing in "thin" ways about any living situation. He is worried that such "thin" knowing can lead to arrogance about engaging in practice. He does not wish to throw out the value of what he calls "thin" patterns for knowing and acting as they can be used as "aids for the much richer and moving flow that constitutes a person […]" – and I may add, constitutes a situation.

So, attending to "much more" than thin patterns and instrumentality, a judgment-based care requires a sensitivity to transferable, intersubjective phenomena, as well as to unique persons, contexts and practices that are always transcending rules and categories. This says something about the kind of understanding that is needed here: a form of understanding that is relationally alive and open as an ongoing unfinished activity rather than as something we possess. Such understanding does not contain itself; it is not complete as if it can be simply applied in an already formed state. It needs to be mixed with some "not knowing" if it is to be present to the aliveness of living practice situations. And here we come to a consideration of the nature of embodied relational understanding.

2. Embodied Relational Understanding

In this section, I will attempt to clarify what I mean by "embodied relational understanding". In considering the relevance of Husserl's philosophy for the development of psychology as a human science, Giorgi articulated what I see as the crucial rationale for approaching the psychological realm in a non-reductionistic way. He notes how much of psychology is based on assumptions that are taken for granted such as realism or idealism (Giorgi, 1983). He explores the implications of what Husserl meant by "going back to the matters themselves". For psychology, this would require the kind of knowledge that faithfully expresses the phenomenal realm, a realm of relational presences. The articulation of such relational presences within their living context requires the kind of description that retains this quality of phenomenal presence appearing to consciousness (Giorgi, 1986). This requires a suspension of the natural attitude (Husserl's *epoché*) in order to guard the "space" within which the character of phenomenal presence can be respected on its own terms. More than this, because language can express, show and communicate phenomenal presence, it is possible that insights into the general qualities of psychological phenomena can be intuited and articulated.

Giorgi pursued a number of important implications of Husserl's epistemology for the development of a human science approach to psychology. But the one that I want to concentrate on here, and develop further with help from Gadamer and Gendlin, is how and why phenomenological descriptions are particularly helpful sources of understanding when one is relating to the living situations of caring practice in health and social care contexts. The overarching argument for this concerns how phenomenological description can better "sensitize" practitioners in practice: how a good description of a human phenomenon in general, such as anger, learning or forgiveness, can enable a practitioner to see better, and to relate to, the living phenomenon in practice, and to engage intelligently and sensitively with such phenomena in both general and unique ways.

In pursuing the productive relationship between phenomenologically-derived findings and their value for relating to everyday practice situations, I draw further on Husserl's understanding of the lifeworld as a unified totality with horizons of meaning and possibilities that give any understanding its "alive source". I further draw on Gadamer's view of understanding which, in its emphasis on "application", is centrally concerned with how knowledge stays "in touch" with the aliveness of the lifeworld as it moves in practice. I also draw on the philosophy of Gendlin to consider how the lived body is implicated in any act of relational understanding, and so reveals phenomenological insight as a kind of understanding where "knowing" meets "being", and as such, is intimate to practice.

In order to develop all this, I wish to introduce the phrase "being with that" as a phrase that can indicate the concern to "go back to the things themselves", but to do this in a way that also considers the importance of the embodied person when engaged as a practitioner of care. As such, the phrase "being with that" may provide an important clue to the kind of understanding that may be very relevant for the practice of judgment-based care. I will thus briefly tease out what may be indicated in the term: "being with that".

Relationality:

First of all "being with that" describes a concrete relationship between self and other, happening not just theoretically, but actually, as part of a living situation. The term "with" indicates something relational, a happening together and a "being affected". To be "related to" means that what is related, ("self" to "other") has a meaningful connection far richer, and more specific, than a world of objects mindlessly bumping into one another according to simple laws of cause and effect.

"That":

"That" indicates some phenomenon, person or situation beyond oneself – an alterity experienced in the lifeworld. "That", "there", – such as the phenomenon of another's pain or a family situation of conflict – cannot be reduced to what we already know. If we are open to it, "that" is in excess of what we know because it is alive in time and can always surprise with something new, some new nuance, meaning or texture. The flavor of being called by such "otherness" is well expressed by certain Japanese poets and thinkers. For example, Basho says, " Learn about the pine from the pine, Learn about the bamboo from the bamboo" (Basho cited in Hirshfield, 1988, p. 120).

"That" asks us to go beyond ourselves in order to be present to what is showing itself beyond that which we are constructing. Gadamer (1989) is talking about a similar kind of openness, availability and other-orientation when he says: "For it is necessary to keep one's gaze fixed on the thing throughout all the constant distractions that originate in the interpreter himself" (p. 268). This openness to otherness requires a certain attentiveness and personal availability. Hirshfield (1988), when writing about the mind of poetry, puts it this way:

> [...] the basic matter of poetry comes not from the self, but from the world. From things which will speak to us on their own terms and with their own wisdom, but only approached with our full and useful attention. (p. 120)

This is a certain kind of de-centering of the self but not the de-centering of the deconstructionists. To paraphrase Giorgi (1992), it is a de-centering from the side of consciousness rather than a de-centering that pretends to eradicate consciousness or make it unnecessary. With reference to the imagination, Giorgi points out that through a de-centering from the side of consciousness: "[...] one can place oneself in a possible situation that can be actualized through effort" (Giorgi, 1992, p. 430). So "that", as the phenomena, people and situations that constitute the lively world where practice takes place, is what is attended to as part of the task of understanding – to understand "that".

"Being" or "Being There":

But "that" as the direction of understanding is not the only part that makes up the kind of understanding I wish to call embodied relational understanding. Here we come back to the word "being" in "being with that".

I now take a turn that I do not think Giorgi would choose to pursue in his practice of the psychological-phenomenological research method. In his steps of analysis, he wishes to alleviate the tendency of a researcher to project himself into the data (Giorgi, 2006). I am however suggesting that, while descriptive phenomenology should be descriptively robust in all its steps to arrive at an essential structure that focuses on clarifying psychological phenomena in general, it becomes fruitful for a health care practitioner who is utilizing the insights of phenomenological findings to re-project oneself into a living situation when the relevance of the research findings become available to the world of practice.

"Being" in "being-with-that" brings the self to "that". In being present to "that", we are not simply separate from "that". We are not, as human beings' originally non-participant observers processing things deep inside. We are more immediately responsive, before distancing ourselves from the "being with". In emphasizing "being with" we bring ourselves to "that". It is not a "that" that is occurring in the space of some neutral consciousness. It is to an embodied person who is "being there" very specifically, that "that" announces itself. Gadamer, in his exposition of the nature of understanding remembers the "self" that is being there when we are present. In understanding the living situation of "that", we do not disregard ourselves. Indeed, Gadamer asserts that for understanding to be meaningful, "we must bring precisely ourselves" (Gadamer, 1989, p. 305). Gadamer further points out that in trying to understand, without bringing precisely ourselves to "that", there is no bond to that. "Hermeneutics must start from the position that a person seeking to understand something has a bond to the subject matter" (Gadamer, 1989, p. 299).

I would like to emphasize this word "bond" because it merits further reflection. The word "bond" is an embodied relational word. For there to be a "bond" for understanding, a person finds something in "that" with which they can resonate – something in "that" that is familiar to their own historical world of experience that is some variation of "that". And here we come to Gendlin's (1962) emphasis on the importance of embodiment for making understanding significant in a world of persons. Gendlin builds on a certain trend also seen in the work of Merleau-Ponty (1962) in which understanding requires the whole perceiving body as it is related to all the fleshly textures of the world. In this respect, van Manen (2007) notes that the philosopher, Immanuel Kant had already pointed out that we can only think the world because we have already experienced it. For Gendlin, embodied experiencing is central for "bonding" with that. Without this bonding that "comes from" relational embodied existence, we would have a knowledge that objectifies the world in a way that sees "that" –phenomena, people and situations, as alien or foreign.

In my book, *Embodied Enquiry* (Todres, 2007), I elaborate on Gendlin's philosophy and how the lived body provides the fleshly historical experiences that make any human act of understanding meaningful as follows:

> [...] we find a living body that inhabits situations intimately; it interweaves the realms as a matter of being, and is often lost out there in the textures, the senses, the flesh, the histories, and the meanings that come from the flowing excesses of the lifeworld. Yet it also carries personal history and prereflective sediments of historical meanings that shape its openness. One could say that embodying is where being and knowing meet [...]. (Todres, 2007, p. 20)

This is much larger than our traditional conceptions of knowing.

So the "being", or "being there" part of "being with that", emphasizes all the personal and cultural lively textures that the embodied self brings to any event of understanding. Such embodied "being there" or "embodied presence" brings the possibility of intimacy or familiarity to the unfamiliarity and possible strangeness of the "that" and its "otherness"(for example, in the psychotherapy client). As such, our own prior relation to that carries something truthful, the truth of "that" being humanly significant.

In characterizing embodied relational understanding as "being with that" we finally come to Gadamer's notion of understanding as an open and ongoing conversation, a "play" between self and other. I would like to say just a few more words about the nature of this "play of understanding" as it helps to crystallize why embodied relational understanding is so relevant to the complexities and aliveness of practice.

Understanding as Play between "Self" and "That":

One of the implications of my exposition so far is that Gadamer sees understanding, not as an abstract view on things, but as a way of' "being present" (Gadamer, 1998, p. 31). The play of understanding between self and other arises out of an ongoing creative tension between what is familiar and what is unfamiliar, between self and other, between the known and the fresh textures of the unknown, between the existing framework of understanding that one brings, and the new and context-specific "reality that surpasses" such a brought framework (Gadamer, 1989, p. 109); between general understandings from the past and the different understandings that come by being present to the otherness of "that" as it lives. In Gadamer's view, understanding is always, in a sense, a new event and happening that requires the refreshment of a new potential insight or application. This is similar to what Gendlin called a "thick pattern". Understanding would be killed by the "already known" if there were not this play between the excess aliveness of "otherness" and any existing theme or "thought pattern".

This play of understanding is therefore already in practice – its essence requires one to continually bring the known, but to continually give it up in practice. Such understanding itself is a practice in that it connects self with "that otherness" in an embodied way. And this embodied way carries a certain openness in that, to understand, is to understand differently and "more" in living situations. Embodied relational understanding "stands among" rather than "stands apart from". Also, such understanding involves what Gendlin calls "carrying forward". Embodied relational understanding does not conceptually "trap" situations as if they were frozen in the present. To quote Gendlin: "[…] we do not want our efforts to end in a consistent, stable [and] non-contradictory system. […] this means that we must always use concept and experience, never just concepts" (Gendlin, 1974, p. 9). The challenge is how to allow the aliveness of ongoing experience to function "in play" with what we might know in any task of understanding.

And here we come back to the relevance of "embodied relational understanding" for judgment-based caring practice. Judgment-based caring practice requires "embodied relational understanding" as "being with that" for a number of reasons:

- The involvement of being with that, gives "heart" and "empathy" for caring judgments.
- The involvement of "being with that" brings the resources of the self of the practitioner into play so that judgment-based caring practice can draw on the thoughtful resources of the practitioner.
- The involvement of "being with that" gives an openness to the alive otherness of what is being addressed so that existing knowledge opens to the "thickness" and complexity of the openness that judgment-based caring practice requires.
- The involvement of "being with that" gives to understanding the resources for transforming "thin" patterns or summarized themes of knowing into sensitizing frameworks that can enter into productive play with living situations of "that".

So we come to the question of whether the active play of embodied relational understanding can be enhanced by the findings of phenomenologically-derived qualitative research. And by implication, we also come back to the question of how the findings of phenomenologically-derived qualitative research, through facilitating embodied relational understanding, can better support the practice of a judgment-based care.

How can the findings of phenomenologically-derived qualitative research help health and social care practitioners practice "embodied relational understanding"? I will approach this question by offering two ways forward, while acknowledging that there may be others:

3a) First of all, I will progress the assertion that more can be done to express the findings of phenomenologically-derived qualitative research in a way that aids practitioners to go beyond "thin" patterns of knowing so that they can engage in "embodied relational understanding". This involves the task to re-present qualitative research in more evocative ways.

3b) Secondly, I will consider why and how such findings of qualitative research can be used for the education and personal/professional development of health and social care practitioners.

3a. Re-presenting qualitative research in more evocative ways

By drawing on the work of Eugene Gendlin I have already considered how "sense-making" requires a knowing with the body, as it is the lived body that connects language to the world of experience. Such "sense-making" is not just logical and populated by bits of information, but is full of textures, "the senses, the flesh, the histories, and multiple meanings" (Todres 1997, p. 20) that cannot be summarized and is more than words can say. Such multiple meanings are there to be felt and not just to be known in abstract ways; it is not just a matter of the "head" but is also a matter of the "heart". (Hillman, 1984). Portraying experiences of self and other is thus not just a scientific concern that aims for truth or validity, but is also an aesthetic concern, which the world of art and literature knows something about. I have thus become increasingly interested in pursuing ways of re-presenting qualitative findings in a way that can show "that" – human phenomena, situations and people – in ways that can evoke their concrete and embodied occasions. The task of such re-presentation of qualitative research findings then focuses on the communicative concern to show qualities with words that work to evoke the "thick" patterns and the textures to which they point. When this is done well in writing, in literature, in theatre, readers and audiences can begin to embody the understanding that is communicated in a way that includes its experiential possibilities – an understanding from within that carries both the generalities of "what it may be like" as well as the possible unique variations and "othernesses" to which one can stay open. This emphasis in re-presenting qualitative research findings may be referred to as the "textural" dimension of articulating qualitative research findings, summarized in Figure 1 as "textured qualitative research findings".

In a previous study on the nature of self-insight in psychotherapy, (Todres, 2007) I expressed my wish for an evocative emphasis in writing up and presenting my findings as follows:

- "It would be more than a definition or series of statements about therapeutic self-insight".
- It would tell us something that connects with universal human qualities so that the reader can relate personally to the themes.
- It would tell a story which readers could imagine in a personal way.
- It would attempt to contribute to new understanding about therapeutic self insight.
- It would not attempt to exhaust the topic but would attempt to allow it to be seen more clearly: "like shining a light which increases the reader's sense of contact with this phenomenon without fully possessing it" (p. 49).

More recently, building on some of these sensibilities, my colleague Kate Galvin and I have been developing an approach we call "embodied interpretation" (Todres & Galvin, 2006, 2008; Galvin & Todres, 2009). It uses Gendlin's practice of experiential focusing as a form of embodied resonance in order to become present to the worlds of our informants so that we can include a sense of thick experiential patterns in our portrayals of situations such as "caring for a life partner with Alzheimer's disease". In this respect, we found Gendlin's (1992) "philosophy of the implicit" very helpful for taking phenomenology in a more aesthetic direction towards a body-based hermeneutics that could go back and forth between embodied understandings and the "otherness" of "that". His thought helped us to focus much more on the epistemic body, the body that can implicitly "hold" multiple meanings and significances in ways that are more holistic and interrelated than abstract thought. Such holistic felt meanings in the body are more than thoughts and words, but can become the source of thoughts and words, and attempt to do some justice to the "more" of these meanings coming from the excess of the lifeworld of self and others. I cannot pursue here some of the challenges and nuances of this approach, but just wish to highlight a few characteristics of a more evocative focus when using language that "comes from" meanings as felt and not just thought.

It is not surprising that such pointers towards evocative writing come from poets reflecting on their work. In this respect I have been inspired by the poet Ruth Hirshfield (1988), and have modified her contributions in order to highlight two particular demands of evocative writing:

- Wholeness: this involves a concern to indicate more than is there; pointed to by some of the details; pointing towards a greater whole. This sense of the "world in a grain of sand" is also indicated in the following image of interconnectedness: "one moon shines in many dewdrops". The faculty of language to show interconnection is here emphasized. The greater wholeness can never be fully summarized; but its impact can be somewhat felt and held through the evocative power of words. Such words ask the reader or audience for their imaginative participation and to enter the embodied play between self and the otherness of "that". Such invitation to participation means that the writing, though aiming at coherence, does not wish to be written in such a way that it replaces what it is pointing to. To quote Hirshfield (1988) in relation to poetry: "[…] a good poem can never be completely entered, completely known" (pp. 31-32). Such writing is an invitation for further participation, rather than the transport of completed bits of information from one to another.

- Existentiality: this dimension refers to a desire to be faithful to that which Hirshfield (1988) calls, our "primary life", our concrete human existence, "the prospect of aging, the death of a daughter, the first winter storm in November" (p. 105). Highlighting this existential dimension, the places where we might touch our common humanity, requires a style of writing that goes back and forth between rich particular details that are happening to "this" person "there", and language that connects such specificity to its more general existential significance: for example "the vulnerabilities of illness", "the nature of human comfort". There is a certain intensity or density offered in such writing. The words are not the whole thing but, in Hirshfield's perspective, are "entrance tokens to large and often slippery realms of being" (pp. 6-7). We are more likely to feel and remember such intensities, where the existential significance comes closer to us, and thus becomes available for our own responsiveness for caring practice. Such existential intensity may function as a significant personal resource for caring, and may fade less as a source of acting than that of the next policy guideline for caring practice.

By attending to more aesthetic, communicative concerns, representing qualitative research findings may appeal to more embodied and less cognitive dimensions of knowing in order to provide rich resources for the practice of judgment-based care. Attention to such aesthetic dimensions to knowing may support a judgment based care that: "depend(s) on a sense and sensuality of the body, personal presence, relational perceptiveness, tact for knowing what to say and do in contingent situations, thoughtful routines and practices, and other aspects of knowledge that are in part, prereflective, pre-theoretic and pre-linguistic" (Van Manen, 2007, p. 20).

Finally, I wish to touch on a point about the educational potential of qualitative research findings to support the personal/professional development of the practitioner of care.

3b. Practitioners' engagement with qualitative research findings for personal and professional development

This final section raises the possibility that qualitative research findings which communicate both the "head" and the "heart" of things can be transformative for the person of the practitioner of health and social care, if they are engaged with in a particular way. Let us imagine a practitioner engaging with qualitative research findings in an actively relational and embodied way. She is interested in carrying forward the process by which she and "that" intersect. Gadamer noted how such intersection is transformational in that the self does not come out of this intersection in exactly the same way that she went in. For Gadamer, we enter the play of understanding by putting ourselves at risk. To be grabbed by "that" is to allow that to affect self as a "thick pattern" in a way that is engaging and participative. What does it take, to be borne along by the subject matter, to participate in such shown findings with imagination and bodily resonance? With regard to reading relevant qualitative research, how do practitioners of care participate in understanding in personal ways that are more complex than the outcomes and conclusions of theoretical explanation – how can such responsive hospitality be facilitated? These questions raise the possibility that qualitative research findings can become more central to the education and development of health care practitioners. This direction would include a consideration of how qualitative research findings can be used in educational curricula for professionals in transformational ways that enhance emotional intelligence, context sensitivity, and empathic and ethical sensitivity. Progressing this concern requires, in my view, much more attention to facilitating an embodied experiential process by which practitioners engage with the meaning of findings that are consistent with embodied relational understanding.

Jennifer Shultz (2006) offers one interesting process for listening and entering into the meanings of others' writings. I have modified her approach for the purpose of engaging with specifically qualitative research findings. I will briefly point to just one phase of this educative procedure in order to illustrate this direction:

1. In a group situation, participants read or listen to the findings and insights from a study.
2. Each participant highlights words or phrases that resonated bodily for them. At this stage, they just simply underline these words and phrases without stopping to reflect on choices.
3. They spend some time writing further about how they each personally relate to these words and phrases.
4. Each person reads their pieces of personal writing back to the group.

5. Participants listen to each person's piece and each person writes down how she relates to the words offered both personally and bodily. Each person creates a poem out of her own writing.
6. All read their poems back to the group.
7. A final discussion occurs about whether, and how, their understanding of the issue has changed or not.

This is just one example of the potential for facilitating "being with that" in health and social care professionals through encountering qualitative research findings.

Concluding Thoughts

I wished to show a goodness of fit between judgment based care, embodied relational understanding, and qualitative research: how textured qualitative research findings can facilitate embodied relational understanding as "being with that"; and how such understanding sensitizes practitioners for judgment-based care. Consistent with Gendlin, embodied relational understanding draws on ongoing personal resources that are experiential and preconceptual, that are located in the way the body knows, where language is never alone and always mixed with what is more than language. I wish to encourage more attention to the task of formulating our qualitative research findings in a way that can sensitize practitioners to such embodied relational understanding. In facilitating "embodied relational understanding", we are then aspiring towards something larger than propositional knowledge and evidence. It is not a matter of making a picture of something outside of oneself. In conclusion, I believe that one of the distinctive values of phenomenologically-derived qualitative research will be better understood to the degree that we champion its capacity for facilitating judgment based care based on "embodied relational understanding".

References

Gadamer, H-G. (1989) *Truth and Method.* 2nd Revised Edition. Translated by Joel Weinsheimer and Donald g. Marshall. London: Sheed & Ward.

Gadamer, H-G. (1998). *Praise of Theory*, New Haven: Yale University Press.

Galvin, K. T. & Todres, L. (2009). Poetic Enquiry and Phenomenological Research: The Practice of "Embodied Interpretation". In M. Prendergast, C. Leggo & P. Sameshima (Eds.). *Poetic Inquiry: Vibrant Voices in the Social Sciences* (pp. 307-316). Rotterdam: Senses Publishers.

Gendlin, E.T. (1962). *Experiencing and the Creation of Meaning.* Glencoe: Free Press.

Gendlin, E.T. (1974). The role of knowledge in practice. In G.F. Farwell, N. R. Gamsky & F.M. Mathieu-Coughlan (Eds.). *The Counselor's Handbook* (pp.269-294). New York: Intext. From http://www.focusing.org/gendlin/docs/gol-2030.html [Accessed 15/10/06].

Gendlin, E.T. (1992). The primacy of the body, not the primacy of perception: how the body knows the situation and philosophy. *Man and World, 25* (3-4) 341-353. Available from: http://www.focusing.org/pdf/primacy_excerpt.pdf [Accessed 15/10/06].

Giorgi, A. (1983). The Importance of the Phenomenological Attitude for Access to the Psychological Realm. In: Giorgi, A., Barton, A. & Maes, C. (Eds.). *Duquesne Studies in Phenomenological Psychology*. Vol. IV. Pittsburgh, PA: Duquesne University Press, pp. 209-221.

Giorgi, A. (1984). Towards a New Paradigm for Psychology. In Aanstoos, C. (Ed.). *Exploring the Lived World: West Georgia Studies in the Social Sciences.* XXIII, 9-28.

Giorgi, A. (1986). Theoretical Justification for the Use of Descriptions in Psychological Research. In Ashworth, P. D., Giorgi, A., de Koning, A. (Eds.). *Qualitative Research in Psychology*. Pittsburgh PA: Duquesne University Press, pp. 3-22.

Giorgi, A (1992). Whither Humanistic Psychology? *The Humanistic Psychologist. 20* (2-3), 422-438.

Giorgi, A. (2006). Concerning Variations in the Application of the Phenomenological Method. *The Humanistic Psychologist, 34* (4), 305-319.

Hillman, J. (1984). *The Thought of the Heart. Eranos Lectures Series 2.* Dallas: Spring Publications.

Hirshfield, J. (1988). *Nine gates: Entering the Mind of Poetry*. N.Y.: Harper Collins.

Merleau-Ponty M. (1962). *Phenomenology of Perception* (trans. C. Smith). London: Routledge.

Polkinghorne, D. (2004). *Practice and the Human Sciences: The case for a judgment based practice of care.* Albany, NY: SUNY.

Schulz, J. (2006). Pointing the Way to Discovery: Using a Creative Writing Practice in Qualitative Research. *Journal of Phenomenological Psychology, 37* (2), 217-239.

Todres, L., & Galvin, K. (2006). Caring for a partner with Alzheimer's disease: intimacy, loss and the life that is possible. *International Journal of Qualitative Studies on Health and Well-being, 1* (1), 50-61.

Todres, L. & Galvin, K. (2008). Embodied Interpretation: A novel way of evocatively representing meanings in phenomenological research. *Qualitative Research. 8* (5), pp. 568-583.

Todres, L. (2007). *Embodied Enquiry: Phenomenological Touchstones for Research, Psychotherapy and Spirituality.* Basingstoke: Palgrave Macmillan.

Van Manen, M. (2007). Phenomenology of Practice. *Phenomenology & Practice, 1*, 11-30.

Note

[1] Acknowledgements: By permission of SAGE Publications, Les Todres' "Back to the Things Themselves: The Relevance of Embodied Understanding for Caring Practices" in this book is a modified version of an article reprinted from: Todres, L. (2008). Being with that: The relevance of embodied understanding for practice. *Qualitative Health Research. 18* (11), 1566-1573, copyright © 2008. [License agreement number : 2391290332329].

THE METHOD OF EIDETIC ANALYSIS FOR PSYCHOLOGY

Frederick J. Wertz, Ph.D.

Fordham University
United States

Abstract

Amedeo Giorgi has asserted that the two key procedures that make psychological research genuinely phenomenological are: 1) the epochés: *and 2) the intuition of essence. Giorgi's insistence on this point is reviewed and the often-misunderstood method of grasping essences is explored. Attention is given to Husserl's ideas about free imaginative variation and the procedures of eidetic analysis. Examination is made of how Husserl used his method to determine the essence of "psychological phenomena", and of the demands the essential characteristics of psychological subject matter place on the discipline. Implications for the sciences, especially for psychology's use of the phenomenological method, are spelled out. Basic practices in phenomenological psychological research are addressed, including the roles played by the investigator's imagination, by descriptions of others' real lives, and by literary and artistic works in eidetic research. Post-modern critiques of essentialism and of skepticism concerning "essences" are challenged in light of a clarification of the procedure. Finally, it is argued with Giorgi that eidetic analysis is crucial for a genuine science of psychology.*

As post-positivist and post-modernist thought has emerged and taken hold, the idea of "essence" has lost favor. Critiques of foundationalism and essentialism are common in both mainstream and avant-garde approaches to human science. Attempting to know the *essential qualities* of psychological subject matter is thought to involve a false sense of certainty and infallibility, an insensitivity to context and differences among diverse peoples, an ossification of the fluid and dynamic, an intolerance of ambiguity, an assumption of rigid predetermination in human life, and a detachment from existence. Claims about essences are thought to involve problems of dogmatism, universalism, reductionism, idealism, and even biological determinism. On account of inevitable limits of sampling data and of researcher biases and fallibility, assertions of essence are viewed as ignoring such important contexts as gender, culture, and age. Does not essentialism open the door to sexism, racism, ethnocentrism, and ageism? Do not assertions of essence, missing the multiform and changeable character of psychological life, translate politically into totalitarianism and a denial of human freedom?

Giorgi (1989, 2008) has consistently insisted that the intuition of essences is one of the two defining procedures of phenomenological psychological research. It is ironic that a necessary procedure of phenomenology, indeed its methodological *sine qua non*, would be thought to entail the problems of the very *isms* that this approach has so strenuously attempted to resolve. Are the principles and procedures designed to guide the intuition of essences, the method of eidetic analysis, self-deluded or at least *naïve* and *passé*? Some psychologists who are sympathetic with phenomenology have responded by identifying it as a *movement* and by taking the existential and hermeneutic turn with Heidegger, Merleau-Ponty and Sartre; the ethical turn with Lévinas; the narrative turn with Ricoeur, or even a constructionist turn, which make the study of essences a footnote to history. As interest in qualitative research methods grows in the human sciences, fundamental analytic procedures are of great concern. Some contemporary research that presents itself as phenomenological neither mentions nor makes use of the method of eidetic analysis. Is the intuition of essences, as Giorgi suggests, truly necessary for human science?

This chapter addresses the topic of the intuition of essences, which has not been well understood in the qualitative research movement. Here, I will reaffirm Husserl's view that in order to proceed soundly from a scientific, social and ethical standpoint, human scientists must understand and employ the procedure of eidetic analysis throughout their research and theorizing. I will focus on the nature of this procedure and the general importance of eidetic psychology rather than offer an account of the ways that eidetic analysis has been and can be employed in specific psychological research. Another limit of this chapter is that although I will touch on the link between eidetic and empirical research in psychology, the complexities of this relationship and the details of an eidetically grounded *empirical* psychology will not be elaborated.

Background

At mid-century in the *Phenomenology of Perception*, Merleau-Ponty (1945/1962) noted that misunderstandings of the procedure of intuiting essences could lead to the conclusion that phenomenology is a myth or a passing fashion. Recently, Husserlian scholar Rochus Sowa (2008) called "disastrous" Husserl's adoption of the "tradition laden", "vague and ambiguous" term *essence* because of its connotation of irrationalism and esotericism. Although Husserl himself explicitly ruled out "semi-mystical" thoughts concerning essence and *eidos*, Sowa asserts that Husserl's term has triggered totally false associations and obscured an unprejudiced view of this research method.

Sowa (2008) argues that of the two fundamental procedures of phenomenology – eidetic analysis and intentional analysis, the former – the intuition of essences, is the truly scientific method, that which grounds phenomenology's claim to be a science. Thanks to this procedure, Husserl's philosophy, as a rigorous science, radically guides human rationality; fundamentally distinguishes the physical from the human, socio-historical sciences; and provides psychology with a genuinely scientific research method for the first time in its history. Husserl accepted Dilthey's contention that psychology of the late 19th century was unscientific and would remain so as long as it erroneously adopted the methods and theoretical assumptions of natural science instead of developing methods and concepts suited to its own subject matter. For Husserl (1911/1965, pp. 102-103), the true method follows from the nature of things to be investigated, not from our prejudices and preconceptions. He argues that the prejudice of naturalism leads to an inauthentic psychology because it blinds us to the method of seeing essences. At stake for Husserl in identifying and developing the eidetic method is not only the rationality of sciences guided by a rigorous epistemology and ontology, but the overarching ethical imperative that science address the deepest and most far reaching concerns of human society and history with the freedom and responsibility necessary to shape our destiny (Jalberg, 1988).

Development of the Idea

In his focus on "essence", Husserl revives ancient philosophical wisdom in order to address pressing scientific problems. Husserl reaffirms the view that intelligence includes the power to distinguish the essential from the accidental, and that the essential, the *eidos*, is presented objectively (Cobb-Stevens, 1992). That is, the *eidos* (Plato's term [Smith, 2007]) of a subject matter is evident in the way it presents itself. Cobb-Stevens (1990, 1992, 2002) elaborates Husserl's kinship with Aristotle and his application of ancient philosophy to contemporary science. In emphasizing our grasp of objectivity unmediated by mental representations, Husserl reaffirms the primacy of seeing and intellectual insight over hypotheses, language and historical constructions. Grounded in perception and predication, in what Husserl calls *intuition*, knowledge takes up real situations and not mental substitutes. To see and to say that "the paper is white" is not to have a mental idea of "white" but to grasp the paper itself through its "look", the whiteness *belonging to the paper* (Cobb-Stevens, 1990). The *paper is white.* The German word *Wesen* (essence) is derived from *was* (what) and *sein* (is) (Smith, 2007). In Husserl's view, the seeing of essence provides the most fundamental knowledge of *what is.*

Husserl's aim is neither to return to ancient ways nor to diminish the importance of the recent advances of science; his efforts are progressive. Phenomenology is a new and strictly scientific style of philosophy (Husserl, 1929/1969, p. 249). Holding modern science in high esteem, Husserl provides it with a rigorous philosophical grounding and shows how science can, for the first time, be extended to human affairs. In his *Logical Investigations*, Husserl (1901-1902) argues against nominalism and delineates ways of knowing that return, from empty words, abstract models, hypotheses (etc.), to the matters themselves under investigation; the "return to the things themselves" is first principle of Husserl's phenomenology (Lévinas, 1930/1973).

Husserl is committed to the vision of modern science, in which rationality is wedded to the encounter with the real world. Opposing uncritical dogma, Husserl proclaims: "Let us examine the evidence of ordinary experience, to see what it itself can teach us" (Husserl, 1929/1969, p. 261). There he finds that predication, ideality, concepts – knowledge relates to its objective evidence through *intuition*. As opposed to mere thinking and empty speaking about something without any specific details, "intuition" is the presentation of the subject matter in the fullness of its concrete presence (Cobb-Stevens, 1990, p. 43). For instance, as opposed to merely thinking or saying that we should consider a relaxing summer vacation in the country, my intuition – in perception or even imagination – might involve laying on a lakeside dock, feeling the warm rays of the sun and a gentle wind caress on my body as I hear the laughter and splashing of my children and turn to see them playing in the shallow water near the sandy shore.

Our direct, intuitive experience of the world is first an apprehension of individual things. Conceptual thought, language, and abstract constructions are erected and inseparably founded on prior intuitions of individual things (Husserl, 1948/1973). Already at work in the experience of a particular object is a consciousness of its general type, the distinctive familiarity of its look and/or sound, and this may be articulated in speech (naming, describing). However, this familiar, objectively experienced *kind* is not necessarily thematized. The *active* identification of this generality – of these types, kinds, genera – is an elementary, intuitive form of insight. When I see not merely *that* something is present but *what it is* that is present, this objective apprehension of quality is the consciousness of its essence. In seeing a car pass by, I see *what* is passing by –something familiar, typical, of which this particular car in its empirical facticity is an example. Similarly in the case of a plurality of objects like birds (e.g., in a pair or a flock), each individual has the same "look" and we directly apprehend their sameness, their common properties, their mutual affinity, their blending and coincidence of likeness, their kinship of objective being

– their *kind* (Husserl, 1948/1973, p. 322). Although the individuality and commonality of things can be distinguished, both are concrete, immediately given moments of the beings that we apprehend (objectively given beyond consciousness). The thematization of this communality at once illuminates something that pertains to an individual and also to its *general core*, which is an objective moment present in many otherwise varying particular individuals, indeed *all* individuals of that *kind*. The individual thing, as an instance of what is not strictly limited to it, is a moment of an infinite horizon of like objects, a *universal* (Husserl, 1948/1973, 328).

We can intuitively thematize this objectively given universality by passing beyond what is particular into an open horizon of multipilization or possibilizing (Zaner's term, 1973a), toward an infinity of imaginable examples of the kind. Through this process we may form a concept, rudimentary knowledge, of *what all these individuals are* in common. On the basis of such ordinary acquisition of empirical or actual generalities, we understand what we refer to as "animals", "plants", "houses" or "cities". When we see a particular dog, its sense or meaning includes a common way of eating, playing, running, jumping, and even certain kind of teeth, whether or not we actually see them, all implicit in what we mean by saying "dog" (Husserl, 1948/1973). Essences are given everywhere in our experience of reality prior to active ideation, language, and conceptual knowledge, through which they can be thematized and articulated. It is only the theoretical dogma of naturalism that, by reducing the world to individual physical facts devoid of meanings, blinds us to essences.

Ordinary experience of the world involves "typification" (Schutz, 1973) and shifts between our regarding affairs in their particular factuality (this dirty, old Chevy), typicality (a car), and higher generality (a material thing). Husserl traces the path from passively preconstituted typifications to actively formed general concepts in everyday life and in science. The active *thematization* of essence involves a shift of consciousness that Zaner (1973a) names "exemplication". One can see anything in two ways – in itself, for its own sake, in its unique individuality, or *as an example of something.* Husserl offers procedures for making this shift of attentive seeing rigorously methodical and thereby scientifically generative (Zaner, 1973b). As indicated above, eidetic consciousness is *prior to all concepts* and verbal significations. Knowing and naming are founded on this primary consciousness that takes place in ordinary experience. To be truly meaningful, to refer to what is (being talked about), predications must articulate an *eidos*. Regarding eidetic intuition, Merleau-Ponty writes, "In the silence of primary consciousness can be seen not only what words mean, but also what things mean: the core of primary meaning round which the acts of naming and expression take shape" (1962, p. xv).

Most important is to understand that essences are not inferred, deductively or inductively, and they cannot be derived from an abstract system or model. They originate and are given in intuition. In this sense consciousness of essence is akin to perception, the primary awareness of transcendent reality. Essences are not hypotheses, mental constructs, inferences, abstractions, interpretations, or mental phenomena at all but are instead objective characteristics of transcendent objects (Husserl, 1913/1982, p. 42). "Like other objects, they can be intended to correctly, at times falsely, as, e.g., in false geometrical thinking. Though the intuition of and seizing upon essences is a complex act, specifically *seeing essences is an originary and presentative act* [...] the *analogue of sensuous perceiving* and *not of imagining*" (Husserl, 1913/1982, p. 44). Universal intuition (called "ideation"), founded on individual intuition, is a consciousness of the exemplary character of singularities, through perceptual, memorial, or imaginal intuitions that involve a generic judgment ("insight") that is itself intuitive. Essences are found in the very own being of the individual as *what that individual is*. Presence to evidence, not deduction, makes this form of rationality scientific (Lévinas 1930/1973, p. 111).

A Key Distinction: Formal versus Material Essences

One may intuit the essence of anything – "every kind of state of affairs" (Husserl, 1948/1973, p. 359). In a given individual, many different essences, even different types of essences, and different levels of eidetic generality may be grasped. A sea shell found on the beach is "hard", "shiny", "beautifully colored", "elegantly shaped", "6 inches in circumference", "useful as an ash tray", "a former home", "abalone", "a shell", "organic matter", "a material thing" and "God's creation". Husserl distinguishes formal essences from material essences. For instance, numbers – 1, 3, 100 – are formal essences. Mathematics and logic are formal eidetic sciences. The truth of the simple equation "2 + 3 = 5" is an eidetic truth, as is the logical law of non-contradiction. Two cats and 3 cats are 5 cats; 2 cats and 3 insects are five animals; 2 rocks and 3 animals are 5 material objects. This eidetic truth is universal inasmuch as it is repeatable again and again through an infinity of exemplary individuals, by different mathematicians, and remains intuitably identical in all instances. The distinctive characteristic of formal essences is the exactness of their ideality. The great achievements of ideation can be seen in Galileo's mathematization of nature, and in Newton's specification of the universal law of gravity, which explains both terrestrial and celestial movement of bodies with the same formula. Standardized measurement and quantitative analysis offer tremendous advantage to physics and the other sciences of nature. Exact quantitative idealization of the physical world by measurement is possible because material things are extended in space, independent of each other, and *akin in their kind of being* to the instruments that calibrate measurement, as the floor is to a ruler or the rotation of a planet is to a clock.

Eidetic thinking is not limited to mathematics and formal logic. Ideation, in addition to the exact idealization of the formal disciplines, is capable of grasping essences of things that are not exactly determinable and even those whose being is not akin to physical things. Whereas mathematics uses the method of idealization, other methods of ideation grasp "vague configurational types" that cannot be determined with exactitude. Husserl calls these material essences *morphological*, in contrast to the formal. The vagueness and fluidity of concepts concerning such essences is not a defect; they are indispensable and "in those spheres are the only legitimate concepts" (Husserl, 1913/1982, p. 166). Each kind of subject matter must be taken as it is given, even if given precisely as fluid. Vague, inexact, changing, continuous matters give rise to morphological notions like "toothed", "fluted", "lenticular", "flowing" or "transformational" that cannot be mathematized (Husserl, 1913/1982). Another intrinsic limit of morphological essences is that they can only be grasped imperfectly and "one-sidedly" in a given moment of apprehension, and although they may show many-sidedness in a sequence of intuitions, they cannot be grasped non-perspectivally as one does when one idealizes formal essences like numbers.

Regional Ontologies

Knowing the essences of various kinds or regions of being makes possible the rational establishment of distinct sciences. Husserl calls this task *regional ontology*, which also delineates the overlapping and interweaving of different sciences, for instance the physical sciences and psychology, psychology and history (Husserl, 1913/1982, p. 32). Material or morphological essences of the highest genera such as "physical thing" and "person" ground the distinction of the natural and human sciences. Distinct regional essences pertain to material object, plants life, animality, humankind, society or history. Regional ontologies articulate the essences of various scientific subject matters in their concreteness and yield necessary insights about their differences without the exactness of geometric and mathematical concepts. A distinct kind of being belongs to each of these regions according to their essences. Because essential characteristics of ontological regions pervade all factual manifestations within them, eidetic sciences can guide factual ones. Galileo's application of geometry and mathematics to physical nature enabled great progress in modern physics. However, if psychological subject matter is essentially different from material nature, it would be a mistake to assume that this same method applies. To say that a planet's orbit is elliptical, that a lake is 30 meters deep, that a heart beats 78 times a minute, that a car travels 50 miles an hour involves knowledge of what these matters essentially are (though not necessarily all of what they are). Geometric and mathematical knowledge of things extended in space, physical reality, has enabled the natural sciences to make impressive theoretical and technological progress. Measurement, calculation, causal inferences, model building and practical applications have enabled natural scientists to know and to shape nature with far reaching consequence. Husserl claims that psychology has not achieved comparable success because it has borrowed methods from natural science rather than developing methods in keeping with the essential qualities and structure of its own subject matter.

According to Husserl's regional ontology, materiality founds psychological processes, which in turn found cultural and historical realities, but each level contains something novel that cannot be reduced to its founding levels. The interwovenness of different regions poses difficult problems. The physical thing is related to an experiencing subject and to the intersubjective constitution of the objective physical thing-world. Communities and their institutions are novel objectivities of a higher order, which defy both naturalistic and psychologistic determinations. Objects of practical importance and value in the hard reality of our life, such as the state, the law, customs, and the church are essentially different structures compared with those of material nature and psychological processes (Husserl, 1913/1982, p. 365). And yet they are related to what is physical in space and human experiential processes, on which they are founded. Of utmost importance for science is that each region is clarified with insight into its own essential structure, which would rigorously determine, with methodological and conceptual authenticity, its own appropriate theory of reason (Husserl, 1913/1982). Before turning to Husserl's delineation of the essential characteristics of mental life, we will delineate in greater detail the method of eidetic analysis on which these insights are based.

Methodical Procedure: Toward Scientific Method

Husserl developed a procedure of ideation for performing the basic work of regional ontology and also for use in scientific psychological research. As we discussed above, essences are given in the intuitive consciousness of individuals, but they require active thematization, clarification, and propositional expression (see Mohanty, 1991). In this process there is a "shift of attitude" or focus from the individual as such to the individual as an example, in keeping with the intention to grasp "what-is-exemplified" (Zaner, 1973a, p. 32). The grasp of universal qualities requires more than a comparison of various empirical examples. Husserl stresses that whether the individual that serves as a starting point is factical or imaginal, insight into its essence requires free imaginative variation of the individual example, transforming it into different examples in which *what is possible (and impossible)* regarding the essence can be discerned. The procedure of imaginative variation is one feature of eidetic analysis that distinguishes it from induction, which is limited to empirically given facts and actual commonalities (Mohanty, 1991). The general essence, the *eidos* is found in those features that are invariant through all possible individual variations, as the general form necessary in order for individuals to be examples of the essence in question. The *eidos* is the congruent and identical content without which the object cannot possibly be an example, a variant of the kind (Husserl, 1948/1973). Although thematically grasping an essence is founded on the consideration of individuals, the essence itself is not strictly individual as it shows itself across infinite variations of different individuals. Indeed, it holds not merely for a large population of empirically real individuals, as do the results of induction, but for the infinity of possible individuals (Mohanty, 1991). Husserl clearly distinguishes this procedure from empirical generalization by: (1) its use of *fantasy*, and (2) its concern with what extends infinitely through all *possible* variations (Husserl, 1911/1965, p. 112).

Although an essence is intuitively grasped and immediately seen, its rigorous articulation is neither automatic, instantaneous, or easy. This procedure involves judgment that is labor intensive – a step-wise, progressive, sorting, comparing procedure. Eidetic intuition is fallible in that essences can be vaguely represented, represented in symbol, and falsely posited (Husserl, 1911/1925, p. 112). Prior to the thematization of the essence of "dog", one may be familiar with dogs, and if one has any concept and speaks about dogs, one's concept may be superficial, incomplete – with indeterminate horizons, or even wrong. The foundation, or better, the point of departure for an essential intuition can be a perception, a recollection, a judgment or an imagination. By seeing various different dogs, we may encounter new attributes and may discover more about what "dog" is. Any given idea of "dog" in the course of this process is "open, ever to be corrected" (Husserl, 1948/1973, p. 333). Husserl insists that this method is a process of *clarification* that demands a close, careful, and full presence of individuals and their possible variations so that the matters under investigation can be grasped in their essences and stated as completely and precisely as they themselves are. Any ideas that are not born out with concrete evidence in all exemplary singulars of a subject matter must be discarded.

Although an *eidos* can be presented in the data of memory and perception as well pure fantasy (Husserl, 1913/1982, p. 11), Husserl contends that originally presentative perception has primacies for knowledge of factual being as well as for eidetic findings. Factual reality provides great clarity through steady singularizations that spontaneously show themselves (independent of our prior knowledge) and that resist disruption by reflection. Less effort is needed to apprehend original factual examples than to imagine examples. And yet "[...] there are reasons by virtue of which in phenomenology, as in all other eidetic sciences, presentifications and, more precisely, *free fantasies* acquire *a position of primacy over perceptions* and do so even in the *phenomenology of perception itself* [...]" (1913/1982, 158-159, italics in original). This privilege resides in the infinite *freedom* of the imagination for shaping and reshaping variations of exemplary singulars. We can produce and vary in free fantasy spatial formations, melodies, social practices, liking or disliking, willing and, on the basis of ideation, see essences, the particular kind exemplified. The spontaneity of imagination provides ideation with far reaching access to an infinite range of possible examples, which necessarily includes within it all empirical instantiations and evidence of the essence.

Free and arbitrary imaginative variation provides a facility for identifying the core or invariant structure of a given *eidos*. When the removal of a certain quality or moment alters the individual such that it is no longer an example of the kind in question, we know that quality or moment is essential to the kind. As long as the individual remains an example of the matter in question even after the feature is imaginatively removed, the investigator knows that feature is not essential. Whereas falsification of empirical laws by imagining counter-examples (that is, by invented facts) would be absurd, imagination is the means par excellence for grasping and verifying eidetic law. Futility of the search for counter-examples in prescientific life, in science, and in the imagination, is a validation of eidetic law (Sowa, 2008). Critical thinking in the performance of this method is decisive for its scientific character. Zaner (1973a) stresses the need for continual return to examples through free imagination, in order to revise, reiterate, refute, extend and improve eidetic knowledge. Empirical and imaginative data collection and variation may utilize extreme and unusual states of affairs with the intent of eidetic critique, which is informed by singular cases that falsify and modify our prior knowledge. Sowa notes that this double testability, by fact and fantasy, renders eidetic analyses scientific by Popper's falsifiability criterion. "(Descriptive eidetics) turns out to be the true and genuine scientific element of Husserl's phenomenology, and legitimates its claim to being a science" (Sowa, 2008, p. 105).

General Essence of the Psychological

Husserl credits Brentano and Dilthey for brilliant intuitive insights that decisively distinguish psychological life from physical nature and thereby provide psychology with a basis for genuinely scientific methods and concepts. First and foremost, Brentano (1874/1973) recognized that human experience is *intentional*, that *consciousness is conscious of something* (other than itself). Human experience transcends itself, in contrast to physical things, which reside within themselves. I open the drawer, take out the book, read the title on the cover, and look for the chapter that will be the subject of a lecture. Because experience (as act, perceiv*ing*, remember*ing*) is not extended in space and is nothing in itself, it cannot be measured. Instead, its meaningful ways of relating to situations (beyond experience) must be described and understood.

Dilthey (1874/1977) recognized that lived experience flows, streams, changes through a plurality of various kinds (perceiving, remembering, anticipating, thinking, feeling), manifesting unities in which different moments interrelate and mutually imply each other by virtue of their *meaning*. Lived experience is essentially temporal, based on a history and reforming, developing, becoming toward a future. Experience includes the first person "I" in embodied, efficacious, practical, value laden, fundamentally social and collective engagement in a meaningful world in which personal experience casts itself and from which it is inseparable. Psychological life is not fragmentable does not contain independent parts, isolated variables that can be exactly measured and known through functional analyses and mathematical models as can physical things. Most importantly, the relations among moments are intelligible by virtue of unities of *meaning*. Because psychic life is not independent of our experience but is lived through, it need not be inferred but is intuitively present and is, even if difficult to know, accessible to description and intelligible in its motivated, ever-changing, meaningful nexus.

Although neither Brentano nor Dilthey reflectively formulated the method of eidetic analysis, Husserl views their profound insights as eidetic because they delineated core features apart from which human mental life is unimaginable and therefore inconceivable. The living human being is not conceivable, even possible, as a self enclosed, static, asocial, inefficacious, indifferent, contextless collection of mutually external and independent parts that can be separated or fragmented. Just as the human being is inconceivable without intentionality, embodiment, efficacy, values, temporality, sociality, holism, motivation, unity, and the potential for change, these features are also mutually implicit and inconceivable apart from each other. Moreover, these multiple qualities and horizons constituting personal experience make psychological life essentially inexhaustible, fundamentally indeterminate and ambiguous in its very meaningful intelligibility. Psychological life by essence changes, is in flux. No mental process can be accurately viewed as static and enclosed within itself; its interdependencies as part of a larger stream must be grasped. Moments of lived experience are bound together in its streaming and flow one into another one, by their very essence. Therefore nothing can be torn away from or separated from the stream, the concrete context. The unity "I as human" is an identity through this manifold, embodied in perceiving, feeling, judging, willing and so on. In each case this "I" encompasses the whole human – body, temperament, habitualities and convictions (Husserl, 1913/1989). Although Husserl emphasizes the unity of experiential life, this does not mean it is homogeneous or even free of conflict and contradictions. Husserl states that experience may show what cannot be united, for instance, in the "consciousness of deception" (Husserl, 1911/1965, p. 113). However, deception is, by its very meaning, the presence of a surreptitious act and a lie with mutually implicative meanings, together within one (a unitary and as such self-contradictory) experiential life.

Motivation, not causation, is the principle of the human being. Things do not cause interest but *arouse* interest on the part of a person, who is always already meaningfully engaged in situations ((Husserl, 1913/1989, p. 227). Objects have meaning by way of their utility and values as concern human desires and aims. The potentiality of motility, the "I move", is constitutive of human freedom. "No causal research, no matter how far reaching, can improve the understanding which is ours when we have understood the motivation of a person" (Husserl, 1913/1989, p. 241). The person is a subject of the surrounding world in an inseparable relation (Husserl, 1913/1989, p. 195). Things immediately excite my desire and frustrate or fulfill my needs. Not given as "stimuli", the surroundings appear through practical intentionalities as useful things –heating materials, choppers, hammers. Husserl writes, "The surrounding world is comprised not of mere things, but of use-Objects (clothes, utensils, guns, tools), works of art, literary products, instruments for religious and judicial activities (seals, official ornaments, coronation insignia, ecclesiastical symbols, etc." (Husserl, 1913/1982, p. 191).

Human experience and selfhood are also essentially and internally social, founded on community with others and unified by means of a bond of reciprocal and shared ays of being and understanding. Individual humans, as is eidetically evident in their behavior, perception, speech, and throughout their psychological life, are dependent on and constituted in communities, social institutions, moral orders. Inconceivably unrelated to others, whether bound or free and creative, human beings are socially related in their essential being (Husserl, 1913/1989, p. 148). For Husserl, even the experience of oneself as an individual human being is founded on social relatedness. He says, "*I fit myself into the family of man* [...] and then for the first time do I become an ego, and the other precisely an other" (1913/1989, p. 254). Human communities, with their moral and juridical regulations and modes of functioning, have their own history and preserve themselves despite the joining or leaving of individual persons. The individual person is not human except as the bearer of such relations as family, marriage, gender, unions and class. As communal, we are also interrelated with Nature: "The earth and sky, the fields and the woods, the room in which 'we' dwell communally, the picture we see [...]. We could not be persons for others if a common surrounding world did not stand there for us in a community, in an intentional linkage of our lives [...] the one is constituted essentially with the other" (Husserl, 1913/1989, p. 201). The individual person is an abstraction from the common, natural world, which is essentially implicated and primary (Husserl, 1913/1989, p. 201).

Human Science Research Methods: Free From Naturalism

The Investigator's Own Experience as a Source of Examples for Research

One immediate consequence of Husserl's liberating human science from naturalism in psychology by returning to the things themselves – to lived experience, is that research scientists can investigate their own personal lives as a legitimate part of their scientific enterprise. The preconceptual spontaneity and immediacy of the researcher's own lived experience is an invaluable source of psychological data and insight, as Freud and others have profoundly shown without explicit, scientific justification. It is possible to take one's own experience as exemplifying a particular psychological subject matter, as a basis for ideation and objective knowledge. Provided that one has lived through a topic of investigation, one's own experience can provide examples on the basis of which essential psychological insights can be achieved through rigorous, methodical ideation. Whether the investigator's own original sphere of experience is a valuable, sufficient, or even necessary source of examples for research depends on the nature of the research problem and the aims of research. Eidetic investigation requires imaginatively varying these original examples rather than remaining limited to the investigator's actual experience. Also already within the investigator's experience are examples of other people living through psychological subject matters under investigation, and these may also be valuable and even necessary sources of examples to be imaginatively varied. Zaner characterizes the freedom of the investigator as "roaming the fields" (1973a, p. 35). One may begin anywhere, move from one example to another, travel from what one has actually lived through to fantasy. One is free to stop, return, reiterate or continue. All the while remaining strictly within the relevancies and scope of the research problem, one is free from the facticity and empirical limits of one's life as from all ideographic singularity. Essential meanings and structures of psychological life may be brought to light with objective evidence through careful conceptualization, articulate discourse, and concrete exemplifications.

Empathic Communication with Others as Source of Examples for Research

The researcher's essential sociality as a person has implications for necessary extensions of human science method. Husserl says, "The psychologist has the problematics of intentionality through his own original sphere, but this is never isolable for him. Through the empathy of his original sphere of consciousness, through what arises out of it, as a component which is never lacking, he also already has a universal intersubjective horizon [...]" (Husserl, 1936/1954, p. 243). The psychological investigator can and often must enter and understand the lives of other people whose communicative expressions serve as an original source of access to psychological realities. It is most often valuable and necessary for psychologists, given the broad empirical diversity and scope of their subject matter, to go beyond what they themselves have lived through in their quest for insight and knowledge. A psychologist need not have actually experienced "schizophrenia", "torture", or "artistic creativity" in order to investigate such phenomena. Husserl says, "In an amazing fashion, (the person's) intentionality reaches into that of others and vice versa" (Husserl, 1936/1954, p. 254). Phenomenological research can be carried out in communication with others as research participants and partners because others are not outside one's experience, as two physical objects are mutually external; self and other exist in reciprocal mutuality. People are...

> [...] not a multiplicity of separated souls, each reduced to pure interiority, but rather: Just as there is a sole universal nature as a self-enclosed framework of unity, so there is a sole psychic framework, a total framework of all souls, which are united not externally but internally, namely, through the intentional interpenetration [*Ineindander*] which is the communalization of their lives [...]. There is no separation of mutual externality at all for souls in their own essential nature. What is a mutual externality from the point of view of naïve positivity or objectivity is, when seen from the inside, an intentional mutual internality. (Husserl, 1936/1954, p. 255)

I grasp the other's intentions, according to Husserl, "with intuitive flair" (1913/1989, p. 286). I can put myself in the place of others by empathy, enter the way they experience their situations (their level of education, age), assume their passions, co-perform their psychological acts, and share their meanings.

> I not only empathize with (an other person's) thinking, feeling, and actions but I must also *follow* him in them, his motives becoming my quasi-motives, ones which, however, motivate, with insight in the mode of intuitively fulfilling empathy. I co-share his temptations. I co-participate in his fallacies; in the co- there lies an inner co-living. (Husserl, 1913/1989, p. 287)

> We capture the development of a person if we reconstruct the course of his life and make it intuitive in such a way that the entirety of his development as a man becomes comprehensible in an experiential way [...]. That is "knowing a person", "the science of the soul", "psychology". (Husserl, 1913/1989, p. 285)

Empathic access to the lives of others provides a second and often necessary source of examples for rigorous psychological ideation. The deliberate, self-critical, and careful collection of diverse examples from the lives of others, freely varied in imagination and analyzed according to their meaningful processes and structures, is crucial to the yield of objective psychological knowledge.

Cultural Objects and Media as a Source of Examples for Psychological Research

Eidetic methodology also legitimates and appropriates the full spectrum of cultural expressions in the arts, humanities and popular media as additional bases and reference points for psychological research and insight. The social and imaginative works in the arts and letters suggest their great value for human science research. Some of the most excellent and abundant expressions of psychological life, sources of concrete examples of human life, are found in artistic creations, literary productions, media sources, cultural artifacts, and historical records. Fact and fantasy alike, inasmuch as they provide rich descriptions of human lived experiences, fertilize eidetic knowledge.

> It is necessary to exercise one's fantasy abundantly in the required activity of perfect clarification [...]. It is also necessary to fertilize one's fantasy by observations in originary intuition, which are as abundant and excellent as possible [...]. Extraordinary profit can be drawn from the offerings of history, in even more abundant measure from those of art, and especially from poetry, which are, to be sure imaginative but which, in the originality of their invention of forms, the abundance of their single features and the unbrokenness of their motivations, tower high above the products of our own fantasies and, in addition, when they are apprehended understandingly, become converted into perfectly clear fantasies with particular ease owing to the suggestive power exerted by artistic means of presentation [...]. If one is fond of paradoxical phrases, one can actually say, and if one means the ambiguous phrase in the right sense, one can say in strict truth, that *feigning* [*Fiktion*] *makes up the vital element of phenomenology as of every other eidetic science*, that feigning is the source from which the cognition of "eternal truths" is fed. (Husserl, 1913/1982, p. 160)

In a footnote to the last statement, Husserl writes with wry humor: "This sentence, as a quotation, should be especially suited for a naturalistic ridiculing of the eidetic mode of cognition" (1913/1982, p. 160).

It should be noted that scientific practice remains distinct from art, not collapsed into it. Art, literature, media, history and cultural artifacts may well provide revelatory examples of meaningful human life, but their original thematic disciplinary aim is not ideation, knowledge. Whereas artistic activities and cultural products remain within imaginative, observational, and expressive forms, scientist practice aims at theory. The thematic goal and outcome of scientific research, in utilizing art and literature as a source of *examples*, is knowledge proper – the conceptual articulation of essences, in this case the invariant psychological structures. Good poems, novels, biographies, anecdotes and stories, though excellent starting points for science, are not themselves psychology (Husserl, 1925/1977, p. 6). Incidentally, cultural objects of the arts, letters and media may play a similar role in history, sociology, literary study, and other human sciences, which in their own respective ways ("attitudes") thematize, conceptualize and communicate distinctive disciplinary knowledge of human beings. Scientific practice is above all characterized by its unique rationality, its use of imaginative variation in the service of ideation, knowledge proper. In illuminating the fundamental unity of human life in its manifold strata and delineating the theory of reason appropriate to each, phenomenology grounds and guides authentic interdisciplinary collaboration, dialogue and knowledge.

The Cultural Context of Research: Culture-Bound Essences

We have noted above that human life and human science take place within a cultural context, a "we-horizon". "In communicative society, each member sees what I see and hears what I hear, or at least *can* do so" (Husserl, 1913/1989, p. 208). Empathy grounds co-existence in the flesh. Because one's mental life can be experienced by another (and vice versa), human lived experience takes shape within specific cultures and civilizations, which can communicate with and understand each other (Husserl, 1936/1954). Science is a fundamentally social activity (Husserl, 1913/1989).

Psychological research can illuminate and address these cultural horizons. Such investigations may reveal essential differences among peoples' lived experiences and thereby provide a variegated knowledge of psychological phenomena. Solokowski notes, "(E)*ide* may indeed be culture-bound; perhaps other traditions do not break up a color continuum or even the animal kingdom the way ours does. The *eide* are not taken metaphysically, but as moments that can come to be registered as phenomena, and some *eide* may arise as only for a consciousness that articulates certain distinctions and not others" (1974, p. 75). In other words, *what something is* psychologically is culturally constituted and may be essentially limited to the human life in one or more cultures. A culture-bound psychological phenomenon is unimaginable, inconceivable, and impossible in other cultural contexts, for it is incompossible with the communal lifeworld and institutions of other cultures. Therefore, knowledge of culture-bound psychological structures requires comparative understanding and knowledge of cultures.

For instance, the "mental disorder" *bulimia nervosa* was first observed in the Western world in the last half of the 20th century. Beyond behavioral earmarks of binging and purging, essential to this disorder is a persistent concern about female bodily appearance including the desire to be thin. Although examples of binging and purging behaviors have been found in other cultures and historical periods, they have a different meaning, consistent with contrasting cultural values and structures, such as social status and pleasure – hedonistic privilege. Prior to the introduction of Western television on the island of Fiji, bulimia nervosa was nonexistent. Fijian culture's indigenous values of beauty did not include female thinness, which is unimaginable within that culture's intentionality of desire during that time in history. With the introduction of television, incidents of bulimia emerged and increased as youth began to live a new cultural ideal of thinness (Becker, Burwell, Gilman, Herzog, & Hamburg, 2002). Bulimic binging and purging is essentially related to emergent cultural ideals of female beauty and is therefore a culture-bound phenomenon in that "what it is" involves certain meanings, values, and aims that are shared in some cultures but not others. To assert knowledge of the essential constitution of a culture is not to suggest that culture is static or unchangeable, or that cultures are necessarily separate, as we see in the case of 20th century European and Fijian cultures. From the standpoint of eidetic analysis, "culture" concerns essential meanings and the structures of compossibility in collectively shared intentionalities, not merely a de facto collection of people with comparatively high behavioral frequencies.

The Community of Scientists: Broader Accountability and Scientific Progress

Zaner states that the grasping of the other as an alter ego can "have the import of a creative mutuality" because the *thou* is truly other and free (1973b, p. 209). In this respect, eidetic intuition is open to criticism, entails social collaboration and responsibility between the investigator, other scientists, and lay communities. Zaner appropriates Gabriel Marcel's (1965) notions of availability, evocation and appeal to characterize this social horizon of human science research (Zaner, 1973b, 210). Lévinas (1961/1969) similarly insists that research ethics demand accountability to others, who are essentially beyond our knowledge and representations. Therefore, knowledge of the essence of psychological life is an appeal to others, who are free to exercise their own potential for presenting counter-examples, imaginatively varying examples, performing their own comparisons, and insightfully describing essences. Eidetic claims can be contested and remain tentative appeals to critical communication (Zaner, 1973b, p. 211). Zaner, in considering those who have moved beyond Husserl's actual work (e.g., Heidegger, Sartre, Merleau-Ponty, Schutz, Lévinas, Ricoeur, and Derrida) likens Husserl to a "mid-wife" of profound and lively children (1973b, p. 212).

Within the context of psychological research proper, eidetic knowledge requires correction and improvement, an inclusive and diasporic communal movement. Husserl calls into question any rigid absolutist a priori by emphasizing that, "every eidetic claim is subject to deception, modification, revision, and even denial – in short, continual criticism" (Husserl, 1911/1965, p. 216). Husserl, for whom evidence involves an "encounter" (1929/1969, p. 36), rejects every absolutism and holds that in the positive sciences, it is an error to interpret knowledge as adequate because the subject matter cannot be known completely (Husserl, 1929/1969, p. 277; Zaner, 1973a, p. 37; Mohanty, 1991, p. 265). Husserl asserts that even the most highly developed science "remains involved in relativities by its essence" (1929/1969, p. 278). We start out with naïve judging, reflect, return to living sources with continual openness to criticism and acceptance of accountability. This availability on the part of the psychological researcher, in its inclusive appeal, sharply contrasts with the deductive stance that in sovereignity asserts abstract axioms/models and inductively calculates empirical probabilities. Social responsibility, justice, and ethical relatedness are at the heart of the scientific objectivity of eidetic method. Cobb-Stevens (1972) asserts that Husserl's appropriation of the scientific ideal of universal truth in infinity is ultimately an expression of "hope" (Cobb-Stevens, 1992, p. 275).

Eidetic Generality in Contrast to Empirical Generalization

Mainstream psychologists express reservations about the generalizability of qualitative research with *naïve* reference to the relatively few number of participants who provide data in some studies. Phenomenology, apart from its utilization of a large number of examples and imaginative variations, involves *a special kind of generality* distinct from empirical generalization. Generalization, in scientific parlance, refers to the extension of facts through empirical populations. Phenomenology, even in analyzing the details of one individual experience, aims at the essence of which it is an example. Essence is by nature universal. Eidetic generalities therefore refer to *qualitative kinds* as such. Although eidetic qualitative knowledge claims and laws apply universally to empirical examples of the kind under investigation, they make no claims about the factual extent of that kind in empirical reality. How common or rare examples of an essence are requires quantitative empirical investigation of the kind. Knowledge of essence is fundamentally different from knowledge of empirical frequency or prevalence.

Higher levels of essential generality, with their greater scope than lower levels, are not to be confused with empirical, quantitative scope, for they concern the extent, the range-restriction, of *kinds in comparison to more qualitatively inclusive kinds* (Husserl, 1948/1973). The individual example of a phenomenon, as a limit point at the lowest level, admits of a certain (the most restricted scope of) essential generality, for we can imagine various individuals that are exactly the same--independent individuals that are completely alike. Husserl calls this a *concretum* and points out that because two (and an infinite number of) completely alike individuals are imaginable, the concretum itself has an essence, manifests a kind, a concrete or specific universal which extends beyond the individual to all like it, whether any actually exist in empirical reality or not. Husserl puts it: "This universal, born of the repetition of like independent objects is the lowest generality [...]" (Husserl, 1948/1973, p. 335). Because psychologists are not usually interested in singular examples of a matter under investigation, research requires study of different individuals in order to achieve higher levels of generality. Thus there are limits to and gradations in levels of qualitative generality, which do not refer to empirical scope or extent but to other kinds and other levels of generality. Each *eidos* has universal extension through its empirical and imaginable exemplifications and limited scope in comparison with other *eide* and more general *eide*.

As we have seen, each eidetic analysis is conducted within a determinate scope that restricts the examples and thereby limits the qualitative generality of eidetic claims. When we elaborated the essence of the psychic as such and distinguished it from the formal and the physical, our scope of analysis was at a very high level of generality – the characteristics of all psychological phenomena. Eidetic knowledge, nevertheless universal, can reach low levels of generality with more restricted, local, context-bound scopes of qualitative compass. Less general, more specific essences require investigations under the titles of the full variety of psychological subject matters. Because psychological phenomena are essentially context bound and involve multiple strata and dependencies, phenomena under one title can often be fruitfully differentiated according to lower-level, context-bound essences. For instance, it is possible to analyze "hallucination" and to make eidetic claims that cover all hallucinations, but these statements may be less important for psychology than investigations at lower levels of qualitative generality that focus, with more restricted scope, on alcohol-induced hallucination, paranoid schizophrenic hallucination, and hallucination in the context of religious ritual which admit of qualitatively different eidetic structures. Similarly, in the "the psychology of moral reasoning", essentially different typical structures are dependent on various developmental levels. Social psychology offers eidetic insight into "leadership" that concerns the broadest scope of all examples of leadership and also knowledge of less general styles of leadership (e.g., autocratic, consultative). Detailed knowledge of qualitative kinds is important in every subfield of psychology from learning to cognition, perception, abnormal and developmental. It is characteristic of other human sciences also to investigate such mid-level, context-bound general structures, as Durkheim (1897) does in distinguishing egoistic, altruistic, anomic, and fatalistic kinds of suicide. Again, the empirical prevalence of such kinds is another kind of knowledge that requires other methods.

Various levels of generality may be relevant to the psychologist, depending on the research interest, which may be determined by theoretical or practical aims. For instance, in *The Divided Self*, Laing (1960) presents an analysis of schizophrenia that is essentially limited. He claims to elaborate only *one* (among others) paths to, style of, structure of, "type" of schizophrenia. He presumes there are other types, which he does not elaborate and examples of schizophrenia that do not manifest the eidetic structures he delineates. Laing elaborates the essence of this particular way of becoming schizophrenic on the basis of many examples and their imaginative variations, including ones he finds in the clinic, in the psychological literature, in fictional literature, and in film. His analysis applies universally, that is, to *all schizophrenics of this type*, irrespective of how frequently such examples are manifest in the empirical population of schizophrenics. Eidetic intuition and analysis produces eidetically limited and yet universal generality, which is not to be confused with empirical or quantitatively extended generalization.

Relations of the Eidetic and the Empirical

Husserl's reference to the intuition of essences as "pure" concerns its freedom from all positing of actuality. However, the discerning thinker recognizes that the essence of actuality itself can be grasped, that is, that one can limit the scope of imaginable variations to the realm of real human beings, to what is actually possible. Husserl writes, "If we vary freely but secretly stipulate that the variants must be optional tones *in the world*, tones heard or able to be heard *by human beings on earth*, then we have indeed something universal or an eidos, but one related to our *factually actual world* and restricted to this all-inclusive fact" (Husserl, 1925/1973, p. 55, parentheses mine). Cobb-Stevens (1992) points out that, unlike many contemporary philosophers, Husserl does not extend the method of free variation to improbable scenarios in possible worlds.

Husserl distinguishes "pure" essences, which may serve specifically philosophical purposes, from such *impure eide* as are relevant for psychology, which concerns actual human beings in this world and therefore methodically restricts its focus and scope to what is possible and essential to *human beings as empirical realities* (Husserl, 1948/1973, p. 374). Hence, although phenomenological psychology is an eidetic discipline and strictly speaking makes no assertions about quantitative empirical extensiveness, its knowledge of essence deliberately focuses on, restricts itself to the structural possibilities of actual human life. Though this discipline is impurely eidetic, it is not empirical. Psychology imaginatively varies examples of psychological life through potentially infinite variations in order to grasp the essential structural *possibilities of humans as actually they exist in the real world.*

Zaner (1973a) complains that Husserl's rigid dichotomy between the eidetic and the empirical is not justified. However, Husserl himself acknowledges an intimate connection of eidetic analysis to empirical reality: "The experienced world is granted to us as the universal permanent ground of being and as the universal field of all our activities. As the firmest and most universal of all our habitualities, the world is valid and remains valid in its actual validity for us, no matter what interests we may pursue; like all interests, those involving eidetic cognition are also related to it" (1948/1973, p. 350; also in 1925/1977, p. 55). Husserl speaks of a "bond of being" between essence and facticity and insists, " [...] every fact and every eidos remains related to the factual world, belonging to this world [...]" (Husserl, 1925/1977, p. 55; 1948/1973, p. 351). It is possible to methodically put this "bond of being" out of play, to achieve perfect purity as does phenomenological philosophy: "Then we find ourselves, so to speak, in a pure world of the imagination, a world of absolutely pure possibility" (Husserl, 1925/1977, p. 55; 1948/1973, p. 351). Such knowing of *pure eidos* is also practiced in geometry, for instance in the idealization of the exact essence of "circle", which cannot appear intuitively in empirical reality, and in formulating the Pythagorean theorem. All essences, whether pure or empirically restricted, hold for all individual examples (if there are any!) in the empirical world. For good reasons, the psychological researcher seeks morphological knowledge restricted in its extension to actual human life and therefore psychological ideation (theory) deliberately ties itself to empirical reality. Merleau-Ponty says, "The eidetic method is the method of a phenomenological positivism which bases the possible on the real" (1962, XVI-XVII). Husserl, with his profoundly expanded notion of objectivity, says: "If by "positivism" we are to mean the absolutely unbiased grounding of all science on what is "positive", i.e., what can be primordially apprehended, then *it is we who are the genuine positivists*" (Husserl, 1913/1982, pp. 39-40, italics mine).

Phenomenological, eidetic psychology is an indispensable methodological and conceptual foundation for empirical psychological investigations, just as mathematics has been for physics (Husserl, 1913/1982). For instance, a psychologist investigating the *prevalence* of "child abuse" in various populations, in order to perform valid measurement, requires guidance by knowledge of *what child abuse is*, that is, by an essential understanding of the meaning(s) of child abuse that covers all individual examples. Similarly, a psychologist investigating "intelligence" in school age children or the neurological or genetic substrate of adult intelligence must have a sound qualitative understanding of *what intelligence is*. Historically psychology has skipped over this necessary descriptive, qualitative stage, for instance when it conceptualized intelligence only by means of empirical measurement, assuming that intelligence is equivalent to the IQ without having conducted critical investigation of qualitatively different examples of intelligence. Recently psychologists have gained the essential insight that there are various kinds of intelligence, including the social-emotional and practical in addition to the cognitive. Colaizzi's (1967) phenomenological replication of a classic learning experiment concludes that the method of paired associates, which involves cued verbalization of previously presented nonsense syllables, is not an example of learning in that participants simply perform previously acquired memorization strategies in this experimental task, and therefore experimenters were not studying examples of learning. The genuineness and qualitative generality of quantitative-empirical psychology fundamentally rests on critically established eidetic psychological science. Without eidetic knowledge, empirical psychologists literally do not know what they are studying.

The lack of development and systematic employment of eidetic methodology, based on rich, full, and diverse concrete examples of psychological phenomena, has held psychology back from the rigorous clarification of its basic scientific concepts. Husserl says, "[...] it is the fundamental error of modern psychology, preventing it from being psychology in the true, full scientific sense, that it has not recognized and developed this phenomenological method" (Husserl, 1913/1982, p. 189). The eidetic method, which phenomenology provides psychology, is necessary for its scientificity. According to Husserl, "[...] the spell of the naturalistic point of view, to which all of us are at the outset subject [...] has blocked the road to a great science unparalleled in fecundity [...]" (1913/1982, p. 110). This spell makes it difficult to see essences "or rather, since in fact we do, so to speak, constantly see them, for us to let them have the peculiar value which is theirs instead of absurdly naturalizing them. Intuiting essences conceals no more difficulties or "mystical" secrets than does perception" (Husserl, 1911/1965, p. 110).

Conclusions

Far from being a dogmatic over-reach of knowledge, eidetic analysis involves a fresh, open attitude that is evidence-based, methodical, and self-critical. By beginning with systematically collected examples and varying them imaginatively, psychological conceptualization can be carefully shaped and can faithfully reflect the data, with no prior norms or demands placed on its insights, which follow from an encounter with concrete realities. Far from deriving intelligibility from a realm outside of existence and claiming an apodictic and eternal truth, eidetic analysis engages with the complexities and ambiguities of our pre-conceptually familiar yet intellectually obscure existence. The uncertainties of our knowledge are gradually overcome by grounded and extended intuitive contact with and thinking about psychological subject matters. When distinct concepts are finally formed and articulated through this rigorous encounter, they are asserted only within the limits of their achievement, which calls for tentativeness and humility given the possibilities of error and inadequacy at every step: the collection of examples, the extent and restriction of imaginative variations, the insightful grasping of eidetic law, and the discourse in which insights are communicated (Mohanty, 1991).

Psychological reality, by its very essence, can be known only partially and imperfectly. Therefore eidetic methods must be self-critical and resist final conclusions. Because concepts in psychology are necessarily inexact, they never achieve the formal perfection of mathematics or the exactitude of geometry. Psychological knowledge can always be improved. The essential characteristics of mental life – its change through time, its context boundedness, its inexhaustibility, its openness to possibility, and its transcendence (non-manipulability) – require humility, accountability, and collaborative accommodation on the part of scientists. The phenomenological notion of "essence" is anything but idealistic, for essential structures are restricted to the possibilities of actual psychological life; they are intuitively grasped in and must accept counter-evidence in the real world and revise propositions accordingly. The very procedure of eidetic analysis is designed to rigorously move beyond preconceptual familiarity, preliminary concepts, and empty assertions by engaging continually considering all concrete examples of the subject matter that are relevant to the adopted scope of investigation. This form of ideation draws conclusions from the real rather than by imposing any pre-established intellectual order.

We have stressed that the intuition of essences, eidetic analysis, is corrigible, is accountable, and involves social responsibility. Critical dialog has its rational basis, on the part of both researcher and critic, in intuitions of the matters under investigation. The rational principles and methodical procedures of eidetic analysis scientifically ground and guide social scientific processes of agreement, disagreement, criticism, and corrective revision of knowledge, whether enacted individually, dialogically, or collectively. Whether an investigation proceeds alone, interpersonally or with a group, the truth of its knowledge claims rests on the objective evidence brought forth by its initial exemplifications, free imaginative variations, and identification of invariants through essential insight. Whether employing our knowledge in the contexts of practice or seeking to improve our knowledge in research, we must remain perpetual beginners, continually returning to concrete intuition as a wellspring of infinite encounter.

References

Becker, A.E., Burwell, R.A., Gilman, S. E., Herzog, D. B., & Hamburg, P. (2002). Eating behaviors and attitudes following prolonged exposure to television among ethnic Fijian adolescent girls. *British Journal of Psychiatry, 180*, 509–514

Brentano, F. (1973). *Psychology from an empirical standpoint* (A.C. Rancurello, D. B. Terrell, & L. L. McAlister, Trans.). New York: Humanities Press. (Original work published 1874)

Cobb-Stevens, R. (1990). Being and categorical intuition. *Review of Metaphysics, 44*, 43-66.

Cobb-Stevens, R. (1992). Husserl on eidetic intuition and historical interpretation. *American Catholic Philosophical Quarterly, 66* (2). 261-275.

Cobb-Stevens, R. (2002). Husserlian hermeneutics: Mathematics and *theoria*. In B.E. Babich (Ed.). *Hermeneutic philosophy of science, Van Gogh's eyes, and God: Essays in honor of Patrick A. Heelan, S. J.*, pp. 153-161. Dordrecht: Kluwer.

Colaizzi, P. (1967). An analysis of the learner's perception of the learning material at various stages of the learning process. *Review of Existential Psychiatry and Psychology, 7*, 95-105.

Dilthey, W. (1977). Ideas concerning a descriptive and analytical psychology (1894). (R. M. Zaner, Trans.). In W. Dilthey (Ed.). *Descriptive Psychology and Historical Understanding.* The Hague: Martinus Nijhoff. (Original work published 1924)

Durkheim, E. (1897/1997). Suicide. New York: The Free Press.

Giorgi, A. (1989). Some theoretical and practical issues regarding the phenomenological psychological method. *Saybrook Review, 7*, 71-85;

Giorgi, A. (2008). Concerning a Serious Misunderstanding of the Essence of the Phenomenological Method in Psychology, *Journal of Phenomenological Psychology, 39* (1), 1-26

Husserl, E. (1913/1982). *Ideas Pertaining to a Pure Phenomenology and to a phenomenological philosophy. First Book: General Introduction to a Pure Phenomenology* (tr. F Kersten). The Hague: Martinus Nijhoff Publishers,

Husserl, E. (1913/1989). *Ideas pertaining to a pure phenomenology and to a phenomenological philosophy. Second book: Studies in the phenomenology of constitution.* Tr. R Rojcewicz and A. Schuwer. Dordrecht, The Netherlands: Kluwer Academic Publishers.

Husserl, E. (1929/1969). *Formal and transcendental logic.* (Tr. D. Cairns.). The Hague: Martinus Nijhoff.

Husserl, E. (1948/1973). *Experience and judgment: Investigations in a genealogy of logic.* (Ed. L. Landgrebe, Tr. J.S. Churchill and K. Ameriks.). Evanston, IL: Northwestern University Press.

Husserl. E. (1931/1960). *Cartesian meditations* (D. Cairns, trans.). The Hague: Nijhoff.

Husserl, E. (1962/1977). *Phenomenological psychology: Lectures, summer semester, 1925.* (J. Scanlon, Trans.). Boston: Martinus Nijhoff. _

Husserl, E. (1936/1954). *The crisis of European sciences and transcendental phenomenology.* (D. Carr, Trans.). Evanston: Northwestern University Press. (Original work published 1939).

Husserl. E. (1900-1/1970). *Logical investigations* (J.N. Findlay, Trans.). London: Routledge & Kegan Paul Ltd.

Husserl. E. (1911/1965). Philosophy as a rigorous science. In *Phenomenology and the crisis of philosophy* (Q. Lauer, trans.). New York: Harper.

Jalbert, H. E. (1988). Husserl's position between Dilthey and the Windelband-Rickert school of Neo-Kantianism. *Journal of the History of Philosophy*, *26*, 279-296.

Laing, R. D. (1960). *The divided self.* London: Tavistock.

Lévinas, E. (1930/1973). *The theory of intuition in Husserl's phenomenology* (A. Orianne, Trans.). Evanston: Northwestern University Press.

Marcel, G. (1965). *Being & Having: An existentialist diary.* New York: Harper & Row.

Merleau Ponty, M. (1961/1964). Phenomenology and the sciences of man. In *The primacy of perception.* Evanston, IL: Northwestern University Press.

Merleau-Ponty, M. (1945/1962). *Phenomenology of perception.* (C. Smith, Trans.). London: Routledge & Kegan Paul.

Mohanty, J. N. (1991). Method of imaginative variation in phenomenology.In T. Horowitz and G.J. Massey (Eds.). *Thought experiments in science and philosophy.* Savage, MD: Rowman and Littlefield Publishers, Inc. 261-272.

Schutz, A. (1973). Collected Papers, Volume 1. The Hague: Martinus Nijhoff.

Smith, D. W. (2007). *Husserl.* New York: Routledge.

Sokolowski, R. (1974). *Husserlian meditations: How words present things.* Evanston, Northwestern University Press.

Sowa, R. (2008). Essences and eidetic laws in Edmund Husserl's descriptive eidetics. *The New Yearbook for Phenomenology and Phenomenological Philosophy*, *7*, 77-108.

Zaner, R. M. (1973a). Examples and possibles: A criticism of Husserl's theory of free-phantasy variation. *Research in Phenomenology*, *3*, 29-43.

Zaner, R. (1973b). The art of free fantasy in rigorous phenomenological science. In *Phenomenology. Continuation and criticism; Essays in memory of Dorion Cairns.* The Hague: Martinus Nijhoff, pp. 192-219.

A PHENOMENOLOGICAL EXPLICATION OF A MASTER TEACHER'S QUESTIONING PRACTICES AND ITS IMPLICATIONS FOR THE EXPLANATION/UNDERSTANDING ISSUE IN PSYCHOLOGY AS A HUMAN SCIENCE

Akihiro Yoshida, Ph.D.

Shukutoku University & Tokyo University (Emeritus)
Japan

Abstract

Situated in his personal circumstances in Japanese history, culture and society, the author explicates the implicit meanings of a Japanese master teacher's practices of teaching literary works of art. From his records, there emerge the implicit contrast between the "Why-question" and the "What-question" with respect to the behavior/experience of the character(s) in novels. The contrast turns out to correspond to the "Explanation/Understanding" contrast in the Human Sciences, and is seen to permeate through the various distinct levels from "school classrooms", through "Psychology as a Human Science", to the "Philosophy of the Human Sciences". Some explication of two-way implications among these various levels has been attempted.

This essay is an attempt to explicate the meanings of a Japanese master teacher's questioning practices by examining his published teaching records. In Japan, there is a historically long tradition among teachers to keep descriptive records of their own teaching practices and to publish and exchange them just the same way as, for instance, clinical psychological therapists have been doing for years. I, the author of this chapter, was trained as an educational psychologist. I have wished to contribute three things, occurring simultaneously, to the creation of an authentic educational psychology: (1) grasping the rich concrete living human psychology, (2) obtaining the powerful insights to help teachers in their educational efforts, and (3) achieving a systematic rigorous psychological science. However, after I got involved with the activities of the expert practicing teachers in 1971, I had to experience a series of serious disillusionments with my own discipline for its remoteness from real life and for its powerlessness in helping teachers' efforts. In short, I found that "I am not to teach teachers, but to learn from them". Thus, I began to search for a better way.

In 1977, I encountered Amedeo Giorgi's *Psychology as a Human Science* (1970). Three years later, I found myself studying for a year (1980-81) at Duquesne

University, in Pittsburgh, as a Fulbright visiting scholar. I became acquainted with the Duquesne school of phenomenological psychology. Ermarth's book (1978) was the text of one of Giorgi's graduate classes. Some difficulties of communicating "phenomenological thought" mentioned by Giorgi (1985, p. 23) are: (1) its intrinsic difficulty, (2) Husserl's work as still evolving and changing, and (3) among Husserl's followers, there are as many "deviants" as "true followers". After 30 years since 1977 when I first read Giorgi's book (1970), I now feel myself to be among the "deviants" and not to have yet fulfilled my three wishes above, particularly the third wish. I have become increasingly aware that I am more strongly oriented toward my first and second wishes, which I have been slowly but steadily fulfilling, at least partially. My intended readers in Japan are more among practicing teachers than among those mainstream academic psychologists who are self-satisfied with, and proud of, their own discipline as an established "objective science". I am situated in my life history, as everyone is.

For me that "situatedness" is in the Japanese history, culture and society. Accordingly, this essay is born in, and emerges from, these same Japanese situations, which, I believe I know, would be quite different from those of my colleague friends in the United States and elsewhere in the world. My lived situations have already been published (Yoshida, 2001). However, quite recently, it happens that I was invited to give an academic address at the Plenary Meeting of the Japanese Association of Qualitative Psychology on November 30th, 2008. This may be a significant sign of the changing situations in Japan.

On the Central Importance of Questioning and Questions in Teaching-Learning

"Man is a questioning being" (Bollnow, 1978, p. 181; Straus, 1966, p. 166). From this perspective, human knowledge, being composed of sentences, will be the system of answers that have historically been attempted and claimed as true in response to questions once raised. And, "the meaning of a sentence is relative to the question to which it is a reply, i.e., [also] it necessarily goes beyond what is said in it. The logic of the human sciences is [...] a logic of the question" (Gadamer, 1975, p. 333). Teaching a system of knowledge would be a process of helping every learner acquire a system of answers-with-questions and the ability to ask questions and find answers on his/her own, far more than the mere transmission of a fixed knowledge system as "the mere recreation of someone else's meaning" (Gadamer, *ibid*, p. 338). When learners learn from a teacher, they initially learn knowledge as answers. Then they learn what questions to ask, how to ask them, and how to find the answers. They will learn to ask questions and to find answers on their own, and, they will learn even to discover possible and/or probable questions to the given "texts", as they perceive the "texts" as attempted answers to the questions. Thus, true teaching-learning is expected to help learners liberate themselves to become autonomous learners being able to ask their own vital questions. A Japanese master teacher Tsuneo Takeda (1929-1986) went so far as to say "To teach is to question" (Takeda, 1990/1971, p. 134) and "To teach is not to teach" (*ibid*, p. 43), emphasizing the importance of the development of the autonomy in learners, even in elementary school children. For instance, when the teaching-learning a literary work of art is successful, the horizon of each learner will be fused in an expanded and enriched way with the horizons of the teacher and other learners, of the characters in the work of art, and/or of the artists (Gadamer, *ibid*, p. 337). Questions and questioning are vitally important in the psychology of teaching-learning. In addition, the psychology of teaching-learning and the teaching-learning of psychology mutually include each other.

Some Teaching Records on Questioning: Cases by Tsuneo Takeda (1929-1986)

The Japanese master teacher Tsuneo Takeda has left us many of his teaching records published in Japan. The following descriptive records are on cases of his teaching experiences in an elementary school. [Note: Takeda's original is written in Japanese and the translation into English is by Yoshida.] Let me invite you into the Takeda's lived-world of the elementary school classrooms sometime during the period of 1950-1975. This lived-world is now going to be made available in the narrative form to the English world.

CASE 1) TEACHING RECORD ON "SEIBEI AND THE GOURDS" (Takeda, 1973)

The class was the 5th grade, and the work of art being taught was the novelette "*Seibei and the Gourds*" (Shiga, 1968), a masterpiece by the Japanese Novelist Naoya Shiga (1883-1971).

Record: In the earlier part of the novelette, there is described an extraordinary fascination that a boy, called Seibei, has with his collection of artistic gourds. One day, when walking on the street, he mistook an old man's baldhead to be a gourd and became deeply impressed with it as a splendid one. When he became aware of his own mistake, he felt it so funny that he burst into laughter, started running and ran for half a block or so, but "he could not stop still laughing".

I [Takeda] thought this example was a good one to study in class.

Why did Seibei start running, I cannot know for sure. Perhaps, he still could not stop laughing at the wildness of his own misperception and could not bear the feeling and started running. Or, it may have been a behavior motivated by the unconscious wish to remove himself as soon as possible from the place where he committed such an absurd, wild and funny mistake of which he was so much ashamed – even though no one witnessed his mistake. However many such inferences we may give, we would still not be able to reach any decisive conclusion whatsoever. It may be so, but it may not be so. The important point here would not be the reason why he started running but the content of Seibei's funny feeling in which he could not but start running, so I thought.

Thus, I asked squarely the straightforward question: "*Why did Seibei laugh?*" in the seventh hour since my class began studying the novelette. "*Because it was funny.*" children answered. Such a natural answer that sounded almost foolish. "*Why was it funny?*" "*Because he mistook the baldhead to be a gourd.*"

I got stuck. My questions and the children's answers were both amazingly simple and clear. And yet, if I ask myself whether there were any elements in our exchange that stimulated the children's thinking or imagination, I have to admit that there were no such elements at all.

I did not pick up this spot intending to make such an idle exchange. What I intended was to look into the inner life of Seibei, together with my children. The inner life of Seibei is his extraordinary fascination with artistic gourds, which is depicted behind this little episode, and his seemingly abnormal behaviors in which his fascination sometimes finds its expressions.

The old man's splendid baldhead is not the cause of Seibei's laughter. Of course, it cannot be said to be totally irrelevant. However, what attracted Seibei so strongly was the intensity of his own fascination with gourds, that led him to make the mistake and to get so deeply impressed, and also the intolerable funniness of his own state of being less than normal, to say the least. Nevertheless, there is here none of the abnormal dark shadow, which is commonly observed with an engrossed monomania. Seibei's fascination is bright and healthy through and through, always filled with the *naïveté* of a young boy.

Seibei must have thought that something was a little wrong with him to have mistaken the baldhead for a gourd, but also that the old man's baldhead, nevertheless, was a splendid one. Both of these thoughts grew into such an intolerable funniness that they made him burst into bright loud laughter. I wished to help children read the inner image of Seibei: his almost abnormal fascination with the gourds, which is at the same time always filled with bright healthiness...

In teaching a literary work of art, it is one thing to grasp clearly the passage that should be considered as specially important, and it is quite another to present, as a concrete problem to children, the same incident in the same form as it is originally given. The core of the teaching material is not the core of the development in teaching.

The next day, I raised my questions on the same spot.

"Seibei ran half a block or so and eventually stopped running. And yet he could not stop laughing. He must have been so amused. However, at some point, his laughing must have calmed down. There must have been a time when he stopped laughing. What on earth did Seibei think at that moment?"

This time, children did not answer so immediately…

- *"Something must be wrong with me, he thought."*
- *"He felt his face a little abashed, thinking that he is a little too much fascinated with gourds, even if he loves them so much."*
- *"I think that Seibei began laughing because the way the old man's baldhead went into the side-street was so funny. And, when he stopped laughing, I also think, he thought himself to be a little abnormal, of course. Yet, the funny feeling of the baldhead remains still. I would say there were both of these feelings."*
- *"When Seibei calmed down, I would think, Seibei was reflecting upon everything from the moment of discovering the baldhead to the moment of stopping after the running. And, he must have thought more about the abnormality of his own fascination with gourds than about the funniness of the baldhead."*

The responses of children in this session were so different from the preceding one. It was because children's thinking and imagination are dependent upon the content of the problems the teacher raises, the sharpness of the angles of the questions and the clarity of the images behind them (Takeda, 1973: extracted from pp. 183-190).

Why-Question (Why-qn) and What-Question (What-qn)

This author would like to request you, my respectable reader, to re-read carefully the extracted but detailed record above to get the sense of the atmosphere and the implicit meanings of the exchanges between the teacher and the learners, Takeda and his children, and also to consider it all for itself.

Described implicitly in the record are two different ways of understanding, i.e. clarifying, to oneself and/or to others, the meanings of some other person's (in this case Seibei's) act/behavior and experience. Simply put, these two ways can be formulated as corresponding to the two distinct ways of asking questions. "Why-question", e.g. "*Why did Seibei laugh*?" or, "*Why was it funny*?" on the one hand, and "What-question", e.g. "*What on earth did Seibei think at that moment?*" on the other. Hereafter, let us denote, to save the space, "Why-question" as "Why-qn" and "What-question" as "What-qn", respectively.

Granted, this differentiation is certainly rather a simplistic one, based only upon the superficial difference of the linguistic expressions of the questions, nevertheless it is still a good start for our further explication. Still staying with the linguistic expression, let me formulate the contrast between the two ways of asking questions as follows. "Why-qn" typically asks "Why did this person do this?", whereas "What-qn" asks "What did this person perceive/feel/think when he did this?" Thus simply formulated, the author has discovered over time that, whether implicitly or explicitly, this contrast between the two appeared repeatedly in the other cases of teaching records, such as the following by Takeda. Let me sketchily review a few of such other cases.

CASE 2) TEACHING RECORD ON "A GIRL WHO BECAME MUTE" (1964, pp. 45-73)

Takeda asked his children: "*Why did Morii become mute?*" Morii is the name of a girl whose father was executed by the feudal landlord because of her own careless disclosure of the father's theft, a theft done in order to feed her while ill in bed. After knowing the particulars of her father's death, she abruptly became mute. Against Takeda's expectation, the above question failed in the class, to bring about, in his own comment, "even a piece of satisfaction after the fighting [of ideas among the teacher and the children in the classroom teaching-learning]" (*ibid*, p. 73).

CASE 3) TEACHING RECORD ON "THE FATHER OF THE SALT PANS" (1964, pp. 112-116)

Takeda asked: "*Why did he [the father] think so?*" which again failed. Takeda himself gave a severely critical comment on that particular teaching of his own as being "the worst one" (*ibid*, p. 114).

CASE 4) TEACHING RECORD ON "RUN, MELOS!" (1964, pp.117-177)

This record is, in my judgment, the most remarkable one, in which Takeda worked so hard as to prepare a series of well-thought-out and tightly related twenty-five questions aimed at leading and guiding children into re-living of the lived-worlds of the characters of the novel, by means of explicating the implicit meanings of the text of only about a page's length. These questions were prepared to invite and help children to focus on the details of the lived-worlds of Melos, and of Philostratus, the main two characters being presented in the page. Among the typical What-qns asked were, for example: "*[While waiting for*

Melos], what was Philostratus looking at?" / "*What was the feeling of Philostratus, a minute or a second before Melos showed up?*" / "*While waiting for Melos, what was Philostratus thinking?*" Please, notice that these variants of the question are based upon "perceive/feel/think". Another What-qn: "*While thinking of his friend [who was almost going to be executed as his hostage] being mocked and taunted [by the tyrannical King Dionysius] in front of the crowd, what kind of thoughts did occur to Melos's mind?*" In addition, Takeda included in the series of the 25 questions the only one Why-qn: "*Why did Philostratus say only "Ah, Mr. Melos" [and no further]?*"

After reading these teaching records in the original, the first question that a reader would ask may be: "Why does such a great difference come about between the children's responses to the two kinds of questions by the teacher?" Or, "What is the cause of the great difference in their answers?" A simple answer to the question might be: "Because, the questions were different." Then, the reader might ask further, "Why children's responses differ so much while these two questions seem to differ so little?" A simple answer could be: "Because, even the naive children sincerely attempted to answer in response to different questions." Or one might respond, "If possible, why don't you ask the children the reason-why of their different answers?" These imaginary exchanges, this author hopes, will remind us of the following paragraph by Takeda in the teaching record given above of Case #1: "I got stuck. My questions and children's answers were both amazingly simple and clear. And yet, if I ask myself whether there were any elements in our exchange that stimulated children's [the readers' and this author's, at this time] thinking or imagination, I have to admit that there were no such elements at all. I did not pick up this spot intending to make such an idle exchange." Similarly, this author did not pick up this teaching record while intending to make such an idle exchange above. Our idle exchange started with a Why-qn. What happens if we shift to ask a "What-qn", instead of the "Why-qn", in the similar manner to Takeda's shift in Case #1? What-qns in our situation could be, for example: "What did children perceive/feel/think, when asked a "What-question"?" More specifically, "What did the children, not Seibei, imagine, when and if asked: "*When he stopped laughing, what on earth did Seibel think at that moment?*"

Allow me to propose to use hereafter, the coinage of word *perfink* by J. S. Bruner (1998/1986, at the end of chap. 4) to represent the simultaneity of "perceive, feel, and think". Indeed, the new term *perfink* could properly be represented by the traditional term "experience", but the *perfink* preferably enables us to remain watchful of the analyzability, the simultaneity and the wholeness of "perceive/feel/think". Here, I would venture to be so wild as to include as many variations as possible: such as, naturally, "see", "hear", "taste", "smell", "touch", but even "imagine", "remember seeing", "anticipate hearing" and so on. *Perfink* is supposed to be a short-hand to help ourselves remain free-imaginatively varying a specific concrete *perfink* experience.

Comparison Between Why-qn and What-qn

Now, let us begin to make comparisons between the "Why-qn" and "What-qn", by means of explicating the actualities and the possibilities of what children would *perfink*, when they were asked either Why-qn or What-qn. Please, notice that the following comparison is performed by asking the author himself not Why-qns but What-qns regarding the possible experiential lived-worlds of the children, in the situation when and where they are possibly asked either of the questions.

(1) *Specification of Time and Space (Why-qn is without, What-qn is with)*:

Regarding the time and the space, Why-qn can be asked without concretely specifying the particulars; e.g., "*Why did Seibei laugh?*" which does sufficiently make sense to ask, and the children can answer the question accordingly: e.g. "*Because it was funny.*" Given a description of a behavior/experience, a Why-qn can be asked, without further adding the specification of time and space. Indeed, you could add, if you wish, "when" to a Why-qn, for instance, "*Why did he laugh, when he laughed?*" which, however, would not at all help us in answering the Why-qn. On the other hand, a What-qn tends to invite, even to force, children to think more concretely by imagining within the specified particular time and space. To the What-qn "*When he stopped laughing, what on earth did Seibel think at that moment?*" with the specification "at that moment", the children must answer the question accordingly. If the teacher were to ask a What-qn, without specifying the situation, e.g., ""*What on earth did Seibel think?*" the children, even not knowing the reason why, would find it difficult to answer the question, unless they assume, even on their own, some particular time-space situation. From this observation, a little insight is obtained that a What-qn invites children to think specifically as to time and space, while a Why-qn does not necessarily do so. Casey (2000/1976), while explicating the "Imagining as Intentional", presented a classification of imagining in two ways; i.e. in (1) "Act Phase", "sensory and nonsensory", and in (2) "Object Phase", "single object or event", "state of affairs *simpliciter*" and "state of affairs involving the imaginer (or surrogate) as agent"(*ibid*, p. 48). In addition, he points out, as the "nonthematically present" and "non-nuclear components of imagined content", what he calls a "world-frame" (*ibid*, p. 50). He writes that specific "*imagined space* and *imagined time*" are derived from "the spatializing and temporalizing powers of world-frames" (*ibid*, p. 51). In these terms, we may say, a What-qn invites children to imagine among the three kinds of "Object" along with a "world-frame", which necessarily and non-thematically makes space and time present.

(2) *Forced and Imposed Ways of Thinking (More vs. Less)*:

A Why-qn tends to force some ways of *perfink-ing*, somewhat a presumed "frame of reference" or a "type", upon the children, while a What-qn does not necessarily do so. The word "Why" tends to invite children forcefully to think in terms of (a) "because motives"; e.g., "*Because he felt so funny*", or (b) "in-order-to motives" (Schutz, A. & Luckmann, T., 1973/1975), e.g., "*In order to escape from the pressure*", or (c) causality; i.e., in terms of "cause and effect", e.g., "*Because the baldhead caused him to laugh*". On the other hand, a What-qn can be asked and answered without assuming any such presumed patterned ways, or types, of *perfinking*. For the question "*What was Philostratus looking at?*", for instance, the children can simply answer what Philostratus, based upon their own imaginative reading of the story, must have been looking at. Nothing more is necessary. The readers, who have been absorbed in reading the story, naturally even implicitly imaginatively re-experiencing the "inner life history" of the character, would have no other way than to imagine that, in the given situation, s/he must be looking at what must have been so meaningful and significant for her/him as almost impossible not to look at. They were, for Philostratus, the sun while the sunset shall be the time of execution of his master, and the direction from which Melos will be coming to rescue his master detained as a hostage. In short, a What-qn would tend to invite children to imagine, far more than a Why-qn would, freely and concretely the particulars of the character's *perfink*, consequently of the character's lived-world.

(3) *The Invited Perspectives (Others' vs. the Person's)*:

A Why-qn would tend to leave children free to take a perspective *other* than the perspective of the person in question. For instance, "*Why did Seibei laugh?*" would tend to invite children take the perspective external to Seibei himself, the perspective of a person other than Seibei, the other person being somebody who may perhaps be expected further to explain to somebody else the reason why Seibei laughed. This expected explanation will be made by appealing to some common sense "type", shared among people – in other terms, structure, pattern, constraint, regularity, principle, rule, law, and what not – regarding Seibei's, and also regarding some other common people's acts and experiences. Such an implicit *naïve* primitive "type" regarding laughter might be: "*People laugh, when funny*" or "*People laugh, because funny*". As Husserl points out, "The factual world of experience is experienced as a typified world" (Husserl, 1973, p. 331). In contrast, a What-qn would tend to invite children to take the internal perspective of the person in question. For instance, "*When he stopped laughing, what on earth did Seibel think at that moment?*" would tend to invite children to take anew the perspective of Seibei himself. With respect to a conceivable question for Case #2, for example, "*What did Morii perfink, when she was severely beaten up by the landlord's wife, who mockingly accused Morii of her naïve but careless disclosure of the secret of her father's theft which had led to his execution?*', children would also tend to take the perspective of Morii herself. In responding to a What-qn, children would attempt to put themselves, in their imagination, into the perspective, or into the lived-world, of the person/character, e.g., Morii, in this situation, so as to *perfink* imaginatively in the way the person would. However, if they can imagine the situation for the person vividly enough, no need would be felt to depend on such an external "type" as "People cry, when sad". In sum, a Why-qn would invite one to an *external* perspective, whereas a What-qn would invite one to an *internal* one.

Incidentally, a movie, we may notice, would depict a person multi-perspectively: as the "I" and/or an "I" among many "I's", as a "you" in relations to some other "I", as "s/he", as a person among "they", even as an "it" among objects. Furthermore, a movie might depict "*What Seibei, Melos, or Morii, would have seen*" In this sense, the movie directors have already actualized, perhaps prior to the majority of psychologists, the collaboration of the external and the internal perspectives, which are associated with Why-qns and What-qns respectively.

Let me quickly mention that an "immanent critique", a critique with empathetic understanding, would become possible only through the activation of the internal perspective.

(4) *The Range of Exploration (Limitedly Focused vs. Openly Liberated)*:

A Why-qn tends to limit the range of children's exploration of the meanings of the behavior/experience within those corresponding to the way of thinking, "type", which the Why-qn tends to force upon. These "types" are, for instance, because-motive, in-order-motive, and/or causality. This limitation will correspond to what children would implicitly assume to be what is expected of them in their response to a Why-qn. This feeling, felt by the children, of the expectation on the part of the person who asks the Why-qn, e.g., the teacher, seems to be evident. In contrast, a What-qn tends to impose no such limit upon children's imagination, and even more, tends to liberate them to allow them to explore freely the lived-world of the person in question. Children could freely imagine whatever could present itself, in their imagination, in the imagined lived-world of the person. Children would feel far more freedom and far less restriction as to the range of imagining, so long as staying within the perspective of the fictive person.

To summarize the points made in (1), (2), (3) and (4) so far, a Why-qn looks, on the surface, as if it were to leave children freely to respond, but implicitly it forces upon children a frame of thinking, "type", to respond according to the implicitly assumed expectation of the teacher. For example, expectation might be to take the external perspective and to use the "types" such as the causality. On the other hand, a What-qn looks, on the surface, as if the scope of perspective were limited and imposed upon, from the very start, by the teacher. However, so long as staying within that imposed limited scope, children are left free to imagine the unknown of the lived-world of the person in question, e.g., the lived-world of Seibei in the given context of the story. One might even be tempted to say that children's *noema* and *noesis* are more focused and limited with a Why-qn than with a What-qn, even though on the level of the linguistic expressions, it looks like as if the opposite would be case.

One might imagine a situation where, at a police station meeting, detectives are exchanging views and insights regarding a suspect's suspicious act: "*Why did s/he do that?*" (Why-qn) vs "*What did s/he see, or even smell, (i.e. perfink) when s/he did that?*" (What-qn). The views and insights encouraged by each question would greatly differ in the similar manner to our Seibei's Case #1. Please notice that Sherlock Holmes asks What-qns more frequently than Why-qns.

(5) *Disclosure and Strengthening of the Children's Pre-Existing Explanatory Repertoire vs. Disclosure and Development of the Lived World of Children*:

A Why-qn serves to disclose and reveal, when children succeed to offer their own answers to the Why-qn, their pre-existing repertoire of "because". The experiences of successful answers to Why-qns would strengthen the confidence in, and also the tendency for, using the particularly successful repertoire, even after the particular exchange is over. On the other hand, a What-qn would serve to disclose the lived-world of children. While imagining the lived-world of the character, e.g., Seibei, the children would attempt to put themselves in the place and the perspective of Seibei in the context, but, needless to say, the lived-world they can possibly imagine would most probably be limited by their own actual lived-world. Children sometimes would imagine themselves to be the hero of a story, for instance, as if the children in reality were suddenly transferred into the world of the story, while remaining just as they are along with their everyday taken-for-grantedness. A child might think, "*If I were Seibei, I would think and do this way or that*", however, what s/he thinks in this manner would reveal just the way s/he now lives his/her everyday real life, but not at all the way Seibei would live Seibei's own life in the story. In psychological jargons, one might say that the child makes a "projection" upon Seibei. The child, in other words, would take Seibei only as "an analogue of something included in my peculiar ownness", or "an "intentional modification" of myself" (Husserl, 1977, p. 115). On the other hand, some children could sometimes get into the world of the story, and be so deeply involved as to re-experience or re-live the life of the character, Seibei, so as to experience the human situation confronting Seibei in the story. In such a case, children experience what they could not possibly experience in their own everyday real life. One of the important meanings of the teaching literary works of art, I believe, is to offer the possible opportunity for children to imaginatively experience such a life of others, e.g., of Seibei, and, more generally, to experience and live vicariously the lives of others different from their own. This vicarious living-experience will enrich the lived worlds of children, by allowing them to explore to discover the unexpected unknown lived meanings of the things, persons, self and the world, so different from their own. At this point, allow me to make a little digression.

The Meanings of Teaching-Learning the Fictive Stories for Children

We could ask either a Why-qn "Why are fictive stories to be taught to children?" or a What-qn "What do children possibly perfink, when fictive stories are being taught?" Max van Manen (1990, p. 70) enumerated the significance of story for human science as follows: (1) the story provides us with *possible human experiences*; (2) the story enables us to experience life situations, feelings, emotions, and events *that we would not normally experience*; (3) the story allows us to broaden the horizons of our normal existential landscape by creating *possible worlds*; (4) the story tends to appeal to us and involve us *in a personal way*; (5) the story is an artistic device that lets us turn back to *life as lived*, whether fictional or real; (6) the story evokes the quality of vividness in *detailing unique and particular aspects of a life* that could be my life or your life; (7) and yet, great novels or stories *transcend the particularity of their plots* and protagonists, etc., which makes them subject to thematic analysis and criticism. These points offered by Manen for human science would hold, strangely and surprisingly enough, also with the significance of stories for education of adults as well as children. In the same vein, some other valuable views are also expressed.

The Japanese novelist Kenzaburo Ooe (1935-) emphasized the "de-familiarization/ estrangement" which destroys "automatization" by means of "persistent negation": i.e. by the negation "No, the reality is not such as that, but it is such as this" (1978, p. 9). Kanji Hatano (1905-2001), my mentor, taught that the values of teaching the first class literature would consist in: to let the learners: (1) understand the complexity of human nature and human acts; (2) understand the struggles among values and valuing; (3) understand the tragedy; and (4) understand the beauty and the deep meaning in the ordinary and the common – the reversal of values, e.g., discover the beauty in what is commonly considered ugly. Takehiko Saigo (1920-), my respectable friend, asserts that "[...] only fiction enables us to grasp the deep meanings of life" (1991/1971, p. 154). Fiction offers, in his view, "World and I" that are seen through the integration of "one's own ordinary everyday realistic subjective eyes, on the one hand, and the other eyes of different quality, of extraordinary eyes of the other and of the third person, on the other". "It is the very conflict, being made possible by the richness of imagination, between one's own eyes and the other's eyes that reveals the deep meanings of World and I" (*ibid*, p. 154). All in all, the What-qn seems to play a key role for children by opening up fictive or possible worlds, the possible worlds offered through the eyes of the characters in fictions, stories, novels and poems. Now, let us return to our next comparison (6), taking henceforth into consideration the discussion above on the meanings of teaching-learning literary works of art.

Comparison Between Why-qn and What-qn: Resumed and Continued

(6) *Seen From the Questioning Side (the Side of the Teacher), the Degree of Possibility for Generating the Variations of the Questions Differs (Relatively Closed and Limited vs. Widely Open and Far Less Limited)*:

Corresponding to the characteristics of the Why-qn given in (4) and (5) above, the possibility for generating the variations of a Why-qn is relatively closed and limited. This is because the limitation upon the range of possibly acceptable answers proper to a Why-qn retroacts to limit the range of possible questions. This becomes even more evident when we consider the widely open unlimited possibility of variations of the What-qn. The What-qn could be varied at least according to a variety of dimensions, for instance: (1) the time, e.g., "*at that moment*", "*when Morii heard this*" and so on, choosing "any moment" at will from all the possible temporal points of the story, and even before or after, or beyond, the story; (2) the space, choosing "any place" at will, even imaginary, from all the scenes in the story; (3) the *perfink* in the What-qn questions could be varied from "perceive/feel/think" to the whole range of experiences including such as taste and smell etc.; recall, retrospect, anticipate, predict, present to, etc.; imagine, fancy, dream, etc.; and so on. What-qn can be asked, while remaining faithfull to the possible or potential experiences of the characters, far beyond the givens in the story. One reason for this would be that the What-qns, in their nature, are to help one to concretize the story's multiple "places of indeterminacy" (Ingarden, 1973, pp. 50-55).

(7) *Power of Guiding Children Into the Worlds of the Fictive Characters (Strong vs. Weak)*:

In the same vein, with a What-qn, a teacher can guide children into the "lived worlds" of the characters of a story, far more effectively than with a Why-qn.

(8) *Seen From the Answering Side, the Degree of the Strength of the Assumption Being Made by Children that the Teacher Knows the Correct Answer (Strong vs. Weak)*:

The tendency of a Why-qn to let children assume the correct answer to be known to the teacher would be stronger, than the tendency of a What-qn.

A What-qn would allow children to explore the possibilities that are assumed, by the children, to be unknown even to the teacher. In the classroom teaching, children would generally tend to assume that, when the teacher asks them a question, s/he already knows some correct answer. This is because "the schoolmaster's question" is, usually in most classrooms, perceived as "a question asked of someone who doesn't know by some one who does" (Merleau-Ponty, 1964, p. 167). The teacher must have the answer, because s/he must have already and thoroughly studied before asking the question in the class, so children would assume with a Why-qn. However, with a What-qn, while seeking to answer it themselves, the children would even implicitly become aware that (2), (3), (4), (5) are the case, and, while listening to other children's openly liberated answers, they will be encouraged to explore the answer on their own, gradually liberated from the original strong concern to guess what the teacher's supposed, therefore expected, "correct" answer will be.

(9) *The Degree of the Danger that the Quality Level of Children Would Unavoidably Decide the Quality of the Exchanges Between the Teacher and Children (Great vs. small)*:

In Case #4 on "*Run Melos!*", regarding the Why-qn "*Why did he groan?*", Takeda wrote, "This kind of question contains the danger of resulting either in stereotype answers or in answers of deepened understanding. The result, however, is entirely left to and depends upon how children interpret the question"(Takeda, 1964, p. 128). Thus, Takeda called a Why-qn as a "vacant question" through which the teacher leans exclusively and also too much upon the goodness of the children, with the easy expectation that his "good" children would probably interpret for the better. Implicit within these comments is Takeda's expressed belief that teaching is a lonely activity in which the teacher should not allow himself or herself to be spoiled in leaning upon the goodness of the children.

(10) *The Atmosphere of the Exchanges (Dialogue vs. Monologue)*:

A Why-qn initiates a dialogue, at least on the surface, at the time when the teacher asks "Why", and the children answer "Because" in response. On the other hand, a What-qn sounds as if it invites a monologue in each of the children, when, in response to the teacher's "What", each child begins to ask and imagine, on his/her own. However, in the case of a Why-qn, the exchange would tend to be closed, in principle, with the supposedly "correct" response from a child and with the approval given by the teacher. On the other hand, the exchange would rather open up, in the case of a What-qn, a series of indeed seemingly monological responses expressing what each child *perfink*, e.g., "I would think [...]", while placing himself in the perspective of the person in question, e.g., Seibei, Morii, or Melos. In this case, what looks like a monologue by a child, in fact, invites other children and the teacher, listening to the monologue, to share the image expressed in it. The teacher will enjoy encountering unexpectedly surprising responses from each of the children, because every child unknowingly lives in different lived-worlds and will tend to generate different images out from each of those different worlds, certainly different from the world of the teacher himself or herself. If the sharing of the variety of the images, in this way, were actualized in the class, then, the seemingly "monological" exchanges in the class initiated by a What-qn would become authentically "dialogical", whereas those initiated with a Why-qn might better be characterized as closed as "semi-monological" in its essence, since, in the seemingly "dialogical" superficial exchanges, both parties do nothing more than just to apply and confirm the pre-patterned presumed way, the preconceived "type", of thinking, and nothing really new emerges from there.

(11) *The Imaginative Presence to the Scene of the Generation (The Generation of Explanation and Understanding)*:

When and if we ask "What do children *perfink*, when they are asked either a Why-qn or a What-qn, and when they succeed answering each of them?", then we are unwittingly and imaginatively brought to the scene of the generation of "explanation" and "understanding", even though perhaps in the simplest primitive forms. This is not the place to prove the statement above, which will need a vast bulk of discussions, but the place just to point out the essential meanings of what is happening in the classroom. The children's answers to either of a Why-qn or a What-qn are the simplest prototypes, so to speak, of "Explanation" or "Understanding", which will turn out to be a great issue and debate in the human sciences, (see Apel, 1984; Strasser, 1985). The comparison between a Why-qn and a What-qn, as the horizons open up, could continue infinitely in principle without any visible terminus at this moment. However, let us stop here just for convenience sake.

Continuity and Discontinuity Between the Why-qn and the What-qn

What about the transition from the Why-qn to the What-qn? And from the What-qn to the Why-qn? What do children come to *perfink*, when they begin to ask What-qns, on their own, even when a Why-qn is asked by the teacher? I now present some thoughts regarding the generation and development of the classroom culture.

In Case #1, a Why-qn preceded a What-qn, and the order was chosen by the teacher. However, the teacher could have reasonably chosen a What-qn prior to a Why-qn. In such a case, for instance, the teacher could have asked a Why-qn such as : "*Knowing so much about what Seibei would have thought after he stopped laughing, could we now say something about why he laughed*?" or simply,

"*Now, let me ask, why did Seibei laugh?*" In other words, the sequence between a Why-qn and a What-qn would not at all be absolutely fixed. Moreover, with the classroom history of teaching-learning, both the teacher and the children would also experience and learn both the sequence of "Why-qn then What-qn" and the reverse. Children are usually quick to learn this, it is said, and sometimes they go even so far as to anticipate the teacher's forthcoming questioning. At such a stage, the meanings of both the Why-qn and the What-qn will change accordingly. When What-qn then Why-qn, the Why-qn will become a question urging children to summarize, in relatively abstract terms, the whole series of explicative answers in response to the preceding What-qns. However, when Why-qn then What-qns, in the way described in the teaching record of Case #1, the Why-qn given at the beginning possibly plays the role of urging children the series of explications, but sometimes end up as a "vacant question", as Takeda characterized it, because it obviously can never summarize the non-existent preceding explications. At this point, the situation reminds us of the well-known dictum of F. Hegel: "[…] just as a proverb in the mouth of a youth who understands it quite accurately, yet fails of the significance and scope which it has in the mind of a man of years and experience, for whom it expresses the full force of its content" (Hegel, 1929/1812, p. 69). Here emerges the possibility of continuity between the Why-qn and the What-qn, beyond their usually presumed and admitted discontinuity. This is seen quite simply, if we think of the generation and the development of a so-called "classroom culture", possibly "Empirico-typical generality" in later Husserl's term (Husserl, 1973, pp. 331-334), or "Objective Mind" in Dilthey's term (Ermarth, 1978, pp. 278-291), which will be explained in a moment.

First, as Case #1 has shown, the children's responses to a Why-qn and a What-qn will tend to differ. However, there could be a situation in which the responses would possibly merge. Suppose, for instance, that the teaching such as in Case #1 has been experienced and shared by both the teacher and the children in a class. Now, suppose further that the meanings of these experiences of teaching-learning are explicated in details and the explication is also shared by all the members, and also that the experiences are named adequately, e.g., P, Q, R, and so on, just for the purpose of further reference to the coming classes. Now, suppose again that, in the same class with the same members, the similar interpretive problems arises for the second time on a new character in another story and, also that the teacher asked a Why-qn regarding a crying or a weeping, this time not a laughing, of the character. Then, children might answer, "*Because P, Q, R, and so on*", which is to be taken as referring back to the explicative experiences shared in the past class. Then, even though the question turned out to look as if a "vacant question", what the members would *perfink* with P, Q, R, and so on, are in fact referring back to the former experiences and the terms P, Q, R, etc., are taken *not* as fixed application of some pre-formed presumed rigid "type" of stereotypical thinking prior to the shared teaching experiences. They are now taken as the abbreviations, as the shorthands, of the "reactivation" of the shared detailed explicative experiences in the previous classroom teachings. The results would be that every member of the class will vividly re-experience the shared explications in response to the question and the terms P, Q, R. In such a situation, the exchanges based upon a Why-qn between the teacher and the children would approach the possible exchanges when the What-qns are actually asked in the similar manner as in the former class, e.g. such as described in our Case #1. Here, we might recall the points made by Husserl in his "Origin of Geometry": "There is a distinction between passively understanding the expression and making it self-evident by *reactivating* its meaning" (Husserl, 1970/1954, p. 361, italics mine). In the exchanges based upon a Why-qn between the teacher and the children, which would have originally been "passively understanding the expression" would then be transformed into "making it self-evident by *reactivating* its meaning". The reactivating then would be the reactivation of the expression "*Because it is funny*", when "funny" in the Seibei' lived world had already been explicated in details and named, e.g., "*Funny as Seibei perfinked*", as summarizing the whole series of the explications of the Seibei's world in response to such What-qns as "*What did Seibei perfink, when [...]?*" with sufficient kinds of variations of "*when [...]*".

Second, after experiencing the type of teaching-learning in the classes, well-educated children would come to be able to ask adequately explicative What-qns, on their own, even when the teacher asks only a blunt Why-qn, which, if asked earlier, would have remained a "vacant question". Such a change can be regarded as the betterment of the "quality of children", in Takeda's terms, and be viewed as the objective that the classroom teaching should aim at.

Third, suppose that, after the new situation has been established, a newcomer, a transfer pupil from some other school, joined the class. Naturally, the newcomer will be ignorant of the already experienced typical teaching-learning of the class. The teacher asks a blunt Why-qn in the class, the children, in response to the Why-qn, except the newcomer, may begin to ask and think about many What-qns. The newcomer would observe, in his or her wonder, what is going on in the class. After a while, the newcomer will become able to understand the way other pupils *perfink* and to begin to *perfink* in the same manner. At that moment, the "typification" has successfully been transmitted to and assimilated by the newcomer, and the "classroom culture" has been maintained as "lasting", at least partially, as "objective mind". According to Ermarth (1978, p. 277), "objective mind" (*objektiver Geist*), in Dilthey's view, is "a cultural coherence which is contained in its lasting products", "a cultural possession", "a kind of cultural environment or climate" in which the individual is immersed from birth without ever ceasing to try to appropiate it (*ibid*, 278).

Asking Why-qn and What-qn on the behavior/experience of the teacher and the children

We may now notice that we could also ask Why-qn and What-qn regarding the behavior/experience of the teacher and children, very much the same way as the teacher had asked Why-qn and What-qn regarding the behavior/experience of the character of the story, e.g. Seibei, Morii, and/or Melos. In other words, we can proceed to regard the teaching records as stories of essentially the same nature as fictive novels. First, the possibility to ask a Why-qn and a What-qn regarding the persons in the records, e.g. the teacher and the children, cannot be denied. And, in many "scientific" instructional researches on the teaching-learning based on the teaching records, such as Takeda's records, Why-qs are observed too often to have been asked, seeking to discover the so-called "law" of the teaching-learning. What change of perspective could be expected, however, if many What-qns, in combination with the Why-qn, were asked regarding the persons coming onto the stage in the teaching records? For instance, in the Takeda's teaching record Case #1, we could ask such questions as "Why did not Takeda ask the What-qn, immediately after he found that the Why-qn did not work satisfactorily, and why he waited even a whole day to ask the What-qn?" You could give answers, to this Why-qn question, which may be true but may not be true. The Why-qn could remain a "vacant question". Ask What-qns, if you will, such as "What did the teacher perfink, when he found the children's responses were unsatisfactory to explicate the lived world of Seibei?", or "What did the teacher perfink when he was preparing at home for the next day's class after the failure with the vacant question?" etc. We find that the What-qns could be asked to explicate the lived-worlds of the teacher and the children, just as many and varied as the What-qns for explicating the lived-world of the fictive character Melos. This reminds us of Husserl's dictum: "Pay in small coins!", which would mean in our case, "Describe what is experienced in details, with small concrete lively words but not with big abstract dead words. Do keep to the phenomenological spirit – To the things themselves!"

Some people may understandably express their dissatisfaction with the explications so far. They may say that the explications regarding the Why-qn and the What-qn do not give the necessity of the relationship between the questions and answers, but only the possibility, or the probability at best, which, they may point out, is disclosed in the frequently used expression "tend to". We grant this. Regarding the behavior/experience of other persons, the necessity in such senses as sought by the "rigorous radical behaviorism" is hard to obtain, to say the least, but the possibility/probability based upon understanding is to be sought and obtained. I cannot help but recall the interesting comment on the experiments on human subjects carried out by the method of conditioned reflexes, cited by Leontiev (1961), of Pavlov, the Russian physiologist. The comment was: "But did he (the subject) not wonder what all this was about?" Even Pavlov would agree that the children, in response to the teacher's questions, are going to respond from their own perspectives, in Pavlov's own words, "not like a dog" – in Pavlov's perspective – but as a human being, according to "how he was concerned in the matter" (Leontiev, 1961, p. 245).

Children always have their own existential freedom to choose. [A wise dog – in Konrad Lorenz' perspective, for instance – would also be in this perspective.] In addition, the quality of children will no doubt determine the quality of answers. Ask a baby a What-qn, s/he will mumble, but ask Virginia Wolf, James Joyce or Fyodor Dostoevsky of the same question, s/he might write a book. The ordinary reality sits somewhere in-between.

Besides, "The expression is "creative" because its meaning may exceed the intended meaning of the author: its meaning for us is not identical to its meaning for its originator. *Verstehen* in the human sciences, therefore, entails more than approximating the author's self-understanding of his own actions, intentions, or works" (Ermarth, 1978, p. 280). This is a beautiful statement, and it allows me to rest contented.

In addition, the knowledge of possibilities is as valuable as that of realities, so long as the two are not confused and they are adequately related. Whether or not you would value the knowledge of possibilities would depend upon whether you would be a "realist" with the sense of reality, or a "possibilist" with the sense of possibility, in the terms of Robert Musil (1995/1952, pp. 10-13). We could and should learn from the possibilities as well as the realities, because *we learn at the present from the past for the future.* We might recall the passage on *Bildung* from Gadamer: Bildung is "[…] to keep oneself open to what is other, to other, more universal points of view […]. To distance oneself from oneself and from one' private purposes means to look at these in the way that others see them. […] The universal viewpoints to which the cultivated man (*gebildet*) keeps himself open are not a fixed applicable yardstick, but are present to him only as the viewpoints of possible others" (Gadamer, 1975, pp. 17-18). This idea would lead to the idea of the "Transcendental Subjectivity" treating "Intersubjectivity" as "a transcendental philosophical notion of utmost importance" (Zahavi, 2003, p. 246). Akira Kurosawa's classical film "Rashomon", which depicts the possible multi-perspective views upon a single event, may bring into relief the importance of both possibility and intersubjectivity.

Someone with a strong positivistic orientation might also make an objection; "Seibei and the gourds" is a novel and a fiction, whereas Takeda's record is a documentary record of a fact. He may exclaim that a fiction and a factual record should never be confused. This is granted. However, now that Takeda passed away years ago, how could we know what he had actually and factually thought at the various points of *when* in the records, even if he could have told of them and even if we disregard the complex problems of forgetting, distortion, exaggeration, lying, pretense and/or make-believe. Historical case studies are widely known to have this same problem in common. Fiction and the fact are much the same, from the perspectives of the readers. "What do want to know, to explicate, when we study a fictive story and/or when we study a record of a fact, respectively?" This will lead to an enormous discussion, regarding the relationship between the factual and the fictive, which exceeds the limits of the current discussion. I refer the reader to the philosophies of history, art and human sciences.

Further Steps with Why-qn and What-qn Into the Lived-Worlds of Psychologists, Research Methodologists, Philosophers of History, Art, Science, and...

After re-examining the record many times, we could come to be able to agree that there can be differentiated at least several levels of the psychological events, at each of which we could direct similarly the two kinds of questions: i.e., with respect to the Why-qn and to the What-qn.

Level 1) A teacher and children ask a Why-qn and/or a What-qn, regarding the behaviors/ experiences of the characters, e.g., Seibei, described in the fictive stories being taught in the class.

Level 2) A teacher, e.g., Takeda, and the children could ask a Why-qn and/or a What-qn, regarding the behaviors/experiences of each other: i.e., the teacher and/or children in their actual real co-experienced classroom situations.

Level 3) A researcher, psychological and/or sociological or otherwise, e.g., Yoshida (1992, 2005), could ask a Why-qn and/or a What-qn, regarding the behaviors/experiences, on the Level 1) and/ or Level 2), described in the teaching-learning records by the teacher, e.g., Takeda (1974), or by the children, or even by the participant observers, in their actual real classroom situations.

Level 4) A researcher, in the field of psychological research methodology or otherwise, could ask a Why-qn and/or a What-qn, regarding the behaviors/ experiences of the psychological researchers, on the

Level 3) which are described in the descriptive research reports.

Level 5) A philosophically-oriented researcher, e.g., Strasser (1985) or Apel (1984) – existential, phenomenological, hermeneutical, epistemological, logical, linguistic, or otherwise – could ask a Why-qn and/or a What-qn, regarding the behaviors/ experiences of the researcher(s), on the Level 4), being described in the research reports on research methodology...

In principle, the extension, in a fashion similar to the above, of the multi-layered Levels could be made as far as one likes. However, it is sufficient if the above description establishes that the Why-qn and/or the What-qn can surely be asked on every one of the levels, as long as, on each level, the subject thematizes the behaviors/ experiences of the person(s) on the respectively preceding Level. Needless to add, these questions and answers do not necessarily have to be exchanged by different persons each belonging to the respective level. In a conceivably extreme case, all of them could be asked and answered even by a single person, by a philosopher-novelist teacher like Tolstoy (1828-1910), and, certainly, the intermediate cases would also be possible.

Implications of the Why-qn and What-qn Comparison to the Issue of Explanation/ Understanding in Psychology as a Human Science

The difference between Why-qn and What-qn in teaching literary works of art reminds us of a similar difference between "Explanation/Understanding" in "Psychology as a Natural Science" vs. "Psychology as a Human Science". The issue of Explanation/Understanding has its long history, the extensive elaboration of which would be beyond my capacity here, even beyond such a work as Strasser (1985) or Apel (1984), which has sufficiently demonstrated the existence of multitude of views on the issue (Yoshida, 1992, pp. 42-43).

The Japanese psychopathologist Hiroshi Yasunaga (1929-), for instance, has expressed his dissatisfaction with the Karl Jaspers' classical conception of "Explanation" and "Understanding": (1) the contact point, or the relationship, between Understanding and Explanation is unclear; and (2) how the Understanding as Science should be advanced is unclear. In Yasunaga's view, Jaspers explains that "Explanation has no limit, whereas, in contrast, Understanding has limits everywhere", and that, "when Understanding stumbles upon its own limit, then Explanatory method must be relied upon" (Yasunaga, 1992, p. 28). In this way of saying by Jaspers, comments Yasunaga (*ibid*, 29), "Understanding and Explanation come from entirely unrelated different origins". In contrast, Yasunaga summarizes his own view: "Explanation is a specialized operation derived from within the Understanding in a broader sense", and "The relationship between Understanding and Explanation is a close and inseparable one like the head and tail of a coin, while mutually inter-permeating" (*ibid*, 38). Thus, Yasunaga, adopting and following the Wauchope's view of "Explanation" in the broadest sense, summarizes Wauchope's "Explanation of Explanation" as follows: "When we attempt to explain something, whatever it is, we presuppose some Understanding of "consciousness", along with Understanding of what is supposed to be explained. The Understanding presupposed is, first of all, Understanding within one's own consciousness, and the Explanation aims at the other consciousnesses, which are expected to accept the Explanation, to let the other consciousness understand the Understanding [within one's own consciousness]" (Yasunaga, 1987, p. 18). Wauchope writes "Comprehension is momentary" (Wauchope, 1948, p. 17) and, at the moment of comprehension, the pattern A/B, such as subject/object, quality/quantity, whole/parts, life/death, self/others, is understood. "A pattern is a whole having parts, the parts equalling the whole" (*ibid*, p. 15). In short, the thought on the complementary inseparability of "Understanding and Explanation", just like the head and tail of a coin, is elaborated in details.

The too well known simplistic dictum attributed to Wilhelm Dilthey may be recalled: "We explain nature, we understand mind" (Ermarth, 1978, p. 246). The common criticisms against Dilthey for the rigid separation above between Explanation and Understanding are interpreted by Ermarth as the hasty mis-interpretations based upon too few of Dilthey's published works. He points out the immensely comprehensive view of Dilthey (*ibid*, 245-267). "Life itself – as we live through it – is a constant pattern of interpretive efforts at many different levels" (*ibid*, p. 247). In this sense, the teacher-children exchanges, with Why-qn and What-qn, can be regarded as a prototype of "Explanation and Understanding" in Human Sciences.

Viewed in such a light, the classroom teaching-learning could be considered as an "experimental scene" in a micro-scale and micro-history in the class for the birth and development of "Explanation and Understanding" in the macro-scale and macro-history in Human Sciences. The debate of the issue in Human Sciences, for instance, could be considered as a development of, and as structurally similar to, the teaching-learning experiences in the infinite number of classrooms all over the world in the history of mankind, from the elementary to graduate school levels, and further into the debates among academic scholars, who once were children sometime and somewhere on this globe. "Little brooks make great rivers", at the same time "little brooks" are structurally similar to "great rivers". Both are mutually implicative to each other.

Both teacher and child rarely use philosophical technical terms. However, they often times touch upon the essential points of the philosophical issues in simple everyday ordinary language, which situation we could discover with surprise, if we are perceptive enough to do so. The teacher's comments on Seibei's laughing could be interpreted as revealing some important points on laughing, which are common with Plessner (1970). For example, Takeda writes "Both of these thoughts grew into such an intolerable funniness that they made him *burst into* a bright loud laughter", which would lead to the Plessner's explication on laughing and crying as the "uncontrolled and unformed *eruptions* of the body" (Plessner, 1970, p. 31, both italics mine).

Here, I must refer the readers of English to the prominent references published in English. I believe in and trust their perceptiveness.

We should remember that the language itself is based upon its "type" that enables us: (1) to *perfink* and experience the "World and I" as structured and meaningful; and (2) to express our own experiences of "World and I" in order to share with others these experiences as structured and meaningful. And the language itself evolves in that historical-social-cultural context. "Language is a system of typifying schemata of experience, which rests on idealizations and anonymizations of immediate subjective experience" (Schutz, 1973, p. 233).

Conclusion

While I was working with the Japanese master teachers many years ago, I encountered the following words which struck me with their powerful rich stimulating implications: "Watching trained practitioners in their approach to the phenomena, usually by studying their subsequent accounts, may further sensitize one's own intuiting "(Spiegelberg, 1971: 660). The reason why I was struck was that I found myself struggling to find out how I, a psychologist could contribute to the improvement of the teaching practices of expert teachers, many of whom had been seeking to improve, for one thing, their own intuiting capacity. On the sites of classroom teaching, the teachers were following the advices of their respectable master teacher Kihaku Saito (1911-1981), who had been emphasizing the vital importance for teachers of "seeing" and/or "intuiting". I could say that this study was originally inspired by H. Spiegelberg's words above. Now, let me present a summary of this little study for the teachers: "*Ask not 'either Why-qn or What-qn', but ask 'both Why-qn and What-qn', in their creative collaborations*". Explanation and Understanding will work together at all levels, including at every level of the "Human Sciences" in general, at that of the "Psychology as a Human Science" and, also that of the "Teaching Literary Works of Art" in the elementary school classrooms, in particular.

Personal Observations

Let me jot down a few comments on the nature of the teaching records. First, Takeda (1929-1986), the teacher, was one of my closest personal friends for more than ten years in his later years. He was a most serious, conscientious, studious, sensitive and devoted teacher, from whom, fortunately, I was able to learn in person many delicate secrets concerning teaching children and the lived-worlds of teachers. From my own personal experiences with him, I could never have any doubt on the trustworthiness and authenticity of his classroom teaching records. Second, Takeda was a very sophisticated reader of the literary works of art, particularly of modern Japanese novels. He even published a little commentary book on the representative modern Japanese novelists. However, as far as known to me from many of our personal conversations, the names of philosophers such as Schleiermacher, Dilthey, Jaspers, Husserl, and others were totally unfamiliar to him, and the long debated issue of Explanation/Understanding was entirely unknown to him. His refined sense of reading literature seemed to have had been nurtured solely through his long personal experiences of reading many literary works of art. This much would be sufficient, I believe, to assure the reader of: (1) the trustworthiness of his own factual teaching record; (2) the unawareness, on his part, of the possible relevance to his lived-world of teaching practices, of such an issue as the "Explanation/ Understanding" debate in Western Philosophy; and (3) his spontaneous originality with respect to the implicit distinction in practices between the two types of questions. The distinction was implicitly borne out of Takeda's own teaching practices and was explicated and tentatively named, after his death in 1986, by this author (1988) as "Why-What Phenomenon".

Postscript: I would like to express my deep gratitude to Prof. Thomas Cloonan for his editorial assistance in improving this essay.

References

Apel, K. O. (1984). *Understanding and Explanation: A Transcendental-Pragmatic Perspective* (Georgia Warnke, Trans.). Cambridge, MA: The MIT Press.

Bollnow, O. F. (1978). *Toi heno kyouiku* (T. Morita & K. Ohtsuka, Trans.). Tokyo: Kawashima-shoten.

Bruner, J. S. (1998). *Kanousekai no shinri* (Kazuhiko Tanaka, Trans.). Tokyo: Misuzu-shobo. (Original work published 1986)

Casey, E. S. (2000). *Imagining: A Phenomenological Study* (2nd ed.). Bloomington, IN: Indiana University Press.

Dazai, O. (1988). *Run, melos! And Other Stories* (R. F. McCarthy, Trans.). Tokyo: Kodan-sha.

Ermarth, M. (1978). *Wilhelm Dilthey: The Critique of Historical Reason.* Chicago: University of Chicago Press.

Giorgi, A. (1970). *Psychology as a Human Science: A Phenomenologically Based Approach.* New York: Harper & Row.

Giorgi, A. (Ed). (1985). *Phenomenology and Psychological Research.* Pittsburgh: PA: Duquesne University Press.

Gadamer, H. G. (1975). *Truth and Method* (G. Barden & J. Cumming, Trans.). New York: The Seabury Press. (Original work published 1965)

Hegel, G. W. F. (1929). *The Science of Logic.* 2 vols. (W. H. Johnston & L. G. Struthers, Trans.). London: George Allen & Unwin. (Original work published 1812-16)

Husserl, E. (1970). *The Crisis of European Sciences and Transcendental Phenomenology* (D. Carr, Trans.). Evanston, IL: Northwestern University Press. (Original work published 1954)

Husserl, E. (1973). *Experience and Judgment* (J. S. Churchill & K. Ameriks, Trans.). Evanston, IL: Northwestern University Press. (Original work published 1948)

Husserl, E. (1977). *Cartesian Meditation.* (D.Cairns, Trans.). Dordrecht: Martinus Nijhoff. (Original work published 1931)

Ingarden, R. (1973). *The Cognition of the Literary Works of Art* (R. A. Crowley & K. R. Olson, Trans.). Evanston, IL: Northwestern University Press. (Original work published 1968)

Jaspers, K. (1953). *Seishinbyorigaku-Soron* (U. Uchimura et al., Trans.). Tokyo: Iwanami-shoten. (Original work published 1923)

Leontiev, A. N. (1961). Learning as a Problem in Psychology. In N. O'Connor (Ed.), *Recent Soviet Psychology* (pp. 227-246). Oxford: Pergamon.

Merleau-Ponty, M. (1964). *The Primacy of Perception* (J. M. Edie, Ed.). Evanston, IL: Northwestern University Press.

Musil, R. (1995). *The Man Without Qualities. I* (S. Wilkins, Trans.). New York: Alfred A. Knopf. (Original work published 1952)

Ooe, K. (1978). *Shosetsu no Houhou.* Tokyo: Iwanami-shoten.

Plessner, H. (1970). *Laughing and Crying: A Study of the Limits of Human Behavior.* (J. S. Churchill & M. Greene, Trans.). Evanston, IL: Northwestern University Press. (Original work published 1961)

Saigo, T. (1991). *Kyokou toshiteno bungaku.* Tokyo: Meiji-tosho. (Original work published 1971)

Schutz, A. & Luckmann, T. (1975). *The Structures of the Lifeworld* (R. M .Zaner & H. T. Engelhardt, Trans.). Evanston, IL: Northwestern University Press. (Original work published 1973)

Shiga, N. (1968). *Seibei to Hyotan.* Tokyo: Shincho-sha.

Spiegelberg, H. (1971). *The Phenomenological Movement. Vol. II.* Dordrecht: Martinus Nijhoff.

Strasser, S. (1985). *Understanding and Explanation: Basic Ideas Concerning the Humanity of the Human Sciences.* Pittsburgh, PA: Duquesne University Press.

Takeda, T. (1964). *Bungaku no jugyou.* Tokyo: Meiji-tosho.

Takeda, T. (1973). *Bungaku no jugyou: Imehji wo sodateru.* Tokyo: Kokudo-sha.

Takeda, T. (1990). *Shinno jugyousha wo mezashite.* Tokyo: Kokudo-sha. With a Forward by Akihiro Yoshida. (Original work published 1971)

Van Manen, M. (1990). *Researching Lived Experience: Human Science for an Action Sensitive Pedagogy.* Albany, NY: SUNY Press.

Wauchope, O. S. (1984). *Mono no kangaekata: Gourisei heno itsudatsu* (M. Fukase, Trans.). Tokyo: Kodan-sha. (Original work published 1951)

Yasunaga, H. (1987). *Seishin no kikagaku.* Tokyo: Iwanami-shoten.

Yasunaga, H. (1992). *Houhouron to rinshougainen.* Tokyo: Kongo-shuppan. (Yasunaga's Homepage in English: www.yas73.jp/index.htm)

Yoshida, A. (1988) On the Why-What Phenomenon. Oral presentation at 24th International Congress of Psychology, Sydney, Australia.

Yoshida, A. (1992). On the Why-What Phenomenon: A Phenomenological Explication of the Art of Asking Questions. *Human Studies, 15*, 35-46.

Yoshida, A. (2001) My Life in Psychology: Making a Place for Fiction in a World of Science. *Journal of Phenomenological Psychology, 32*, 188-202.

Yoshida, A. (2005). The Explanation-Inducing Questions and the Understanding-Inducing Questions: A Phenomenological Explication of a Master Teacher's Practices (in Japanese). In *Shukutoku University Graduate School Bulletin*, (*12*, pp. 39-82). Chiba, Japan: Shukutoku University.

Zahavi, D. (2003). Husserl's Intersubjective Transformation of Transcendental Philosophy. In D. Welton (Ed.). *The New Husserl: A Critical Reader* (pp. 233-251). Bloomington, IN: Indiana University Press.

Biographical Sketches of the Contributors

CHRISTOPHER M. AANSTOOS (Ph.D., Duquesne University) is Professor of Psychology at the University of West Georgia. His dissertation, under Amedeo Giorgi's mentorship, examined the phenomenology of thinking as a critical dialogue with cognitive psychology. That critique initiated his ongoing interest in the conceptual foundations of psychology. Many of Aanstoos' publications are in this area, including his editorship of *Exploring the Lived World: Readings in Phenomenological Psychology* and *Studies in Humanistic Psychology*. He has also contributed chapters to such books as *Qualitative Research in Psychology*, *Advances in Qualitative Psychology*, *Measurement and Personality Assessment*, *Imagination and Phenomenological Psychology*, and *Duquesne Studies in Phenomenological Psychology (Volume 4)*. He has served as program chair and on the executive boards of the Human Science Research Association and the American Psychological Association. He has also been president of APA's Division 32, and was the founding editor of that Division's journal, *The Humanistic Psychologist*.

MARC APPLEBAUM'S PhD is from Saybrook University. He completed his doctoral dissertation there under the direction of Amedeo Giorgi. His Master's and Doctoral work, both supervised by Amedeo Giorgi, have focused on the application of phenomenological psychology and philosophy to the field of cultural psychology, with a particular emphasis on relations between the Muslim-majority societies of the Greater Middle East and the United States. The dissertation is a study of Muslim civil society leaders' experience of connection to the Prophet Muhammad. His Master's thesis was a comparative study of intuition in the work of Edmund Husserl and Nishida Kitaro, founder of the Kyoto School of Japanese Philosophy. His research interests are in the area of the application of phenomenological psychological methodology to the study of leadership in the areas of cultural and organizational psychology.

THOMAS F. CLOONAN (Tomás P. Ó Cluanáin) is Professor Emeritus of Psychology, Marymount College of Fordham University. He has been Visiting Professor of Psychology at Fordham University (2007-2010). In addition, he has Part-Time Faculty status at Saybrook University. His Ph.D. in Psychology is from Duquesne University where his dissertation was done under the direction of Amedeo Giorgi, whose graduate assistant Cloonan was during his doctoral studies. Cloonan is also a graduate of the National Academy School of Fine Arts in New York City. He will be Editor of the *Journal of Phenomenological Psychology* starting in 2011. He is currently on the Board of Editors of the

Journal of Humanistic Psychology and on the Editorial Board of *PsyCRITIQUES – Contemporary Psychology: APA Review of Books*. His current research interests and publication topics include phenomenological psychology and phenomenological philosophy, and the psychology and philosophy of art and aesthetics.

LARRY DAVIDSON received his Ph.D. from Duquesne University, where Amedeo Giorgi was his dissertation director. He is Professor of Psychiatry and Director of the Program for Recovery and Community Health of the Yale University School of Medicine and Institution for Social and Policy Studies. His research focuses on the development and application of qualitative research methods for understanding processes of recovery from serious mental illnesses and addictions, and on the development and evaluation of innovative community-based interventions based on the implications of these data for practice. Specific foci include the active role of the person, the impact of peer support, and the role of community inclusion in fostering recovery. On these topics, he has published over 150 articles and several books. Most recently, he has been working on translating these research findings into their implications for policy and service system development, and has been engaged in assisting systems of care to transform to a recovery orientation, as promoted by the U.S. President's New Freedom Commission on Mental Health.

MAGNUS ENGLANDER received his Ph.D. in Psychology from Saybrook University. His dissertation was under the direction of Amedeo Giorgi. He is a representative of the new generation of phenomenological psychologists. After his doctorate, Englander worked at various universities in the United States and Sweden. He accepted a permanent position at Malmö University in Malmö, Sweden. Englander currently teaches courses on the phenomenological research method, psychology for social work practice, and social psychology and communication. Although his research is in the area of emotional memories, he has developed a phenomenological approach to social psychology and communication. Englander has also written articles on the application of the phenomenological research method to nursing science.

BARBRO M. GIORGI (1957-2007) was born in Molkom, Sweden, and grew up and attended high school in Karlstadt, a nearby city. After high school she moved to Stockholm and attended the University of Stockholm but terminated her studies there before graduation in order to emigrate to Canada. She started over again at York University outside Toronto and graduated with an A.B. in Psychology with Honors and with Distinction, and she remained there to get her M.A. degree. She then matriculated at the Francophone university, *l'Université du Québec à Montréal*, and earned her Ph.D. in research methods and clinical psychology, also with Distinction. Her dissertation was a phenomenological study of pivotal moments in psychotherapy. After Barbro M. Giorgi moved to California, she was hired at JFK University as Director of M.A. Research and she remained in that position for seven years. Toward the end of her tenure at JFK, however, Barbro was getting more involved in teaching at Saybrook University as an Adjunct Professor and was waiting for the initiation of the Psy.D. program at Saybrook in order to transfer to there. Unfortunately, she died before the Psy.D. program was initiated. Her interests centered around the clarification of therapeutic practices by means of a Husserlian phenomenological approach. She has published several articles along those lines. Barbro also practiced therapy as a spiritual counselor because she did not accept the APA criteria for legitimating psychotherapeutic practices.

STEEN HALLING, who received his Ph.D. from Duquesne University, is a licensed psychologist, and a professor at Seattle University, Seattle where he teaches in the MA program in existential-phenomenological psychology as well as in the undergraduate program. His research and publications have focused on topics such as psychology of forgiveness, disillusionment, psychopathology, hopelessness, interpersonal relations, and qualitative research methods. He is editor of *the International Human Science Research Conference Newsletter*, co-editor, with Ronald S. Valle of *Existential-Phenomenological Perspectives in Psychology* (Plenum, 1989), and author of *Intimacy, Transcendence and Psychology: Openness and Closeness in Everyday Life* (Palgrave Macmillan, 2008).

MUFID JAMES HANNUSH, Ph.D., is an Associate Professor of psychology at Rosemont College. He earned his doctorate at Duquesne University, his M.A. from American University of Beirut, and his B.A. from Greenville College. He served as Director of Counseling services at La Roche College and as Assistant to the Dean of Students for Counseling at Duquesne University. He has published many book reviews and scholarly articles, including interviews with Rollo May and James B. Watson, the son of John B. Watson. He serves as Review Editor for the Journal of Phenomenological Psychology and has authored the book, *Becoming Good Parents: An Existential Journey* (SUNY Press).

BERND JAGER studied child psychology at the University of Groningen in his native Holland, and received his Ph.D. from Duquesne University. His research interest concerns phenomenology and the meeting ground between continental philosophy and contemporary psychology. He has taught at UC Santa Cruz, Sonoma State University, *l'Université* de Louvain (Belgium), Rhodes University (South Africa), and the University of Johannesburg (South Africa). At present he teaches at the University of Quebec in Montreal. His recent publications include the translation of Van den Berg's book on historical phenomenology (*"Two Laws of Thermodynamics"*) and "Bachelard et la psychanalyse" in *Les Cahiers Gaston Bachelard.*

GEORGE KUNZ has been Professor of Psychology at Seattle University since 1971, and Chair of its Psychology Department from 1975 to 1981. He received his M.A. from Marquette University and his Ph.D. from Duquesne University. At Duquesne University, he had been awarded a teaching assistantship. His dissertation was done under Amedeo Giorgi and was entitled, "Perceived behavior as a subject matter for a phenomenologically based psychology". With Steen Halling he initiated an M.A. program in Existential-Phenomenological Therapeutic Psychology in1981. He has published *The Paradox of Power and Weakness: Levinas and an alternative paradigm for psychology* (1998), and articles in *Humanistic Psychologist, Journal of Phen. Psych., Journal of Theoretical and Phil. Psych., European Journal of Psychotherapy, Counseling and Health*, and *Psychoanalytic Review.* He has presented keynote addresses at the IHSR in Bournmouth in 2005 and at the North American Levinas Society at Purdue in 2007. Kunz, in addition, has organized and hosted an annual international seminar, "Psychology for the Other: implications of Levinas for psychology".

BERTHA MOOK was born in Holland and studied in South Africa and Canada. She received her Ph.D. from the University of Ottawa, Canada, in 1968. She was Professor in Psychology at the University of Ottawa, and retired from this position in July, 2006. She specialized in the field of clinical psychology and focused on phenomenology, hermeneutics, and psychotherapy. She also has a strong and long-standing interest in metabletics (historical phenomenology) and in family history. She has authored two books, co-edited a third, and has written many book chapters as well as numerous articles in peer-reviewed journals. Her writings include various phenomenological and hermeneutic studies in child, adult and family psychotherapy and metabletic studies on the history of the family and the history of childhood. She is consulting editor for the *Journal of Phenomenological Psychology* and the *Humanistic Psychologist.* As a clinical psychologist, she has also been involved in part-time private practice with children, adults and families for the past thirty years.

JAMES MORLEY received his doctorate in Clinical Psychology from Duquesne University in 1988. He has held teaching positions in Connecticut, India, and England and has recently returned to his alma mater, Ramapo College of New Jersey, where he is a Professor of Clinical Psychology teaching courses in Psychopathology, Phenomenology, and the Psychology of Yoga. Morley's research interests are in the philosophical foundations of psychology as a science and the application of existential-phenomenology to topics such as imagination, human development, and religious experience. He is particularly interested in the thought of Husserl, Heidegger, and especially Merleau-Ponty's ontology of embodied experience as a basis for a reappraisal of the position of the imaginary in psychological theory and practice. He has recently edited an edition of Phenomenology and Cognitive Science on "Imagination" (2005), co-edited a text on Merleau-Ponty and social science (1999) and, with James Phillips, a collection of essays titled Imagination and its Pathologies released by MIT Press (2003).

RICHARD ROJCEWICZ received his Ph.D. in philosophy from Duquesne University, where he was for many years the executive director of the Simon Silverman Phenomenology Center. Thereby he became associated with Amedeo Giorgi, who was the founder and *genius loci* of the Center. Rojcewicz is the author of *The gods and technology: A reading of Heidegger* (SUNY Press, 2006) and has translated several volumes of *Husserliana* and of Heidegger's *Gesamtausgabe.* His main research interests reside in an interpretation of Plato and Aristotle as inspired by Heidegger and in the phenomenology of lived experience as elaborated by Merleau-Ponty.

DAVID L. SMITH, C.S.Sp. earned a Licentiate degree in theology from the University of Fribourg, Switzerland, in 1959, an M.A. in existential-phenomenological psychology from Duquesne University in 1961 under the direction of Adrian van Kaam, and a doctorate in clinical psychology from the University of Montreal in 1968. From 1968 to 1972 he taught at Point Park College, Pittsburgh, PA, and he chaired there the Behavioral Science Department. He is Professor Emeritus of Duquesne University's Department of Human Science Psychology which he chaired from 1976 to 1985. He also served as the Executive-Director of the Simon Silverman Phenomenology Center at Duquesne University from 1994 to 2004. Smith is the author of *Fearfully and wonderfully made: A history of Duquesne Univerity's graduate psychology programs* (2002). More recently, he has published his book, *Born to see… Bound to behold: The history of Duquesne University's Simon Silverman Phenomenology Center,* (2008). He has published in *Duquesne studies in phenomenological psychology, The Humanistic Psychologist, The Journal of Existential Psychology and Psychiatry,the Josephinum Journal of Theology and many reviews in The Journal of Phenomenological Psychology.* He is an ordained Catholic priest and a member of the Congregation of the Holy Spirit.

LES TODRES, Ph.D. (Rhodes University, South Africa), is a clinical psychologist and Professor of Qualitative Research and Psychotherapy at Bournemouth University, UK. His previous occupational roles have included head of a student counselling service and director of a clinical psychology training programme. His career spans both academic and clinical contexts. He is author of the book, *Embodied enquiry: Phenomenological touchstones for research, psychotherapy and spirituality* (Palgrave Macmillan, 2007) and of numerous journal articles and book chapters. Current research interests include older person care, mental health, and quality of life.

FREDERICK J. WERTZ received his Ph.D. in Phenomenological Psychology at Duquesne University in 1982 with Dr. Amedeo Giorgi as his mentor. Currently, he is Professor of Psychology at Fordham University and has been Chair of the Department of Psychology at that university. His teaching includes courses in areas related to clinical psychology, psychoanalysis, qualitative research methods, philosophical foundations of psychology, and the supervision of doctoral students in assessment, psychotherapy, and research. His teaching has won awards from Fordham's College at Lincoln Center (2004) and the Graduate Students Association (2006). He is currently editor of the *Journal of Phenomenological Psychology* and has served as editor of *Bulletin of Theoretical and Philosophical Psychology* as well as a guest editor of *The Humanistic Psychologist.* He edited *The Humanistic Movement: Recovering the Person in Psychology* (1994, Gardner Press) and co-edited *Advances in Qualitative Research in Psychology: Themes and Variations* (1987, Swets North America). He served as President of American Psychological Association's Division of Theoretical and Philosophical Psychology in 1998-1999 and Division of Humanistic Psychology in 1994-1995. He is currently the Fellows Chair of APA's Society for Theoretical and Philosophical Society, which gave him the Outstanding Service Award in 2007. His scholarship has focused on human perception, development, psychopathology, psychotherapy, criminal victimization, phenomenological research methodology, psychoanalysis, cognitive psychology, qualitative research methods, the scientific status of psychology, and the philosophical and cultural foundations of psychology.

AKIHIRO YOSHIDA was born in Tokyo, Japan, on May 25th, 1934. He graduated from the University of Tokyo in 1960 as the valedictorian. He obtained his Ph.D. in Educational Psychology from the University of Illinois in 1967. He has taught at Cornell University (USA); and, in Japan, Ochanomizu University, Tokyo University (1972-1995), Iwate University, and Kawamura University. He is now at Shukutoku University. He is Professor Emeritus of the University of Tokyo. He was Fulbright visiting scholar at Duquesne University in 1980-81. Yoshida's published books include *A Way toward Phenomenology of Teaching, Methods of Teaching*, and *Psychology of Education.* Yoshida is an honorary member of the Japanese Association of Educational Psychology. He is also a member of the International Human Science Research Conference and other professional organizations.